THE WORLD OF PLANTS IN
RENAISSANCE TUSCANY

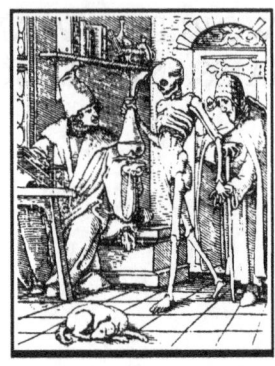

The History of Medicine in Context

Series Editors: Andrew Cunningham and Ole Peter Grell

Department of History and Philosophy of Science
University of Cambridge

Department of History
Open University

Titles in the series include

Uroscopy in Early Modern Europe
Michael Stolberg

The British Pharmacopoeia, 1864 to 2014
Medicines, International Standards and the State
Anthony C. Cartwright

Medicine, Trade and Empire
Garcia de Orta's Colloquies on the Simples and Drugs of India *(1563) in Context*
Edited by Palmira Fontes da Costa

The Fate of Anatomical Collections
Edited by Rina Knoeff and Robert Zwijnenberg

Anatomy and Anatomists in Early Modern Spain
Bjørn Okholm Skaarup

The World of Plants in Renaissance Tuscany

Medicine and Botany

CRISTINA BELLORINI

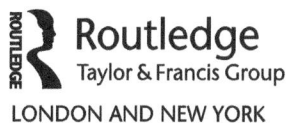

Routledge
Taylor & Francis Group

LONDON AND NEW YORK

First published 2016 by Ashgate Publishing

2 Park Square, Milton Park, Abingdon, Oxon OX14 4RN
605 Third Avenue, New York, NY 10017

Routledge is an imprint of the Taylor & Francis Group, an informa business

First issued in paperback 2021

British Library Cataloguing in Publication Data
A catalogue record for this book is available from the British Library

The Library of Congress has cataloged the printed edition as follows:
Names: Bellorini, Cristina, author.
Title: The world of plants in Renaissance Tuscany : medicine and botany / by Cristina Bellorini.
Description: Farnham, Surrey, England ; Burlington, VT : Ashgate, [2016] | Series: The history of medicine in context | Includes bibliographical references and index.
Identifiers: LCCN 2015027256 | ISBN 9781472466228 (hardcover) |
Subjects: LCSH: Medicinal plants--Italy--Tuscany--History--16th century. | Materia medica, Vegetable--Italy--Tuscany--History. | Botany, Medical--Italy--Tuscany--History.
Classification: LCC RS177.I8 B45 2016 | DDC 615.3/2109455--dc23 LC record available at http://lccn.loc.gov/2015027256

ISBN 978-1-4724-6622-8 (hbk)
ISBN 978-1-03-217957-5 (pbk)
DOI: 10.4324/9781315551395

To Paolo and Tommaso

Contents

List of Figures

List of Tables

Acknowledgements

First and foremost I would like to thank John Henderson who encouraged my project from the beginning, followed its whole development and offered invaluable advice throughout its various stages. He discussed my research progress and listened to my perplexities with sure knowledge and calm assurance, constantly reviving my enthusiasm by suggesting new angles and alternative ways.

I am equally grateful to Filippo de Vivo who helped me develop my research, generously annotating my drafts, challenging my arguments and stimulating my efforts with his perceptive comments and thought-provoking ideas.

I owe a special thanks to Evelyn Welch for her generosity and constructive criticism. She drew my attention to some aspects of my work which needed further investigation, whilst also providing new points of view and suggesting new sources.

I am deeply grateful to David Gentilcore, whose detailed comments and acute observations on the medical topics, and sage advice on the general project were crucial for the preparation of this book.

Sharon Strocchia's insight on the Tuscan pharmaceutical scene, together with her smiling and sympathetic encouragement, was also of great support.

I am indebted to some people who offered their help unexpectedly and with great generosity. Here I can name only a few of them, to whom I am particularly grateful. Giuseppe Olmi, who read and commented on the draft of some of my chapters, offered helpful advice, and suggested new lines of inquiry. Lucia Sandri, who helped me with archival research at the Ospedale degli Innocenti, and kindly let me read some of her essays before publication. Elena Cecchi, who spontaneously shared her knowledge with me when I needed help for the interpretation of some sixteenth-century manuscripts. Alessio Assonitis and Sheila Barker of The Medici Archive Project at the Archivio di Stato in Florence who provided me with information which proved fundamental to my research.

I am also grateful to the people and friends working on various different aspects of the Renaissance who discussed my work, commented on it, asked questions, provided information, and corrected some of my errors. In particular, I would like to thank Sarah Duncan and Sarah Drummond whose presence and assistance were of great importance in the early stages of my research.

Finally, I wish to thank the Tuscan people (those of the past and those of today), who accorded me the privilege of working in places so rich in beauty and glorious in memories.

Introduction

In the sixteenth century the study of plants was considered a branch of medicine, as plants were the basis of therapy. In this same period, however, plants began to be considered not only because they were useful to men, but also in their own right, and a new discipline that later came to be called botany began to take shape.

These two fields have usually been studied separately. Historians of medicine have taken into consideration only the therapeutic use of plants, while the historians of botany have tried to identify and isolate all the elements that could provide evidence of the new interest in plants for themselves, separate from medicine. These two branches, however, did not develop in parallel and independently, but were constantly interweaving and influencing one another, for, apart from some rare exceptions, all the naturalists of the time were medical men.

Moreover, even if we exclude agriculture, which will not be part of my research, the world of plants was much more complex than this. As natural elements, plants were objects of philosophical speculation, and as part of creation, they were evidence of the wisdom of God. Their symbolic meaning formed a recognized language used by poets and painters.

The purpose of this book is to re-establish the interconnections between medicine and botany within the same framework, pointing out their reciprocal influence, trying to reconstruct the world of plants as it was in the sixteenth century, a world completely different from our own.

Historians have to identify a subject to investigate and they are bound to make a series of simplifications to isolate a particular topic and to be able to carry out exhaustive research. There is a point, however, where, after simplification and further simplification, one begins to feel that the picture has been distorted, and that it is necessary to try to reconstruct it and restore it to its complexity.

In the case of plants, which are the subject of this book, the complexity can easily be imagined, as the word 'plant' brings to mind a vast number of meanings and images. We are used to connecting it with different uses and subject fields, some of which (now usually assembled under the comprehensive name of 'plant sciences') obviously did not exist in the sixteenth century. What is less obvious, however, is that we can make the same statement the other way round; that is to say, the realm of vegetables had connotations which do not exist and are hardly conceivable today.

Plants as the primary basis of therapy were listed in herbals where only 'simples' supposed to have medicinal virtues were taken into consideration. The fact that in the sixteenth century a new way of considering plants slowly began to evolve did not change their importance from the therapeutic point of view. The first signs of an appreciation of plants in their own right are to be discovered in these medical texts where sometimes a plant, which was considered interesting because newly discovered or just beautiful, was added almost surreptitiously.

Medicine and botany were linked through natural philosophy. Natural philosophy, as the discipline devoted to the study of nature, was a fundamental part of the curriculum of any faculty of medicine of the time. It encompassed the theoretical principles on which to found the understanding of any aspect of the natural world, including both the human body and the vegetable kingdom. Natural phenomena were investigated by reading, commenting and discussing some of the *libri naturales* of Aristotle.[1] In fact the very idea of the utility of natural philosophy for the medical profession was drawn from some passages of Aristotle himself, later corroborated by Galen. Medicine was a composite discipline and the medical man had to acquire different branches of knowledge. As the physician/philosopher Mainetto Mainetti (a professor at the University of Pisa between 1543 and 1573) put it, 'Medicine coalesces from many sciences, since from the natural philosopher indeed it has drawn anatomy itself, the elements and humours, as well as the knowledge and virtues of plants.' Medical men, he added, must also be familiar with astronomy and mathematics.[2] Although Aristotelianism had been the basis of university philosophy since the Middle Ages, and continued to be throughout the sixteenth and a greater part of the seventeenth century, it was flexible enough to allow a variety of interpretations and positions.[3]

In the sixteenth century, moreover, some Italian humanists fostered the study of Plato alongside Aristotle, and some chairs for a new teaching of Platonic philosophy were established in Pisa (1576), and then in Rome and Ferrara. Philosophical speculation on the natural world was greatly influenced by the Platonic theory of the correspondence between macrocosm and microcosm as was re-interpreted by

---

[1]   Usually the *Physics*, *On the Soul*, and some of the so-called *Parva naturalia*. See the Statutes of 1545 of the University of Pisa in *Storia dell'Università di Pisa* (Pisa, 2000), pp. 615–16.

[2]   Mainetto Mainetti, *Commentarius mire perspicuus in librum Aristotelis De sensu & sensibus* (Florence, 1555), p. 11. Quoted in Charles B. Schmitt, 'Aristotle among the Physicians', in Andrew Wear (ed.), *The Medical Renaissance in the Sixteenth Century* (Cambridge, 1985), p. 11.

[3]   Edward Grant, 'Aristotelianism and the longevity of the medieval world view', *History of Science*, 16 (1978), pp. 93–106. Quoted by Ann Blair, 'Natural Philosophy', *The Cambridge History of Science*, vol. 3: *Early Modern Science*, ed. K. Park and L. Daston (Cambridge, 2006), p. 371.

Marsilio Ficino and the Florentine neo-Platonic school.[4] This approach to nature in general, and to plants in particular, was deeply rooted in a religious vision of the world according to which plants were created by God for the good of mankind. It had many medical implications, as plants were viewed as the cure sent by God to heal all diseases on earth. It went further than that, claiming that God had assigned to plants external signs that indicated their inner medicinal virtues, so that the learned physician could recognize them. This view, that has come to be called the 'doctrine of signatures', offers another insight into the understanding of plants of the time. Although the supporters of this theory claimed that 'signatures' had nothing to do with magic, but were simply an aspect of nature, today it would be difficult not to ascribe this view to magic *tout court*. When reading how Paracelsus used plants in therapy, for example, we cannot help but attribute it to occult forces. If one is patient enough to follow his reasoning, however, it is evident that the procedure he followed was encompassed within his vision of nature.[5]

Plants were not confined to the vegetable kingdom as they are today, but were seen as part of a much wider and composite world. All natural objects were at the centre of a web of symbols and associations without the interpretation of which the knowledge of a particular object could not be considered complete. This view, sometimes referred to as 'emblematic world view' is clearly exemplified by the zoologies of Conrad Gesner (1516–1565) and Ulisse Aldrovandi (1522–1605).[6] The chapter on the peacock in Aldrovandi's treatise, for instance, was divided into thirty-three sections, each one of which had to give account of a special aspect or meaning connected with the bird. As William Ashworth comments, 'The notion that a peacock should be studied in isolation from the rest of the universe, and that inquiry should be limited to anatomy, physiology, and physical description, was a notion completely foreign to Renaissance thought.'[7] The same approach, applied to plants, is to be found in the work of the German physician Joachim Camerarius (1534–1598) *Symbolorum et emblematum ex re herbaria centuria una* (1590).[8]

---

4   Blair, 'Natural Philosophy', pp. 374–9; Jill Kraye, 'La filosofia nelle Università italiane del XVI secolo' and Sebastiano Gentile, 'Il ritorno di Platone, dei platonici e del Corpus ermetico: Filosofia, teologia e astrologia nell'opera di Marsilio Ficino', in Cesare Vasoli (ed.), *Le filosofie del Rinascimento* (Milan, 2002), pp. 350–70 and pp. 193–298.

5   Bruce T. Moran in 'The *Herbarius* of Paracelsus – Translated with an introduction by Bruce T. Moran', *Pharmacy in History*, 35(3) (1993), pp. 99–127.

6   William B. Ashworth Jr., 'Natural History and the Emblematic World View', in David C. Lindberg and Robert S. Westman (eds), *Reappraisals of the Scientific Revolution* (Cambridge, 1980).

7   Ibid., p. 312.

8   Thea Vignau-Wilberg, 'Devotion and Observation of Nature in Art around 1600', in G. Olmi, L. Tongiorgi Tomasi and A. Zanca (eds), *Natura-Cultura: L'interpretazione del mondo fisico nei testi e nelle immagini* (Florence, 2000), pp. 43–57 (pp. 46–8).

Medicine was also seen as a composite discipline because it implied not just a multifaceted and sophisticated learning, but also the actual practice of the profession. All decisions about the kind of therapy a patient ought to be given were in the hands of the physician. University trained medical men rarely had direct knowledge of 'simples' (as medicinal plants were usually referred to), as their education was traditionally based on the theoretical discussion of texts; they usually prescribed a recipe chosen from those of ancient authors, often adapting it for a particular patient, who ordered the preparation from the apothecary.

In the sixteenth century, however, theoretical discussion of the texts was no longer the only way of approaching the natural world. A new attitude began to appear, revealed by the representation of nature in pictures and in the first naturalistic plant illustrations.[9] As far as plants are concerned, this new attitude can be in great part attributed to the impact of humanism. The recovery, translation and new editions of classical authors who had dealt with plants, such as Theophrastus, Pliny, Galen and, above all, Dioscorides were at the basis of this new attitude. All the ancient medical authors, in fact, considered first-hand observation of medicinal plants as one of the physician's tasks.[10] In the first pages of his *Materia medica*, which was the most influential treatise on medicinal plants of the time, Dioscorides spurred physicians to observe plants directly and with great care, in all the stages of their life. The establishment of the first chair of medical botany and of the first botanical gardens, as well as the invention of new techniques and methods for the study of plants, such as *herbaria*, field trips, and realistic plant illustrations, all originated from this new attitude. Although they ended up playing a primary role in the study of plants for themselves, they were all devised and used by medical professors for the teaching of *materia medica*, and for research on medicinal plants. The philological approach to ancient botanical texts was also at the root of the movement that emerged out of concern for the general confusion surrounding the identification and use of simples, whose main object was the retrieval of the herbs Dioscorides had dealt with in his *Materia medica*. The effect of the search for Dioscoridean plants was the stimulus it gave to field trips and the direct observation of nature. It also had the effect of creating a new community of naturalists who shared the same goal. Physicians, learned apothecaries, collectors and amateurs, all shared the same

---

[9]   Otto Pacht, 'Early Italian nature studies and the early calendar landscape', *Journal of the Warburg and Courtauld Institutes*, 13 (1950), pp. 13–47; Wilfrid Blunt, *The Art of Botanical Illustration* (London, 1951).

[10]   Karen Reeds, 'Renaissance humanism and botany', *Annals of Science*, 33 (1976), pp. 519–42.

enthusiasm, and Pietro Andrea Mattioli's commentary on Dioscorides, the so-called *Discorsi*, became the most-read herbal of the time.[11]

The new way of studying plants continued and went beyond the search for the plants contained in the classical texts. Some of the countless new species recently discovered or imported from the New World began to be included and described in the new herbals, often irrespective of their medicinal virtues.

In the course of the sixteenth century, another aspect began to gain in importance. A new conception of garden architecture began to develop, where art and nature coexist and 'incorporated, united and reconciled, they produce stupendous things'.[12] Gardens were an exclusive attribute of grand villas, and once again they were very much inspired by the descriptions of classical gardens by the authors of antiquity. Plants were just one aspect of them, but through gardens one can gain an understanding of plants, which is separate from medicine and from their practical use. In gardens, exotic plants from distant lands were appreciated much more for their beauty and peculiarity than for their therapeutic potential.

The world of plants encompassed all these different aspects and meanings, which coexisted and were often inextricably bound to one another. This book aims to reconstruct a picture where all these aspects are brought together and the world of plants is restored to its diversity and complexity. The building up of this picture will allow us to investigate when and how the study of plants branched out from its traditional focus on pharmacology, and the new discipline of botany had its beginning. Why did the study of plants take a new path, distinct from that of medicine? Which were the circumstances, the cultural context and the conditions which allowed the emergence of the new 'scientific' discipline?

Literature dealing with plants is usually centred either on medicine or botany. Considering the enormous amount of literature on the history of medicine, one cannot help noticing that, although simples are always mentioned as the fundamental sources of therapy, they are seldom the central subject of research.

Both Andrew Wear's and Nancy Siraisi's books on Renaissance and early modern medicine, for example (the first focused on England, the second on Italy), include very comprehensive chapters on remedies.[13] They offer broad surveys of the criteria according to which simples were employed in therapy, expounding at length the Galenic theory of the 'qualities' of medicinal plants, and outlining a series of points in relation to their use. Like any survey, however,

---

[11]   Richard Palmer, 'Medical botany in northern Italy in the Renaissance', *Journal of the Royal Society of Medicine*, 78 (1985), pp. 149–57.

[12]   Bartolomeo Taegio, *La villa* (Milan, 1559), p. 102. Quoted in Claudia Lazzaro, *The Italian Renaissance Garden* (New Haven, CT, and London, 1990), p. 9.

[13]   Andrew Wear, *Knowledge and Practice in English Medicine 1550–1680* (Cambridge, 2000); Nancy Siraisi, *Medieval and Early Renaissance Medicine: An Introduction to Knowledge and Practice* (Chicago, IL, and London, 1990).

they provide general information and at the same time raise questions that can only be investigated by specific studies.

Putting medicinal plants in the centre brings to the fore the issue of their practical use in therapy and the crucial question of the relationship between theory and practice. Research in the field of early modern medicine has explored more the principles on which therapy was based than its practical application. One of the reasons is certainly that sources through which to investigate practice are scarce, difficult to trace, and imply a laborious work of interpretation, often leading to uncertain results. Moreover, while the theory at the basis of therapy was largely shared throughout Europe, the practical use of medicines was likely to present substantial differences in different areas and contexts, and vary according to availability in the market, prices, and personal experience.

As far as Italy is concerned, information about the use of simples is scarce. Italian historians in particular, with some exceptions, have not shown much interest in the matter, and there are only very few recent studies available.[14] The most important is that undertaken by the physician-historian Giovanni Silini on a group of original sources all preserved in the historical archives of the small town of Gandino (Lombardy).[15] These sources include about 4,000 prescriptions written by the town physicians for their patients during the period 1469–1478, and contemporary account books and inventories of the remedies kept in the local pharmacy. The exceptional nature of the sources and the painstaking work of interpretation provide one of the most complete and detailed studies based on quantitative data of the day-to-day use of medicines in an Italian country town.

Recently a series of works has drawn attention to household medical care and has thrown light on the role played by early modern women on the medical scene.[16]

Some essays dealing with the role early modern women played in health and healing are centred on Italy. Very important is, for example, the research conducted by Sharon Strocchia on the apothecary nuns of a Florentine convent,

---

[14] On the state of the art of the Italian historiography in the field of history of medicine see: Alessandro Pastore, 'Medicina, Scienza e storia in età moderna. Lo stato degli studi in Italia', in F. Chacòn et al. (eds), *Spagna e Italia in Età moderna: storiografie a confronto* (Roma, 2009), pp. 253–71.

[15] Giovanni Silini, *Uomini e farmaci: terapia medica tardo-medievale* (Gandino, 2001). Another interesting Italian study is *Una Farmacia preindustriale in Valdelsa: la Spezieria e lo Spedale di Santa Fina nella città di San Gimignano secc. XIV–XVIII* (San Gimignano, 1981).

[16] A series of articles on this theme are collected in *Bulletin of the History of Medicine*, 2008, vol. 82. See also the Introduction to this issue: Mary E. Fissell, 'Women, health, and healing in early Modern Europe', pp. 1–17.

the vast literature on midwives, and that on women 'artisans of the body', according to the definition of Sandra Cavallo.[17]

The most detailed research into medicinal ingredients in Renaissance Italy is that undertaken by Evelyn Welch and James Shaw on the account books of a Florentine apothecary shop, the Speziale al Giglio, kept in the Archivio dell'ospedale degli Innocenti in Florence.[18] The study focuses on the year 1494, and examines all aspects related to the purchase of the various commodities sold by a Florentine *spezieria* of the time. The account books provide a wide range of data, and the section on 'Medicines' in particular contains invaluable information about the simples more frequently used and the preparations they were for.[19]

Another important study is the quantitative analysis carried out by the Spanish historian M. Teresa Huguet-Termes on the first edition of the Florentine pharmacopoeia, the *Nuovo ricettario fiorentino* (1498), which examines all the medicinal ingredients included there.[20] It is worth noting that the new pharmacopoeias which began to be published in Italy in the sixteenth century, have not been the object of study in recent decades. In this regard, the most complete and detailed work is still that of Alfonso Corradi in 1887.[21]

The question of the introduction of American plants into Europe has been variously dealt with. Perhaps the most significant contributions are the studies of a group of Spanish scholars.[22] They examine the first descriptions and the first European herbals where American plants were described, providing information

---

[17]   Sharon T. Strocchia, 'The nun apothecaries of Renaissance Florence: Marketing medicines in the convent', *Renaissance Studies* 25(5) (2011), pp. 627–47. On midwifery see Hilary Marland (ed.), *The Art of Midwifery* (London, 1993); Lianne McTavish, *Childbirth and the Display of Authority in Early Modern France* (Aldershot, 2005); see also the Introduction of Fissell, 'Women, health, and healing in early Modern Europe', p. 3 and note 9. On women performing a professional role see Sandra Cavallo, *Artisans of the Body in Early Modern Italy: Identities, Families and Masculinities* (Manchester and New York, 2007), pp. 160–68.

[18]   Firenze, Archivio dell'Ospedale degli Innocenti, Fondo Estranei, Series 144, 904–6; Series 144, 592–4.

[19]   James Shaw and Evelyn Welch, *Making and Marketing Medicine in Renaissance Florence* (Amsterdam, 2011).

[20]   M. Teresa Huguet-Termes, 'Approximacion historico-farmacologica y studio comparative de los codigos mas representativos de las primeras tendencias a la oficializacion en el contexto de la terapia preparacelsiana en Europa'. Doctoral thesis, Faculty of Pharmacy, University of Barcelona, 1998.

[21]   Alfonso Corradi, *Le prime farmacopee italiane, ed in particolare: Dei Ricettari Fiorentini* (Milan, 1887).

[22]   José Pardo Tomáš and Maria Luz López Terrada, *Las primeras noticias sobre plantas americanas en las relaciones de viajes y cròs de Indias (1493–1553)* (Valencia, 1993); *La influencia Española en la introduccion en Europa de las plantas americanas (1493–1623)* (Valencia, 1997); Teresa Huguet-Termes, 'New World materia medica in Spanish Renaissance medicine: From scholarly reception to practical impact', *Medical History*, 45 (2001), pp. 359–76.

on many new plants. Above all they shed light on how information was conveyed and how and why some of the new plants were taken into consideration by European physicians and naturalists.

All the works mentioned provide a good deal of details on the use of remedies in early modern Europe. Each of them constitutes an important contribution to the understanding of the use of simples, and offers some insights into the relationship between medical theory and practice. However, analyses of this kind are always centred on a particular place and context, often based on different methods, and their results are inevitably partial and not easily comparable. Further studies of this kind are essential to build up a general view of therapeutic practice.

The second branch of literature, that of 'botany', is obviously centred on plants. The general histories of botany, such as the well-known volumes by Julius von Sachs and by Alan Morton cover too long a period to concentrate on a phase when botany was just beginning to take its first steps. They point out the most prominent naturalists of the time, identifying their role in the progress of botany, but they confine themselves to isolating some significant aspects.[23] They both devote, however, great attention and space to the Italian physician-botanist Andrea Cesalpino, and provide an accurate account of his attempt at a general classification of plants. An in-depth study of the Renaissance history of botany is that of Edward Lee Green, who analyses at length and in detail some works of the most important European physician-botanists of the period within the humanistic context.[24] From the point of view of the history of botany, moreover, studies of single botanical gardens like that of Pisa and of Padua are of fundamental importance.[25]

Herbals have sometimes been thoroughly investigated. The greater part of the studies on herbals, however, are meticulous analyses of single books, more from an antiquarian perspective, or from the point of view of the history of books rather than from that of their content.[26] The most complete book on Renaissance herbals is perhaps still that of Agnes Arber, which traces the evolution of printed herbals throughout Europe, with constant references to the humanistic background, analysing a series of different aspects, such as plant description, botanical illustration and plant classification. Arber's interest, however, is very

---

[23]   Julius von Sachs, *History of Botany* (1530–1860) (Oxford, 1890); Alan G. Morton, *History of Botanical Science: An Account of the Development of Botany from Ancient Times to the Present Day* (London and New York, 1981).

[24]   Edward Lee Greene, *Landmarks of Botanical History* (Stanford, CA, 1983).

[25]   Alessandro Minelli (ed.), *The Botanical Garden of Padua 1545–1995* (Venice, 1995); Fabio Garbari, Lucia Tongiorgi Tomasi and Alessandro Tosi, *Giardino dei semplici – L'orto botanico di Pisa dal XVI al XX secolo* (Pisa, 1991).

[26]   Luisa Cogliati Arano, *The Medieval Health Handbook: Tacuinum Sanitatis* (New York, 1976); Minta Collins, *Medieval Herbals: The Illustrative Traditions* (London, 2000).

much centred on the progress of botany, and neglects the medical content of the herbals she describes, sometimes at the risk of misrepresenting them.[27]

A particular subject that has attracted the attention of scholars is that of botanical illustration. Sixteenth-century botanical illustration is a fascinating subject, as it is relevant to art, science, and philosophical speculation.[28] It is, first of all, proof that natural objects were now looked at in a different way. A comparison between the schematic and crude illustrations of a medieval herbal such as the *Herbarium* of Apuleius Platonicus (published at the end of the fifteenth century) and the perfectly naturalistic drawings of Brunfels's *Herbarum vivae icones* (1530) and Fuchs's *Historia stirpium* (1542) reveals a new attitude towards nature.[29] In a period when nomenclature was scant and imprecise, naturalistic botanical illustration was essential to develop a process of standardization and was a fundamental tool to transmit and to exchange information about the unknown plants from distant lands. Plant illustration, however, was not approved of by all naturalists and was at the centre of a philosophical debate, supported by the authority of Pliny and other ancient authors, about the usefulness of representing natural objects and conveying knowledge by means of pictures.

In order to assemble the various aspects of the realm of plants in a comprehensive survey, I decided to concentrate on a single area, and on a limited

---

[27] Agnes Arber, *Herbals: Their Origin and Evolution* (Cambridge, 1912).

[28] James Ackerman, 'Artists in Renaissance Science', *Science and the Arts in the Renaissance*, in J.W. Shirley and F.D. Hoeniger (eds), *Science and the Arts in the Renaissance* (London and Toronto, 1985); Ilva Beretta, 'Illustration and Representation: Botany in the Renaissance', in F. Meroi, C. Pogliano (eds), *Immagini per Conoscere: Dal Rinascimento alla Rivoluzione scientifica* (Florence, 2001); Blunt, *The Art of Botanical Illustration*; Collins, *Medieval Herbals;* S.Y. Edgerton, 'The Renaissance Development of Scientific Illustration', *Science and the Arts in the Renaissance*, in J.W. Shirley and F.D. Hoeniger (eds) (London and Toronto, 1985); Sachiko Kusukawa, 'Illustrating Nature', *Books and Sciences in History*, in Marina Frasca-Spada and Nick Jardine (eds), *Books and Sciences in History* (Cambridge, 2000), pp. 90–113; Sachiko Kusukawa, *Picturing the Book of Nature: Image Text and Argument in Sixteenth- century Anatomy and Medical Botany* (Chicago,IL, 2012); Claudia Swan, 'Lectura-imago-ostensio: The role of the "Libri Picturati" A.18-A.30 in Medical Instruction at the Leiden University', in G. Olmi, L. Tongiorgi Tomasi and A. Zanca (eds), *Natura-Cultura: l'interpretazione del mondo fisico nei testi e nelle immagini* (Florence, 2000), pp. 189–214; Lucia Tongiorgi Tomasi, 'Dall'essenza vegetale agglutinata all'immagine a stampa', *Museologia Scientifica*, 8 (1991–92), pp. 271–95; Claus Nissen, *Herbals of Five Centuries: A Contribution to Medical History and Bibliography* (Zurich, 1958); Pacht, 'Early Italian nature studies and the early calendar landscape', pp. 13–47; Gabriele Baroncini, 'Note sull'illustrazione scientifica', *Nuncius*, 11(2) (1996), pp. 527–43; Renzo Baldasso, 'The role of visual representation in the scientific revolution: A historiographic inquiry', *Centaurus* 2006, 48, pp. 69–88.

[29] Luca Zucchi, 'Brunfels e Fuchs: l'illustrazione botanica quale ritratto della singola pianta o immagine della specie', *Nuncius, Annali di Storia della Scienza*, 18 (2003), pp. 411–65.

period of time. I have chosen to focus my research on Tuscany in the second half of the sixteenth century. In this period Tuscany offers a particularly fertile ground for investigation into medical botany. The three Medici grand dukes who ruled Tuscany in this period, Cosimo I (1519–1574), Francesco I (1541–1587), and Ferdinando I (1549–1609), were personally interested in plants and medicine, and devoted particular attention to them.[30] There is evidence that they used to carry out experiments on medicaments in their personal laboratories (the so-called *fonderie*),[31] and that they supported the scientific activities connected with the University of Pisa where a new chair of *materia medica* was instituted and the first botanical garden established. The Medici were also interested in plants in their own right, as is shown by their interest in new exotic plants, and the laying out of gardens around their villas.[32]

To focus on the Medici, their court and the circle of intellectuals who surrounded them, gives access to a vast number of sources. The letters written by the Medici and their secretaries, and the letters sent to them have been preserved at the Archivio di Stato of Florence. Biographies, reports, visual and written descriptions, inventories, documents and university lectures have come down to us, either in manuscript or printed form. And naturally we have at our disposal the medical books and the books about plants which were written and read in that period.

The pre-eminent role of the grand dukes within the court, as well as the importance I have attached to the *study* of plants and the activities carried out within the university, has led me to concentrate on an entirely male production of medical and plant knowledge. This does not mean that women did not occupy a large portion of the scene. They were involved in the use of plants in myriad forms, from the making and administering of food to the supplying of medicinal herbs and remedies in their traditional and constant care of the sick, infants and the elderly. As seen above, this role of women within a domestic setting has been the subject of several studies, complemented by others which reveal that women healers sometimes performed semi-professional roles.[33]

---

[30]   Giovanni Targioni Tozzetti, *Notizie sulla storia delle scienze fisiche in Toscana cavate da un manoscritto inedito* (Florence, 1852).

[31]   Alfredo Perifano, *L'Alchimie à la Cour de Côme Ier de Médicis: savoir, culture et politique* (Paris, 1997); Luciano Berti, *Il principe dello studiolo: Francesco I dei Medici e la fine del Rinascimento fiorentino* (Florence, 1967).

[32]   Lucia Tongiorgi Tomasi, *The Flowering of Florence: Botanical Art for the Medici* (Washington, 2002); Lazzaro, *The Italian Renaissance Garden*; Luigi Zangheri, *Pratolino, il giardino delle meraviglie* (Florence, 1987); Suzanne Butters, 'Ferdinand et le jardin du Pincio', in André Chastel and Philip Morel (eds), *La villa Médicis*, 5 vols (Rome, 1989–2010), pp. 350–410; Suzanne Butters, 'Pressed Labor and Pratolino: Social Imagery and Social Reality in a Medici Garden', in Mirka Beneš and Dianne Harris (eds), *Villas and Gardens in Early Modern Italy and France* (Cambridge, 2001), pp. 61–87.

[33]   See above, pp. 6–7.

While the university was an institution from which women were excluded, their role within the court has been variously examined.[34] Italian court women in particular have been the subject of a series of works which investigate their role within the court and their states' cultural policy. These studies, however, are for the most part centred on economic, political and artistic aspects.[35] Nevertheless, a new interest in the role of early modern Italian court women in relation to pharmacy and therapy has recently been developing. In this field much remains to be explored even with regard to figures who have already been the object of scholarly attention, such as Isabella d'Este (1474–1539) who was known to distil plant waters and produce perfumes and cosmetics for herself and her entourage of *donzelle*, and as gifts for other court women and princesses.[36]

A very interesting case is that of a manuscript of medical recipes compiled by Caterina Sforza (1463–1509), wife of Giovanni dalle Bande Nere and grandmother of Cosimo I, which was published by her biographer Pier Desiderio Pasolini in 1894.[37] The figure of Caterina and her book of recipes has been examined anew in two recent works.[38]

An area of inquiry which deserves further investigation is that of the part played by the Medici women in the planning and planting of their villas' gardens, which was certainly a major point of interest for the grand dukes. We know for example that Eleonora di Toledo, wife of Cosimo I, played a fundamental role in the transformation of the land behind the Pitti Palace into the Boboli garden. However, she was concerned more with the layout and iconography of the garden than with the choice and care of the plants, a matter the grand

[34] See for example, Alisha Rankin, *Panaceia's Daughters: Noblewomen as Healers in Early Modern Germany* (Chicago, IL, and London, 2013).

[35] See for example, L. Arcangeli and S. Peyronel (eds), *Donne di potere nel Rinascimento* (Rome, 2008); G. Calvi and R. Spinelli (eds), *Le donne Medici nel sistema europeo delle corti (XVI–XVIII secolo)* (Firenze, 2008); Natalie Tomas, *The Medici Women: Gender and Power in Renaissance Florence* (Aldershot, 2003).

[36] See Daniela Pizzagalli, *La signora del Rinascimento, vita e splendori di Isabella d'Este alla corte di Mantova* (Milan, 2013), pp. 360, 369, 401, 405, 430; Evelyn Welch, *Shopping in the Renaissance: Consumer Culture in Italy 1440–1600* (New Haven, CT, and London, 2005) pp. 267–70, and 'Art on the edge: Hair, hats and hands in Renaissance Italy', *Renaissance Studies*, 23(3) (2009), 241–68, p. 261.

[37] P.D. Pasolini (ed.), *Experimenti de la ex.ma s.ra Caterina da Forlj matre de lo Inllux. mo signor Giovanni de Medici*, (Imola, 1894); Pier Desiderio Pasolini, *Caterina Sforza* (Rome, 1893).

[38] Fabrizia Fiumi and Giovanna Tempesta, 'Gli "experimenti" di Caterina Sforza', *Caterina Sforza, una donna del cinquecento: storia e arte tra Medioevo e Rinascimento* (Imola: La Mandragora, 2000), pp. 139–46; J. De Vries, *Caterina Sforza and the Art of Appearances* (Aldershot, 2010), p. 211; M.K. Ray, 'Experiments with Alchemy: Caterina Sforza in Early Modern Scientific Culture', in *Gender and Scientific Discourse in Early Modern Culture* (Aldershot, 2010), pp. 139–64.

dukes had very much at heart, as I have been most interested in pointing out in my research.[39]

The Medici court and the re-founded University of Pisa, as the loci where intellectual life, penetration of new ideas and dissemination of knowledge took place, will provide the general framework of my inquiry and will be examined in the first three chapters of the book. Although they call up very different images to our minds and have been often seen as two contrasting entities, in the period under discussion they were both very lively and dynamic sites of intellectual enterprise. The vast web of relations that connected them with the rest of Europe, and the circulation of ideas testified to by the vast correspondence and the inventories of books of private and public libraries, widen the scope of the inquiry. The personalities and strong cultural interests of the first dukes, combined with the growing centralization of power, obviously played a major role in the shaping of the court, but also had a decisive influence on the university.

Chapter 1 focuses on the personal interest of Cosimo, Francesco, and Ferdinando de' Medici in medicine and botany, and the cultural role it played within the court. The first part deals with the activities carried out in their laboratories or *fonderie*, where they processed and distilled plants to produce medicaments.

Another side of the interest in plants of the Medici and their court can be seen in the new gardens that were designed and laid out around their villas.[40] The second part of the chapter points out, mainly through letters, how the grand dukes devoted a particular attention to the choice of herbs and plants to be grown in their gardens, and, above all, how they used to follow personally and meticulously their rooting, growth, and development.

The importance the dukes placed on medicine and plants also led to their backing a series of initiatives connected with the university which are discussed in Chapter 2. The faculty of medicine of the University of Pisa, where a new readership for the teaching of medicinal plants (*materia medica*) was established, is in fact a fundamental source of investigation.[41] The focal point of the chapter is the first two professors of this subject Luca Ghini and Andrea Cesalpino who, in a different and complementary way, played a central role in the shaping of the

[39]   See for example, Bruce L. Edelstein, 'La fecundissima Signora Duchessa: The Courtly Persona of Eleonora di Toledo and the Iconography of Abundance', in K. Eisenbichler (ed.), *The Cultural World of Eleonora di Toledo, Duchess of Florence and Siena* (Aldershot, 2004).

[40]   Georgina Masson, *Italian Gardens* (London, 1966); Penelope Hobhouse, *Plants in Garden History* (London, 1977); Lazzaro, *The Italian Renaissance Garden*.

[41]   Charles Schmitt, 'Science in the Italian Universities in the Sixteenth and Early Seventeenth Centuries', in Maurice Crosland (ed.), *The Emergence of Science in Western Europe* (London, 1975); Nancy Siraisi, *Medicine and the Italian Universities* (Leiden, Boston, MA, and Cologne, 2001).

new discipline.[42] Their views, activities and endeavours are examined through a series of manuscripts and printed sources.

The chair of *materia medica* led to a series of new ways of teaching and studying medicinal plants which spread throughout Europe and became decisive for the building up of a community of naturalists. These new techniques and procedures are described in Chapter 3. Duke Cosimo supported Ghini's project to establish the first botanical garden in Pisa, which was attached to the university, and was used to teach *materia medica* to the students, who for the first time were urged to look at plants directly. Other procedures such as field trips, *herbaria* of dried plants, and naturalistic illustrations, were devised to encourage the new way of studying plants. Through these new methods, first-hand observation began to complement the reading of ancient texts, which had traditionally been the basis of the teaching of pharmacology.[43]

Chapter 4 focuses on the reception of American plants. In general terms, it investigates what influence the discovery of a whole new flora had on the understanding of plants of the time. In particular, it deals with the question whether and to what extent the new exotic plants had an impact on the Italian pharmacopoeia. Through herbals, letters and descriptions of gardens, it attempts to determine which plants were accepted because of their medical potential, and which were taken into consideration on the ground of curiosity, and for reasons that had little to do with their utility.

The fifth and the sixth chapters deal with medicinal plants from the point of view of the theory and practice of therapy. Chapter 5 investigates a series of aspects concerning the understanding of therapy. It begins by examining in depth the Florentine pharmacopoeia, the *Nuovo ricettario fiorentino* (1498), which was issued with the purpose of providing apothecaries with ideas, precepts and recipes to which to conform, and limit the mistakes in the choice and use of drugs so often lamented.[44] The second part of the chapter attempts to answer the question whether the *Ricettario* actually reflected the understanding of therapy of the time and it also addresses the question of the penetration of Paracelsian theories and practices into Italy.

Chapter 6 analyses a series of primary sources in order to shed some light on the problematic question of the relationship between theory and practice, and the use of medicinal plants in practice.

---

[42]   N. Galassi, 'Luca Ghini, una vita per la scienza', *Museologia Scientifica*, 8 (1991–92), 187–206; Luigi Sabbatani, 'La cattedra dei semplici fondata a Bologna da Luca Ghini', *Studi e memorie per la storia dell'Università di Bologna*, 9 (1926), pp. 13–53; Garbari, Lucia Tongiorgi Tomasi and Tosi, *Giardino dei semplici*.

[43]   Karen Reeds, *Botany in Medieval and Renaissance Universities* (New York, 1991).

[44]   *Nuovo Receptario composto dal famosissimo chollegio degli eximii doctori della arte et medicina della inclita cipta di Firenze. Impresso nella inclyta ciptà di Firenze per la compagnia del Dragho* (1498).

Taken as a whole, the various aspects examined in these chapters are intended to build up a picture of the multifarious world of plants in Tuscany in the period of time under study. Drawing on this picture, the Conclusion discusses in which contexts, on which grounds, and on the basis of which cultural shifts the study of plants abandoned the traditional field of medicine to take its own path.

Chapter 1
Plants and Medicine at the Court of Cosimo, Francesco, and Ferdinando de' Medici

Although the Medici had been a leading family in Florence since the time of Cosimo the Elder (1389–1464), the fluctuations in their fortunes and the non-institutional character of their leadership never allowed the formation of anything like a court. A court in the proper sense only began to develop after 1537, when Cosimo de' Medici was elected head of the Florentine Republic. The salary rolls provide evidence that between that date and 1570, when Cosimo was accorded the title of Grand Duke of Tuscany, the court had grown to a remarkable size, and continued to increase under the rule of his sons Francesco and Ferdinando. The first salary rolls (1540–43) record about forty names, while on the accession of Cosimo II, on the death of Ferdinando I (1609), the personnel of the court included 359 functionaries.[1] The lists of *salariati*, however, give only a vague idea of the size of the court. The number immediately appears much larger if you include the families of the *salariati*, and even larger if you add the great number of people who constantly surrounded the grand dukes without being employed, such as distant relatives, diplomats, merchants, artists, members of the church, military officers and guests.

If the size of a court is not easily determined, it is even harder to grasp its distinctive characteristics. Contemporary writers have represented courtiers in contrasting ways. On the one hand, Baldassarre Castiglione in his famous *Il cortegiano* (1528) traces the figure of the perfect courtier, a *virtuoso* par excellence, man of letters and arms, and so superior as to be able to sustain any physical or intellectual effort with nonchalance.[2] On the other hand, the literature of the time abounds with courtiers seen as scoundrels and opportunists, ready to prostitute themselves for honours, power and wealth.

---

[1]   R.B. Litchfield, *Florence Ducal Capital 1530–1630* (New York: ACLS E-book, 2008), ch. 2, paras 76–9.

[2]   *Il libro del cortegiano del conte Baldessar Castiglione*. The first edition was published in Venice in 1528. In the same year it was published in Florence (Florence, 1528).

And this latter meaning is certainly the one that has survived, at least in the Italian language.

While the figure of the ideal courtier has often been defined, and courtiers as literary characters variously depicted, the same cannot be said for the 'court' itself. On the contrary, it has been often pointed out, both by early modern and today's writers, that the term 'court' is not easily definable, and that each court had its own features which gave rise to a complex system of attitudes, customs and practices to which its members had to conform.

At least one characteristic, however, shared by all courts, has been identified: 'Whether a court was large or small, the personality and interests of its ruler directed court life and organized its vitality as a cultural site.'[3] In other words, the court is the site where the prince performs his action, and is moulded by his personality and by the ways through which he exercises his power.

This definition seems particularly pertinent to the grand duchy of Tuscany. The relevance of the figure of the prince in creating a cultural climate, and his determination to carry out a specific multifaceted cultural project is here particularly evident. The ways in which the various facets of this project contributed to the reinforcement of his power, were crucial for the shaping of the court identity and for the legitimation of the new state.

The aim of this chapter is to throw light on a particular aspect of Cosimo's cultural policy. It will focus on a series of activities and initiatives which stemmed from his personal interest in *materia medica* and plants, and proved fundamental for the building up of his public image and the prestige of the grand duchy. This side of the grand duke's personality, and the achievements of this particular aspect of his cultural project, so often described with wonder by his contemporaries, has not yet been paid much attention. Cosimo's interest in plants, which was continued and expanded by his sons Francesco and Ferdinando, was carried out on two different fronts. The first was connected with medicine and medical botany; the second with a novel attention to the planting of grand gardens, which involved special care being taken in the research and choice of species, and a constant personal control of their propagation and growth.

---

3   Bruce T. Moran, 'Courts and Academies', *The Cambridge History of Science*, vol. 3: *Early Modern Science* (Cambridge, 2006), pp. 251–2. See also R.J.W. Evans, 'The Court: A Protean Institution and an Elusive Subject', in R.G. Asch and A.M. Birke (eds), *Princes, Patronage and the Nobility* (Oxford, 1990), pp. 481–91, and Marcello Fantoni, *La corte del Granduca – Forma e simboli del potere mediceo fra Cinque e Seicento* (Rome, 1994), p. 16.

The Construction of a Cultural Identity

If the Medici court developed late by comparison with other princely courts in Italy, the Medici had long occupied a dominant place in Florence.[4] The political power they gained, although unofficial (or maybe because unofficial), was constantly reinforced by a special attention to religion, arts and letters. They had left a mark and invented a style that characterized their image and procured fame and prestige to themselves and the city. As soon as the 17-year-old Cosimo established his rule over Florence (1537), he was very active in placing under his control the state administration, and its defence, and in planning the expansion of its domain. He never lost sight, however, of the path traced by his predecessors. He was aware from the start that authority had to be supported by and could not be separated from the image of cultural prestige and *magnificentia* fostered by the early Medici. He surrounded himself with humanists and men of letters, taking under his wing the Accademia degli Umidi and renaming it Accademia fiorentina; he invited to Florence the printer Lorenzo Torrentino who obtained the official title of *'impressore ducale'* (ducal printer) committing himself to submit all books to the grand duke, and the universities of Pisa and Florence.[5] Above all he followed his ancestors in placing great emphasis on the work of his artists. One of Cosimo's first steps was to move the family residence from the house in the via Larga to the Palazzo Vecchio, until then the seat of the Florentine Republic. While the exterior of the palace was left untouched, the interior underwent a restoration that took years, and had not been completed when a new princely palace, that of Luca Pitti on the other side of the River Arno, was bought and chosen as the new residence. All the works Cosimo commissioned from Giorgio Vasari in the Palazzo Vecchio were carried out with the precise purpose of the glorification of the family. The new apartments were each named after one of its illustrious members and decorated with frescoes exalting their deeds and authority. Not long after the first series of works, there was material enough to celebrate the deeds of Cosimo himself, which Vasari did, sparing no effort in extolling his glory.

---

[4]   For example, the courts of the Sforza in Milan, the Gonzaga in Mantova, the Montefeltro in Urbino, the d'Este in Ferrara, and the Aragonese in Naples.

[5]   William Eamon, 'Court, Academy, and Printing House: Patronage and Scientific Careers in Late Renaissance Italy', in Bruce T. Moran (ed.), *Patronage and Institutions: Science, Technology, and Medicine at the European Court 1500–1750* (Rochester, NY, 1991), p. 25.

The Importance of the Name *Medici*: Cosmas and Damian

These aspects of Cosimo's cultural project could well be expected of a Medici. Together with these, and often in close association, however, it expanded in a new direction which included a series of 'scientific' activities addressed principally to the field of medicine. Even if Cosimo's initiatives in this field are also to be attributed to his personal interests, one should not overlook the importance of the family name *Medici* and its link with medicine. Although the origin of the name is uncertain,[6] this link was underlined by Giovanni di Bicci de' Medici (1360–1429) who chose as patron saints Cosmas and Damian, the early Christian twin brothers protectors of physicians and apothecaries. Giovanni called his twin sons Cosma and Damiano, and commissioned from Brunelleschi a chapel in San Lorenzo dedicated to the two saints.[7] Under Cosimo the Elder a great number of works of art began to appear, in which the saints are represented, mainly in the church of San Lorenzo, and the Convent of San Marco, two Medicean sites. Some bas reliefs by Donatello (1443) in the Sagrestia Vecchia and two statues designed by Michelangelo but realized by Montorsoli and Montelupo (*c.*1538), in the Sagrestia Nuova, represent Cosmas and Damian. Most significant, however, is a series of altarpieces where the saints are not represented in separate sections but share the same space as the Virgin and Child. The new kind of altarpieces placed a new emphasis on the representation of the physician saints and convey a clearer message about the prominence of the house of Medici (Figure 1.1).[8] The identification of the wealthy family of the Medici with the two Arab doctors who were called 'anargiri', a word that means 'without reward', referring to the fact that the two saints acted in strict poverty and only for charity, never accepting any remuneration, may appear peculiar.[9] However, it should not be forgotten that the cult of the saints and their representation in pictures were an expression of devotion, and were felt and read as such. Cosmas and Damian were intercessors between the Medici patrons and the Virgin, and the association of the family with their patron saints was itself a demonstration of religious commitment.

---

[6]   See R. Brogan, *A Signature of Power and Patronage: The Medici Coat of Arms 1299–1492* (New York, *c.*1993), pp. 33–4. One of the causes put forth to explain the origin of the name Medici is their belonging to the Arte dei Medici e Speziali, which has never been confirmed, as the Medici, as far as we know, were members of the Arte del Cambio.

[7]   Cosma and Cosimo are variations of the same name.

[8]   Francis Ames-Lewis, 'Fra Angelico, Fra Filippo Lippi, and the Early Medici', in *The Early Medici and their Artists* (London, 1995), pp. 107–24; Dale Kent, *Cosimo de' Medici and the Florence Renaissance, the Patron's Oeuvre* (New Haven, CT, and London, 2000), p. 144.

[9]   For example, see Louis Réau, *Iconographie de l'art crétien* (Paris, 1957), p. 333.

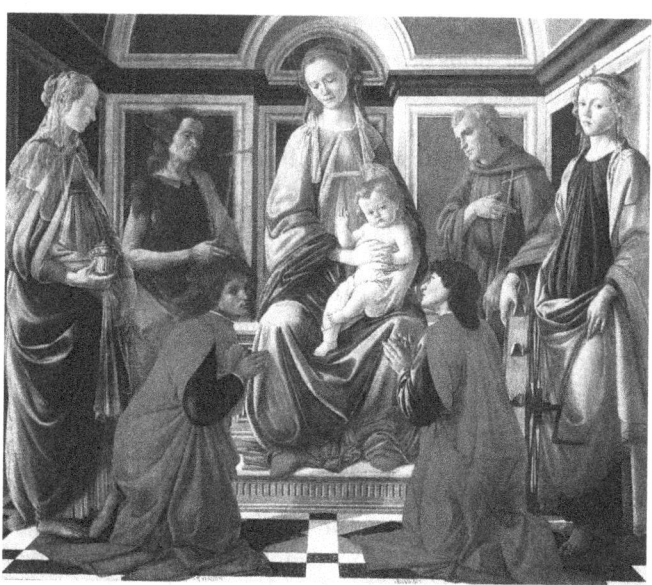

Figure 1.1   Sandro Botticelli, Pala delle Convertite, *c.*1470. Madonna and
Child with Saints Cosmas and Damian in the foreground.
Florence, Galleria degli Uffizi

Saints Cosmas and Damian were not only onomastic saints, as were for
example Saint Peter the Martyr and Saint Lawrence for the members of the
family who bore those names. Although they acquired great importance under
the two Cosimos (Cosimo the Elder and Cosimo I), they had been chosen by
Giovanni di Bicci because of the surname of the whole family, and therefore they
represented all its members. This is confirmed by the fact that Saint Damian
continued to be represented, although his name had not been chosen by the
new generations.

It has to be noted that great importance was then attached to the meaning
of names, the *interpretatio nominum* and to the so-called '*etymologiae*', which
did not concern the linguistic origin of a name, but was based on the belief
that there was a link between the name and the qualities of the person bearing
that name, according to God's will.[10] It is also worth noting that Cosmas and

---

[10]   Valeria Novembri, 'I Santi Cosma e Damiano e la tradizione manoscritta nella
Firenze medicea', *Cosma e Damiano – Dall'Oriente a Firenze*, in Elena Giannarelli (ed.),
Cosma e Damiano: Dall'Oriente a Firenze (Florence, 2002), p. 70. In the *Legenda aurea*, the
best known book about the lives of saints, the life of each saint is preceded by an introduction
about the meaning of his or her name.

Damian's legendary recoveries were attributed more to their skill as physicians than to a generic miraculous power due to their sanctity. It was their medical knowledge and ability that were miraculous. This fact was stressed by their attributes: along with the halo and the palms of martyrdom, they always hold a huge volume (which, when represented open, reveals medicinal plant illustrations), a box of medicaments, and sometimes a *matula*.[11] Moreover they almost always wear the red mantel and the red cap considered the customary dress of physicians.

While the identification of the early Medici with the martyr doctors had probably originated in a play upon the name, Cosimo I's commitment to medicine reinforced the connection by turning the symbolic meaning into a factual one. The Medici were no longer only Medici in name, they had now become *medici* in fact. This novel identification with the two saints is clearly expressed by Vasari in the Palazzo Vecchio, where the two Cosimos are themselves depicted as saints. Vasari transforms two well-known portrayals of Cosimo the Elder and Cosimo I (one by Pontormo and one by Bronzino) into representations of Cosmas and Damian, painting halos behind their heads, and placing in their hands some of their usual attributes: the palms of martyrdom, and the medical books (Figure 1.2).[12]

Under the first grand dukes, the relationship between the Medici and their patron saints was closer not only because they now shared the medical vocation, but also because the grand dukes' interest in the production of medicaments was emphasized by contemporaries as a sign of generosity and charity. The mathematician and explorer Filippo Pigafetta (1533–1604), for example, when describing the fact that the grand duke [Ferdinando] used to take with him various kind of medicaments made in his laboratory to offer them to 'Prelates, Ambassadors, *Signori* and to everybody charitably', concludes: 'so that he proves to be Physician in name and in fact, generous towards the needy, and courteous in every evident cure of the ill ...'.[13] In this sense the grand dukes were acting as 'anargiri', only out of charity, like Cosmas and Damian.

---

[11]   The attributes with which Cosmas and Damian are usually depicted are listed by Ludovica Sebregondi, 'Cosma e Damiano. Santi Medici e Medicei', in Elena Giannarelli (ed.), *Cosma e Damiano: Dall'Oriente a Firenze* (Florence, 2002), pp. 94–7. In the painting by Bernardino Poccetti in the church of S. Lorenzo, the illustrations of medicinal plants are clearly visible.

[12]   Silvia Meloni Trkulja, 'I Medici Santi', in Cristina Giannini (ed.), *Stanze segrete raccolte per caso. I Medici Santi – Gli arredi celati* (Florence, 2003), pp. 25–42.

[13]   Giuseppe Bencivenni Pelli, 'Descrizione della Galleria di Filippo Pigafetta', in *Saggio istorico della Real Galleria di Firenze* (Florence: Gaetano Gambiagi, 1779), vol. 2, pp. 199–200.

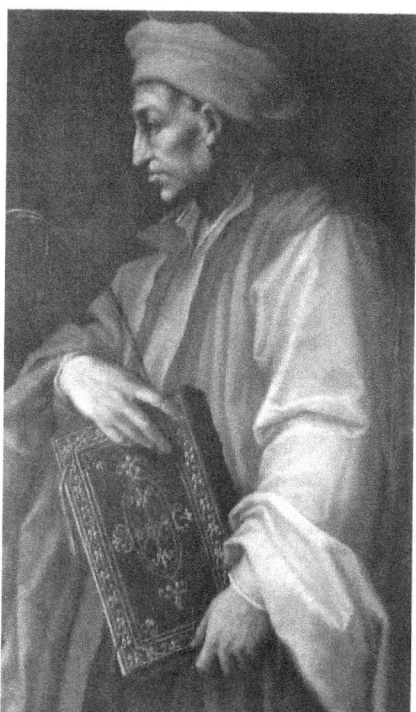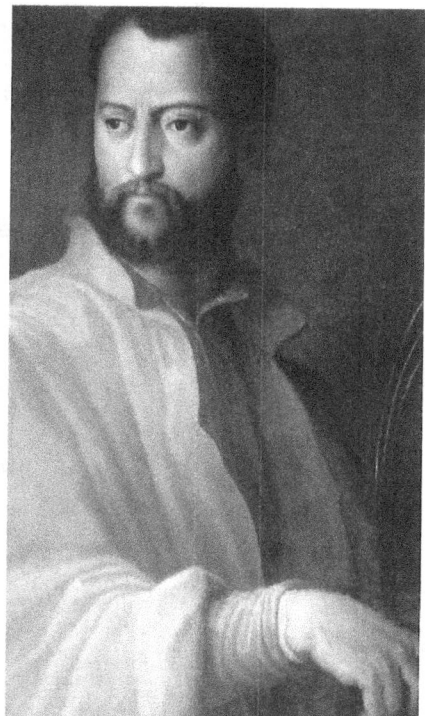

Figure 1.2   Giorgio Vasari, Cosimo I and Cosimo the Elder as Saints Cosmas and Damian, *c.*1558. Florence, Palazzo Vecchio, Chapel of the apartment of Leo X

That the dukes gave medicaments as a present, often in boxes containing several of them, is frequently repeated in the accounts of contemporaries (Figure 1.3).[14]

---

[14]   See for example, the description of Baccio Baldini, reported on p. 40. In Paola Barocchi and Giovanna Gaeta Bertelà, *Collezionismo Mediceo e Storia artistica* (Florence, 2002), p. 473, a letter of the master of *fonderia* Niccolò Sisti is reported, with a list of medicaments for two 'cassette ricche d'ebano'.Valentina Conticelli points out that under grand duke Ferdinando the number of gifts greatly increased. They were boxes of ebony or walnut containing 8, 10, 18, or 24 medicaments with written recipes. They were given to courtiers, ambassadors, monarchs and princes. Valentina Conticelli, in *L'alchimia e le arti: la fonderia degli Uffizi da laboratorio a stanza delle meraviglie* (Florence, 2012), p. 20.

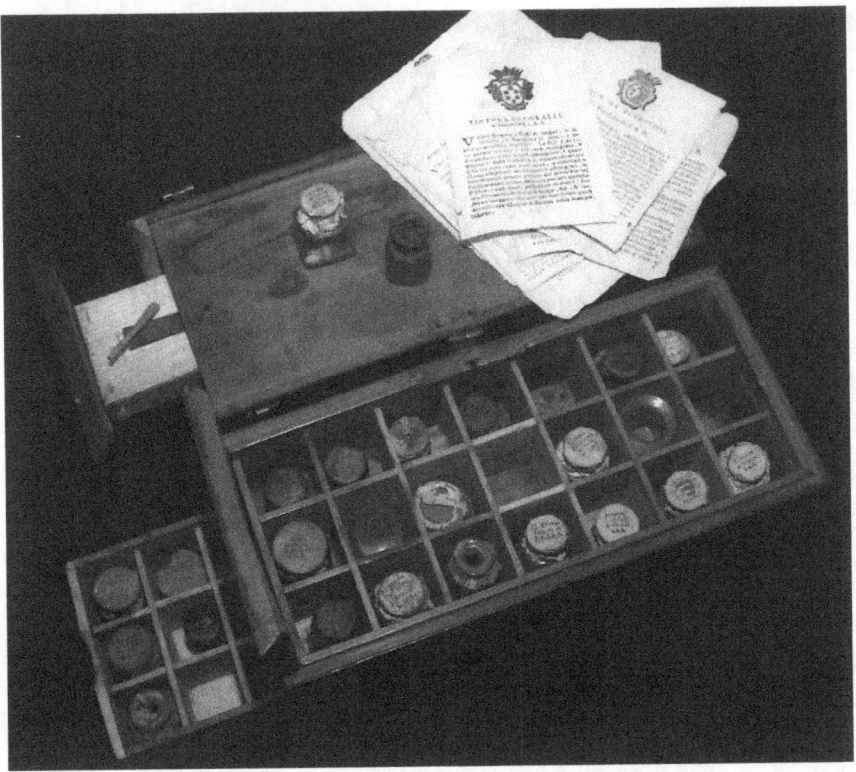

Figure 1.3   Box with medicines and recipes from the ducal *fonderia*. Rome,
Museo Storico Nazionale di Storia dell'Arte Sanitaria, Inv. 757.
Photo Baggieri Boccassini

It has often been pointed out that gifts played a fundamental role in
establishing and maintaining personal bonds within the court; through gift
giving and favours the prince affirmed his superiority and reinforced his
authority over subjects at all levels.[15] From this perspective, it is interesting to
note that medicaments and what is more, medicaments created and made by the
duke himself, constituted very special gifts. They did not only imply generosity:
they also implied skill, and at the same time, charity. Above all, the ability to

---

[15]   Since the anthropologist M. Mauss wrote his *Essay sur le don*, gifts have been object
of many studies in different disciplines. For the period under discussion see Natalie Zemon
Davis, *The Gift in Sixteenth-Century France* (Madison, *c.*2000). For the court of the grand
dukes of Tuscany see Marcello Fantoni, *La corte del Granduca: Forma e simboli del potere
mediceo fra Cinque e Seicento* (Rome,, 1994) ch. 3, 'Il dono: liberalità e potere'.

cure was traditionally associated with the sacralization of power. Although not anointed and not provided with thaumaturgic properties, Cosimo was able to build up and convey an image of providential and charitable prince.[16] The idea that the young Cosimo had been chosen *'fuora dall'aspettativa di ciascuno'* (against anyone's expectation) and almost for divine inspiration was one of the themes *de rigueur*, along with that of his religiosity, in the official panegyrics or 'vitae' of the grand duke.[17] The image of 'Cosmus medicus', conveyed through the identification with Saint Cosmas and Damian, and his donating remedies to courtiers, wealthy or needy, provided a substantial support for this general idea.

The grand dukes' concern for the health of the body was easily transposed to the health of the state, and in the eulogistic writings of contemporaries the similitude was often repeated; there could be no better prince than the one who was equally concerned with the health of their subjects and the prosperity of the State, and had the ability to achieve both.

The Grand Dukes' Commitment to Medicine

Contemporary biographers and writers emphasize the medical interest and activity of Cosimo and draw attention to his knowledge of medicinal plants. Here is the account of the physician Baccio Baldini:

> he [Cosimo] began to use this knowledge he had of plants for the common good and utility of men, and thus he had many kinds of herbs, leaves, and flowers distilled in various ways in all seasons, and obtained the most precious waters and oils; and he produced many different medicaments, both simple and compound, which he gave not only to those of his subjects who needed them, but sent them also all over Europe to anybody who would request them, with the greatest utility for those who used them; a kindness really worthy of great Princes, which more than anything else renders them similar to God, as in this way they provide men almost with the greatest benefit it could be done to them ...[18]

An evident demonstration of the genuine interest of Cosimo in medicine is a copy of the translation and commentary of Dioscorides's *Materia Medica* by Mattioli, preserved in the Biblioteca Nazionale di Firenze, which is crammed

---

[16]   Fantoni, *La corte del Granduca*, p. 16. Although Fantoni never refers to the Medici's devotion to the twin physician saints, the concept of sacralization he outlines can well be applied to it.

[17]   See Carmen Menchini, *Panegirici e vite di Cosimo I de' Medici* (Florence, 2005), pp. 19–20 and *passim*.

[18]   Baccio Baldini, *Vita di Cosimo I Granduca di Toscana* (Florence, 1578), pp. 86–7.

with notes in the grand duke's own hand.[19] The treatise by the Greek Dioscorides was, at the time, the undisputed authority on medicinal plants, and the only text prescribed for the new course on *materia medica* at the University of Pisa.[20] The translation and commentary of the prominent physician Pietro Andrea Mattioli was a great success, and the book went through a great number of editions. This early edition (1544) of Mattioli's *Discorsi*, did not yet include any illustrations, and was not the kind of prestigious book a prince would leaf through. However, we have evidence that the duke read it and, what is more interesting, of how he read it. The notes show that the duke was seriously interested in its contents. That he considered it a subject of study was underlined by the fact that Cosimo concentrated his attention on the original text of Dioscorides, and not on Mattioli's commentary. In fact, all his notes are in the margins of Dioscorides, while the margins of the long commentary of Mattioli are left untouched. There are notes on almost every page of the first, the second, and parts of the third book. Cosimo's annotations concern only the therapeutic properties of the plants, and the diseases that they were supposed to cure; there are no comments on the different species of the plant, on their provenance, or on the medicinal preparations. When he can, he always reports the Tuscan name of the plant described by Dioscorides, which reminds us that nomenclature was a major problem at the time, and a much-discussed question, especially when, as in this case, there were no illustrations to help with the identification. So beside 'Iris' he notes '*giagiolo*', beside '*arbuto*' (strawberry tree) '*corbezzolo*', beside 'siliqua'(locust tree) '*carubbo*', beside 'croco' (crocus) '*zafferano*', and so on.[21] Cosimo then lists the uses for which the plant was appropriate. Just to quote an example, in the margin of Cap. XVIII 'Del Balsamo' (Figure 1.4), he notes:

'Balsam – oil, seeds, and plant'

Removes the ... from eyes – induces menstruation and labour – removes the chills of fever – purges wounds – is good for the chest – for the bite of snakes – for the cough of the lungs – sciatica – the falling sickness – the pains of the body – difficulty in urinating – spasms – takes out the splinters from bones.[22]

---

[19]   BNCF, Banco Rari, 119 – Di Pedacio Dioscoride Anazerbeo *Libri cinque della istoria & materia medicinale tradotti in lingua volgare Italiana da M. Pietro Andrea Matthiolo Sanese Medico* (Venice, 1544).

[20]   See Chapter 2, p. 57.

[21]   Cosimo always reports the Tuscan name, even when it coincides with the translation of Mattioli, who was himself Tuscan. He obviously omits it when the plant is exotic, as in the case of balsam. Also Mattioli, in his commentary, often lists the various names under which the plant is commonly known.

[22]   Pedacio Dioscoride Anazerbeo, *Libri cinque della istoria & materia medicinale*, Book I, ch. 18, p. 20.

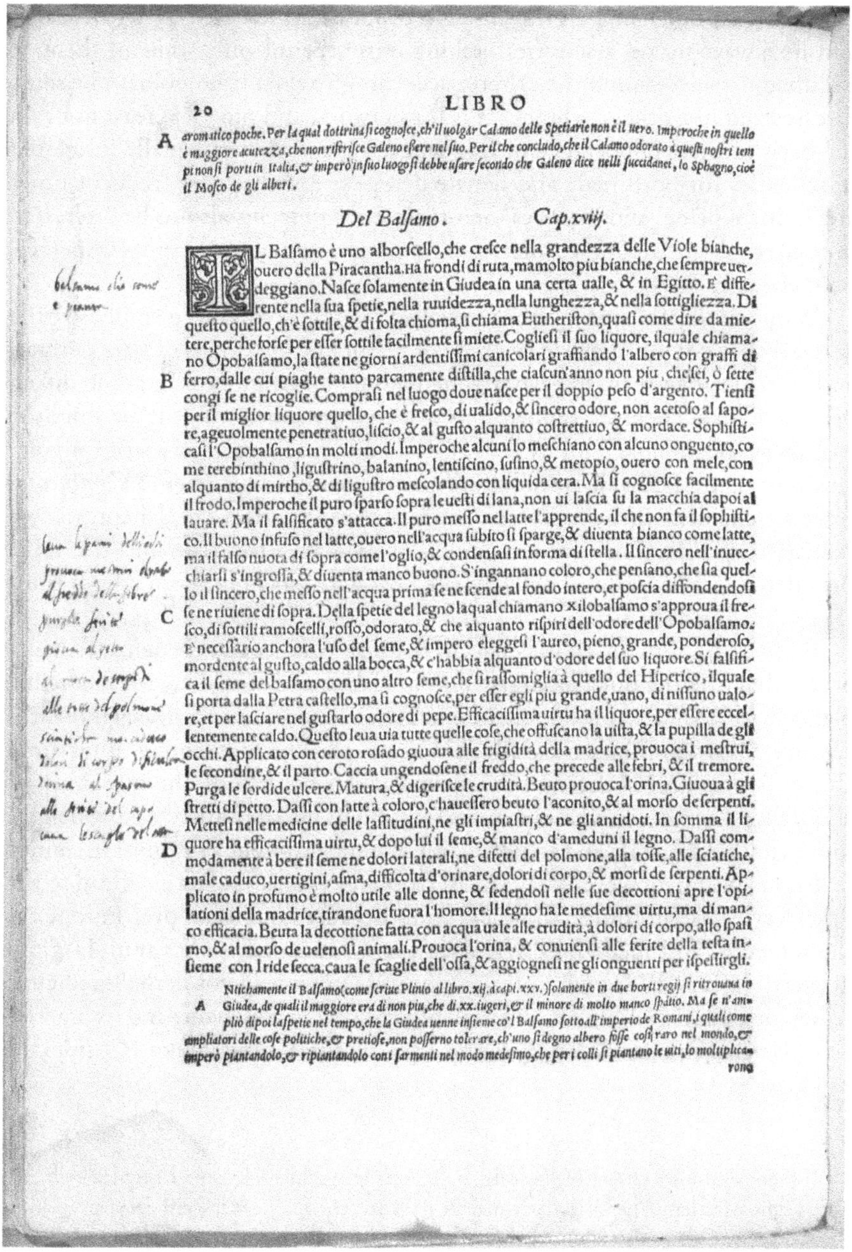

A aromatico poche. Per la qual dottrina fi cognofce, ch'il uolgar Calamo delle Spetiarie non è il uero. Imperoche in quello è maggiore acutezza, che non rifèrifce Galeno eſſere nel ſuo. Per il che concludo, che il Calamo odorato à queſti noſtri tem pi non ſi porti in Italia, & imperò in ſuo luogo ſi debbe uſare ſecondo che Galeno dice nelli ſuccidanei, lo Sphagno, cioè il Moſco de gli alberi.

Del Balſamo.   Cap. xviij.

IL Balſamo è uno alborſcello, che creſce nella grandezza delle Viole bianche, ouero della Piracantha. Ha frondi di ruta, ma molto piu bianche, che ſempre uer deggiano. Naſce ſolamente in Giudea in una certa ualle, & in Egitto. E' diffe rente nella ſua ſpetie, nella ruuidezza, nella lunghezza, & nella ſottigliezza. Di queſto quello, ch'è ſottile, & di folta chioma, ſi chiama Eutheriſton, quaſi come dire da mie tere, perche forſe per eſſer ſottile facilmente ſi miete. Cogliefi il ſuo liquore, il quale chiama

B no Opobalſamo, la ſtate ne giorni ardentiſſimi canicolari graffiando l'albero con graffi di ferro, dalle cui piaghe tanto parcamente diſtilla, che ciaſcun'anno non piu, che ſei, ò ſette congi ſe ne ricoglie. Compraſi nel luogo doue naſce per il doppio peſo d'argento. Tienſi per il miglior liquore quello, che è freſco, di ualido, & ſincero odore, non acetoſo al ſapo re, ageuolmente penetratiuo, liſcio, & al guſto alquanto coſtrettiuo, & mordace. Sophiſti caſi l'Opobalſamo in molti modi. Imperoche alcuni lo meſchiano con alcuno onguento, co me terebinthino, liguſtrino, balanino, lentiſcino, ſuſino, & metopio, ouero con mele, con alquanto di mirtho, & di liguſtro meſcolando con liquida cera. Ma ſi cognoſce facilmente il ſrodo. Imperoche il puro ſparſo ſopra le ueſti di lana, non ui laſcia ſu la macchia dapoi al lauare. Ma il falſificato s'attacca. Il puro meſſo nel latte s'apprende, il che non fa il ſophiſti co. Il buono infuſo nel latte, ouero nell'acqua ſubito ſi ſparge, & diuenta bianco come latte, ma il falſo nuota di ſopra come l'oglio, & condenſaſi in forma di ſtella. Il ſincero nell'inuec chiarſi s'ingroſſa, & diuenta manco buono. S'ingannano coloro, che penſano, che ſia quel lo il ſincero, che meſſo nell'acqua prima ſe ne ſcende al fondo intero, et poſcia diffondendoſi ſe ne riuiene di ſopra. Della ſpetie del legno la qual chiamano Xilobalſamo s'approua il fre

C ſco, di ſottili ramoſcelli, roſſo, odorato, & che alquanto riſpiri dell'odore dell'Opobalſamo. E' neceſſario anchora l'uſo del ſeme, & impero eleggeſi l'aureo, pieno, grande, ponderoſo, mordente al guſto, caldo alla bocca, & c'habbia alquanto d'odore del ſuo liquore. Si falſifi ca il ſeme del balſamo con uno altro ſeme, che ſi raſſomiglia à quello del Hiperico, il quale ſi porta dalla Petra caſtello, ma ſi cognoſce, per eſſer egli piu grande, uano, di niſſuno ualo re, et per laſciare nel guſtarlo odore di pepe. Efficaciſſima uirtu ha il liquore, per eſſere eccel lentemente caldo. Queſto leua uia tutte quelle coſe, che offuſcano la uiſta, & la pupilla de gli occhi. Applicato con ceroto roſado giouua alle frigidità della madrice, prouoca i meſtrui, le ſecondine, & il parto. Caccia ungendoſene il freddo, che precede alle febri, & il tremore. Purga le ſordide ulcere. Matura, & digeriſce le cruditâ. Beuto prouoca l'orina. Giouua à gli ſtretti di petto. Daſſi con latte à coloro, c'haueſſero beuto l'aconito, & al morſo de ſerpenti. Metteſi nelle medicine delle laſſitudini, ne gli impiaſtri, & ne gli antidoti. In ſomma il li

D quore ha efficaciſſima uirtu, & dopo lui il ſeme, & manco d'ameduni il legno. Daſſi com modamente à bere il ſeme ne dolori laterali, ne difetti del polmone, alla toſſe, alle ſciatiche, male caduco, uertigini, aſma, difficolta d'orinare, dolori di corpo, & morſi de ſerpenti. Ap plicato in profumo è molto utile alle donne, & ſedendoſi nelle ſue decottioni apre l'opi lationi della madrice, tirandone fuora l'homore. Il legno ha le medeſime uirtu, ma di man co efficacia. Beuta la decottione fatta con acqua uale alle cruditâ, à dolori di corpo, allo ſpaſi mo, & al morſo de uelenoſi animali. Prouoca l'orina, & conuienſi alle ferite della teſta in ſieme con l'iride ſecca. caua le ſcaglie dell'oſſa, & aggiogneſi ne gli unguenti per iſpeſſirgli.

Ntichamente il Balſamo (come ſcriue Plinio al libro. xij. à capi. xxv.) ſolamente in due horti regij ſi ritrouaua in

A Giudea, de quali il maggiore era di non piu, che di. xx. iugeri, & il minore di molto manco ſpitto. Ma ſe n'am plio dipoi la ſpetie nel tempo, che la Giudea uenne inſieme co'l Balſamo ſotto all'imperio de Romani, i quali come ampliatori delle coſe politiche, & pretioſe, non poſſerno tolerare, ch'uno ſi degno albero foſſe coſi raro nel mondo, & imperò piantandolo, & ripiantandolo con i ſarmenti nel modo medeſimo, che per i colli ſi piantano le uiti, lo moltiplica

                      rono

Figure 1.4 Notes of Duke Cosimo I in the margins of Mattioli's *Discorsi* edition of 1544. Biblioteca Nazionale Centrale di Firenze, Banco Rari, 119

Cosimo does not name all the curative properties indicated by Dioscorides, and he always makes a selection, taking into account only some of them. It is difficult to determine the criteria according to which he points out some diseases and not others, whether it is for personal and practical reasons or on the basis of their importance or frequency. He certainly is equally interested in remedies for both male and female diseases, and the most frequent notes are 'induces urine' and 'induces menstruation'. He seems also to be interested in beauty treatments and cosmetics as he often notes 'removes spots from face' or 'it cures freckles'.[23]

While sixteenth-century historians and biographers tend to emphasize the grand dukes' commitment in the field of medicine, historians of later periods, and even of today, seem to have attached more importance to the grand dukes' penchant for alchemy.[24] Alchemy, as a secret art practised only by initiates, had always been looked on with suspicion and associated with greed for gold, elusiveness and fraud. It is well known that Dante, in his *Divina Commedia*, placed alchemists in hell.[25] In sixteenth-century treatises on alchemy, it was pointed out that there are two kinds of alchemy: the true and the false. Benedetto Varchi in his *Si l'archemia è vera o no quistione*, even adds a third category: the 'sophistic'.[26]

If Cosimo's contemporaries Baccio Baldini, Ambassador Fedeli, and many others describe the duke as engaged in his laboratory mainly with medicinal plants, with a view to producing new beneficial medicaments, the eighteenth-century historian Riguccio Galluzzi (1739–1801), for example, underlines Cosimo's passion for the art of alchemy, which he defines 'the most vain of all' ('*la più vana di tutte*') and depicts Cosimo in his laboratory, taking delight in transmuting metals and in producing the most potent poisons. He cannot help concluding, however, that 'since errors and vanities sometimes lead to the discovery of useful things, this laboratory became famous all over Europe for the remedies and medicines that were there produced'.[27] Giovanni Targioni Tozzetti, (1712–1783) who praises Cosimo's knowledge of herbal medicine, reluctantly admits: 'I cannot and shall not conceal that alchemy and its practice was given credit in Florence in the days of the Grand Duke [Cosimo I],

---

23   For example: ch. 1, 'Della Iride', p. 3: 'leua le machie del viso e lentigi[ni]; ch. 37, 'Dell'Oglio Masticino', p. 33: 'Leua le machie dal viso'; ch. 48, 'Leva li segni del viso'.

24   See for example, Giulio Lensi Orlandi, *Cosimo e Francesco de' Medici alchimisti* (Florence, 1978); Perifano, *L'Alchimie*; Conticelli, *L'alchimia e le arti*.

25   Dante, *Divina Commedia*, Inferno, XXIX, 118–20, 136–9.

26   Benedetto Varchi, *Questione sull'alchimia* (Florence, 1827).

27   Riguccio Galluzzi, *Istoria del Granducato di Toscana sotto il governo di casa Medici* (Florence, 1781), p. 294.

maybe because also the prince delighted in it.'[28] We have evidence that the Grand Duke Francesco, for example, had alchemists (or *filosofi*, as they were called) in his service, who worked in his laboratory. The letters of one of these, Ardicino Castelletti, to the grand duke clearly refer to alchemical writings and alchemical operations.[29] The application of the methods of alchemy and the use of the alchemical language, however, were characteristic of Paracelsian medicine, and in Ardicino's letters there is no mention of the reason why the procedures described were carried out. As far as the grand duke Ferdinando is concerned, an incident, which at the time had a certain resonance, shows that he had confidence in the powers of alchemy. He had invited the Swiss Paracelsian alchemist-physician Leonhart Thurneysser to his court, where he transmuted an iron nail into a golden one.[30]

Certainly the Medici grand dukes and Francesco's son Antonio were interested in alchemy. This, however, does not challenge their commitment to medicine and to producing remedies. Alchemy and medicine are not to be seen as opposed to one another. Alchemy had long been connected with medicine; the philosopher's stone (*lapis philosophorum*) sought after by the alchemist philosophers, and believed to be the substance that could transform base metals into gold, was associated with the elixir of life (*elixir vitae*) capable of transforming the perishable human body, and rendering it eternally young and devoid of illnesses. In the sixteenth century, the original purpose of obtaining gold from other metals began to decline in importance, and alchemy was more and more applied to medicine (it was later called iatrochemistry). Alchemy had the twofold form of philosophical speculation and applied art, and it was mostly in this latter capacity that it became of service to medicine. Even Cosimo's interest in metals was closely associated with remedies, and Andrea Bacci, in his *De Thermis* (1571), highlights Cosimo's interest in 'aurum potabile' (drinkable gold), which was considered a powerful medicine

---

[28] Giovanni Targioni Tozzetti, *Notizie sulla storia delle scienze fisiche in Toscana cavate da un manoscritto inedito* (Florence, 1852), p. 226. And on Francesco, ibid., p. 255.

[29] Ardicino Castelletti is in the rolls of the *stipendiati* employed at the Casino di S. Marco in 1580. Paola Barocchi and Giovanna Gaeta Bertelà, *Collezionismo mediceo – Cosimo I, Francesco I e il Cardinale Ferdinando-Documenti 1540–1587* (Modena, 1993), p. 268. On 1 January 1581 he sent a letter to the grand duke Francesco about the work being done at the *fonderia* with references to Raymond Lull's writings and to various alchemical operations (ASF, MdP, 758, c. 330). Another letter of the same kind was sent by Ardicino on 6 March 1583 (ASF, MdP, 766, c. 156).

[30] The golden nail was preserved in the niche of the Tribuna degli Uffizi. John Evelyn saw the nail in Florence in 1644 and commented on it in his diary. John Evelyn, *Diary and Correspondence*, ed. William Bray (London, 1906), p. 81. Quoted in J.R. Partington, *A History of Chemistry* (London, 1961–70), vol. 2, p. 153.

obtained by distillation.[31] Suzanne Butters, drawing on a great number of sources, shows how botany, alchemy, medicine and metallurgy were all facets of the same cultural interest of Cosimo, and underlines his practical approach to all the activities he undertook. She also points out how contemporary biographers and panegyrists highlighted these aspects of his personality as the attributes of a good ruler.[32]

It can be objected that alchemy was practised secretly and, as Lensi Orlandi says '[alchemy was] an unknown world in which, in the most absolute secrecy, the first dukes of Florence lived, without the knowledge of their courtiers, their contemporaries, and of posterity.'[33] According to this statement, it seems impossible to investigate the matter further. We have evidence, however, that a great part of the grand dukes' activities in their laboratories were aimed at producing medicaments.

The _Fonderie_

It is very likely that the image of the dukes involved in obscure and evil practices was created in association with the laboratories or _fonderie_ (as they were usually referred to), where they performed their experiments. These were equipped exactly like the traditional alchemical sites, with furnaces, stills and retorts that produced fire, smoke, and acrid smells. The tools were the same, even if the purpose was different. Distillation in particular has mainly been associated with metals and minerals, and no one seems to notice that until the end of the sixteenth century it was applied principally to plants.[34] A small manuscript of 1556 consisting of sixteen leaves, is one of the few documents that provide direct evidence of what the ducal laboratory, or _fonderia_, was used for. The title informs us that in the book we will find 'experiments and sure things by the hand of the duke of Florence or in his presence'.[35] The manuscript is centred on distillation, here defined as the 'true way of curing', and deals mainly with 'herbs, roots, gums and seeds'. The 'true way of making waters and then oils' is described and five medical recipes are reported.[36]

---

[31] De Thermis Andreae Baccii Elpidiani, Medici atque Philosophi, civis Romanis, Libri septem (Venezia, 1571), ch. 8, p. 370 (quoted by Perifano, _L'Alchimie_, p. 111).

[32] Suzanne Butters, _The Triumph of Vulcan: Sculptors' Tools, Porphyry, and the Prince in Ducal Florence_, 2 vols (Florence, 1996), ch. 14, pp. 241–67.

[33] Lensi Orlandi, _Cosimo e Francesco de' Medici alchimisti_, pp. 15–16.

[34] See Chapter 5, pp. 202–11.

[35] BNCF, MS Palatinus 1139, [Li]bro nel quale si scriveranno esperimenti e cose certe per mano del duca di Fiorenza o vero in sua presentia, né ci sarà su cosa che non sia certissima per utile comune (1556).

[36] BNCF, MS Palatinus 1139, c. 10r.

The name used for the grand dukes' laboratories, *fonderie*, that is to say 'foundries', contributed to their association with metals. *Fonderia* was in fact the same word as was used to designate the place where metals were smelted and processed, and where coins were minted. Contemporary and later historians very often had to explain the term, adding at least the adjective 'ducal' or some clarifying words after *fonderia*, such as the 'chemical-pharmaceutical laboratory of the duke'.[37]

Contemporaries always describe these laboratories as the places where the grand dukes processed 'with their own hands' plants and minerals in order to produce or experiment on medicaments. The fact that Cosimo's scientific interest in medicine led him to take an active part in its practical application, to the extent of carrying out manual work himself, met with both surprise and admiration. At least as far as the first grand duke is concerned, it was considered an unexpected side of a prince's character. This is very clear in a passage of the report of the Venetian Ambassador Vincenzo Fedeli who states, by way of introduction, that he is going to say 'something rare' (*una cosa rara*) about Cosimo, and then continues:

> [Cosimo] has these simples processed with distilled waters and oils in order to experiment with them on different diseases and wounds; and he has found remedies for the *punta del fianco*, the constriction of urine and the head wounds which in Tuscany were all mortal because of the subtlety of the air, and have now become curable. He makes the *sopravvivo* and the mithridates with great diligence, and with such perfection that they prove to be sure antidotes to poison; and every day the new remedies are seen to be used widely; and the place where so many admirable things are done is called the fonderia of the Duke of Florence, where work is continuously carried out with an infinite variety of fires, forges, furnaces and alembics; and the duke goes there often and works with his own hands to his most great delight; and it is a rare thing to be seen for the order and the great quantity of the remedies found and made for the health of the human body; so that this prince deals with natural things in order to discover the admirable secrets of nature, among which also investigation of metals is included.[38]

Cosimo's laboratories are often referred to by contemporaries. The earliest mention of the *fonderie* is in connection with the Palazzo Vecchio (after Cosimo moved there in 1540 from via Larga). Major works were undertaken on the site,

---

[37]   This is the definition given by Giovanni Targioni Tozzetti in his *Notizie*, p. 208.

[38]   'Relazione di Firenze di Messer Vincenzo Fedeli tornato da quella corte l'anno 1561', *Relazioni degli Ambasciatori Veneti al Senato*, Raccolte, annotate ed edite da Eugenio Alberi, Series 2, vol. 1 (Florence, 1839), pp. 356–7.

and a series of new apartments was commissioned from Vasari, who provides us with the first information relating to Cosimo's laboratory. Vasari mentions the fact that in 1556 he transformed the rooms of the 'old' *fonderia* so that there were in the palace no 'merrier or better' rooms. Vasari reports that the 'new' *fonderia* was right under the room of Clement VII.[39] From his report we understand that it was on the ground floor, located on the corner of the via della Ninna and the via dei Leoni. In 1556 these furnaces set fire to a beam in the pages' apartment, endangering the people and the paintings in Leo X's quarters, which included the room of Clement VII. Vasari urged the duke to remove the *fonderia* from the palace, as we can see from a letter of 12 May 1558.[40] Vasari was concerned that the *fonderia* might damage the paintings in the quarters of Leo X, and does not seem to take the activities carried out there very seriously, as he defines it as a '*bachanalja*', a mess. Although we know that there was a *fonderia* in the Palazzo Vecchio, we do not know exactly what it was like, or of how many rooms it consisted. From the plans of the Palazzo Vecchio we see that beneath the room of Clement VII there were two rooms, which could correspond to the '*officina*' to which Vasari refers. Although a new and larger *fonderia* was later established in the Uffizi, we know that it was still there (although we do not know until when it was in use) at the beginning of the twentieth century as Alfredo Lensi, who wrote his book on the Palazzo Vecchio in 1911, says: 'Not long ago, one could still see the furnaces of this workshop, which were then demolished for the convenience of the communal offices'.[41]

The *fonderia* in the Palazzo Vecchio is the one where Francesco, Cosimo's elder son and second grand duke, inherited the passion for manual work with furnaces and stills. In a letter of 1560 his brother Giovanni, half concerned and half mocking, urges him not to spend too much time in the *fonderia*: 'Be careful not to take too much pleasure in the Fonderia, as here they say that you never go out, especially by day.'[42]

Another *fonderia* was established by Cosimo in the Boboli Garden, when the Palazzo Pitti was chosen as the principal residence of the family. We do not know much about this laboratory, but in the 1650 maps of Pitti Palace by the *sottoguardaroba* Diacinto Maria Marmi, there is the drawing of a roof with the caption 'roof of the *fonderia*'. The drawings are not to scale, but the *fonderia* seems to measure approximately one-fifth of the area of the Ammannati courtyard.[43]

[39]   Quoted in Alfredo Lensi, *Palazzo Vecchio* (Florence, 1911), p. 174.

[40]   Ibid., p. 175.

[41]   Ibid.

[42]   Berti, *Il principe dello studiolo*, p. 28, and Lensi Orlandi, *Cosimo e Francesco de' Medici alchimisti*, p. 135.

[43]   BNCF, Magliab. XIII, 36, 'Appartamenti principali di Palazzo de Pitti di S.A.S. fatto da me D.M. Marmi', c. 10r.

In 1677 the physician Giovanni Cinelli decided to republish Francesco Bocchi's *Le bellezze della città di Firenze* (1591), one of the first guide-books to Florence, supplementing it with new information. Some of his descriptions, however, were never published, and are kept in manuscript at the Biblioteca Nazionale Centrale di Firenze under the title 'Bozze delle bellezze di Firenze – Ampliazione delle Bellezze di Firenze del Bocchi con molte variazioni dale stampate'.[44] Cinelli has left a description of the *fonderia* which was 'between the end of the Uffizi and the beginning of the corridor, towards the river Arno' and consisted of eight rooms and a terrace. As Cinelli wrote his account in the second half of the seventeenth century, it is not surprising he reports that the *fonderia* was intended to produce *only* chemical and 'spagiric' medicaments. Distillation was certainly already one of the main activities undertaken in the Medicean laboratories in the second half of the preceding century, and although there is evidence that mineral substances and chemicals were also employed, it was applied mainly to plants and herbs, as Filippo Pigafetta points out referring to the same *fonderia* in an earlier period: '... where [in the *fonderia*] they continuously distil waters of scented flowers and herbs, and oils from drugs and spices, producing quintessence and ointments, and make electuaries and curative confections, liquors for malignant fevers, plague, and poisons, and powders, and medicines of powerful and prompt virtues'.[45] Cinelli provides us with an accurate description of the rooms which contained alembics and glass vases of all shapes, furnaces and chimneys, and lists a large number of tools and instruments used for distillation.[46] In one of these rooms there were two huge stills, called '*circulatori magni*', 'marvellous instruments' which allowed the production, in a few hours, of a great quantity of aqua vitae (*acqua arzente*) of great perfection. They are carefully described by Cinelli as furnaces with a quadruple ascending line of twelve tin flasks each penetrating the next, and a similar one descending.[47] It is difficult to ascertain if these furnaces were new sophisticated instruments or if they had been there from the time when the *fonderia* of the Uffizi was first set up. The description, however, seems to correspond to one of the illustrations that appeared in the 'Appendix' of Mattioli's *Discorsi* in 1568 (Figure 1.5).[48]

---

[44]   BNCF, Magliab. XIII, 34, Giovanni Cinelli, 'Bozze delle bellezze di Firenze'.

[45]   Bencivenni Pelli, 'Descrizione della Galleria di Filippo Pigafetta', p. 199.

[46]   'Circolatori, separatori, sublimatori, mantenitori, lucerne, colonne, campane, recipienti, storte, bocce' ... And also: 'torculi, strettoi, stufe, fornelli, bagni' (c.123v).

[47]   (c.124v).

[48]   Pietro Andrea Mattioli, 'Appendix', *I discorsi di Pietro Andrea Mattioli sanese, Nelli sei libri di Pedacio Dioscoride Anazarbeo della materia Medicinale* (Venice, 1568).

le acque.

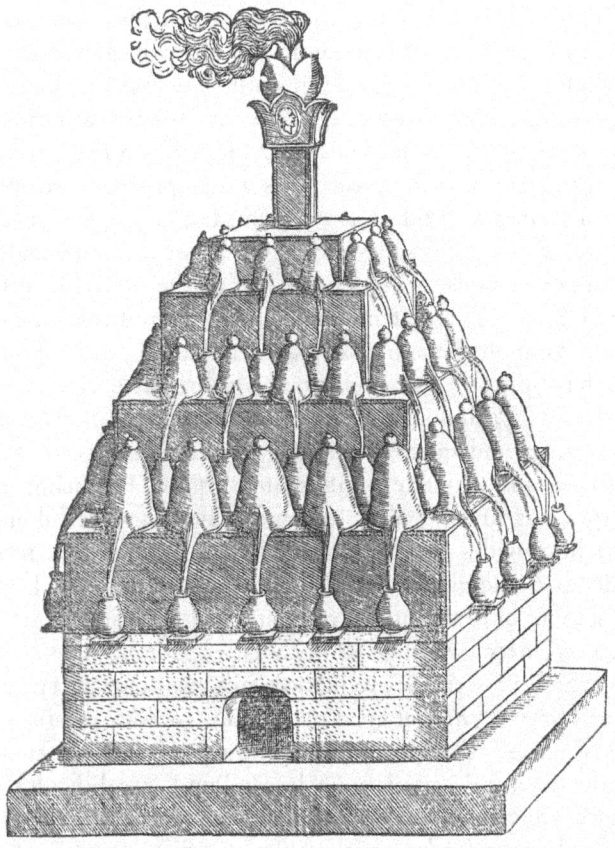

Q Vesta fornace(come appare per il fuo difegno)puo fupplire per lambiccare con xxxxviii.
campa e di piombo, & tutte poffono lambiccare, & lauorare con un fuoco folo:& n'ho uo
luto dare il difegno, ouero modello, non già perche uoglia infegnare à fabricare una fimile fornace, effendo l'acque lambiccate à piombo nociue molto à i corpi humani nell'interiora (co
me habbiamo detto di fopra) & però da lafciarle ftare: ma folamente per dimoftrare, come s'in-
gegnaffero i fucceffori di colui, che ritrouò il modo di lambiccare con le campane di piombo, à
trouar modo con manco fpefa di legna per far fuoco, ò di carbone, à diftillare in un giorno, & in
una notte gran quantità de acqua.

Figure 1.5   Pietro Andrea Mattioli, 'Prima fornace', *Del modo di
distillare le acque*, 'Appendix' to the *Discorsi* of 1568. Milano,
Biblioteca Braidense

The *fonderia* became worthy of a place among the 'beauties' of Florence. Its public image, built up through contemporary descriptions, along with the skilful and meritorious activities performed there, had acquired great prestige and fame within the court and with foreign princes. It is a very different image from that suggested by Vasari when he referred to it as a mess and wanted to get rid of it to prevent the damage its furnaces might cause. Vasari himself certainly came to attach greater importance to the *fonderia*, as in a letter of 1572 he reports to Francesco that the pope had praised it greatly: 'Our Lordship often speaks about you and your virtuous actions, and he is very willing to set up a *fonderia* like that of Your Highness, as he would be pleased to help the sick and the needy with beneficial remedies'.[49] Pope Gregory XIII here probably refers to the *fonderia* Francesco had set up in the so-called Casino di San Marco, on the site where Lorenzo de' Medici had established the Academy of the Arts. The palace, located near the Convent of San Marco within the 'Orti medicei', had been commissioned from Buontalenti by Francesco, who intended to place all his workshops there. Francesco spent a great part of his time there, as we know from the contemporary accounts that have come down to us. One of these, by ambassador Gussoni is worth quoting:

> [Francesco] takes great delight in working with alembics producing many waters and oils apt to treat many diseases, and he has a remedy for almost all of them. And among others he makes an oil of such excellent virtue that using it externally on the wrists, heart, stomach, and throat, protects them and cures any sort of poison, heals the plague-stricken, and is a most efficacious remedy for petechiae and any kind of malignant fever; and I was told that he wanted to experiment with it on persons that had been sentenced to death; he made them drink poison, and then using this oil he cured them.[50]

The prominent Bolognese naturalist Ulisse Aldrovandi, in his letters often refers to the Casino as the place where 'to work night and day and investigate the various secrets of nature', which when tested, with great liberality and kindness, are given to those who are sick and need them; and he defines the Casino 'a house of nature, so to say, where many miraculous experiments are carried out ....'[51]

---

[49] *Il Carteggio di G. Vasari*, ed. K. Frey (Arezzo, 1930), vol. 2, p. 638. Quoted in Berti, *Il Principe dello studiolo*, p. 52.

[50] 'Relazione del clarissimo messer Andrea Gussoni Ambasciator ritornato da Fiorenza l'anno 1576', *Relazioni degli Ambasciatori veneti al Senato* (Bari, 1916), p. 226.

[51] Alessandro Tosi (ed.), *Ulisse Aldrovandi e la Toscana: Carteggio e testimonianze documentarie* (Florence, 1989), p. 26 and p. 246.

Besides the pharmaceutical laboratory, Francesco moved to the Casino di San Marco a series of workshops where various artefacts were experimented on and produced, as Agostino del Riccio informs us: '... at the casino by our convent of San Marco ... where the Grand Duke had an infinite number of artists, or masters as we would call them, some of whom made jewels, and some made miniatures, or china vases; others distilled, or made glasses, or wove cloths and carpets ...'.[52]

The activities performed in the laboratories of the Casino were visually and symbolically represented in the '*studiolo*', a small windowless room the Grand Duke Francesco had commissioned from Vasari in the Palazzo Vecchio. The conceptual frame of the paintings, decorations and sculptures was conceived by Vincenzo Borghini, a man of letters and *spedalingo* of the Ospedale degli Innocenti.[53] The *studiolo* 'must be a place where to keep all the rare and precious things ... each placed in its wardrobe, according to its kind'.[54] Borghini here refers to the objects obtained by art operating on nature, as in the ducal workshops, which are depicted on panels around the room. The pharmacy or 'laboratory of medicines', and the distillery or 'laboratory of alchemy', where Francesco himself is portrayed making some potion, can be seen on one of the walls (Figure 1.6).[55]

---

[52]   Agostino del Riccio, 'Del giardino di un re', *Agricoltura sperimentale*, MS., BNCF, Targioni Tozzetti, 56, III, cc. 42v–93r. Reported in Margherita Azzi Vicentini (ed.), *L'arte dei Giardini, Scritti teorici e pratici dal XIV al XX secolo* (Milano, 1999), pp. 420–45.

[53]   For Vincenzo Borghini see Philip Gavitt, 'Charity and State Building in Cinquecento Florence: Vincenzo Borghini as administrator of the Ospedale degli Innocenti', *Journal of Modern History*, 69(2) (1997), pp. 230–70. The theoretical frame envisaged by Borghini has been associated to the scheme of Isidore of Seville, adopted as a logo by the Warburg Institute. Here is how it is explained in the home page of the Institute: '... [it describes] the interrelation of the four elements of which the world is made, with their two pairs of opposing qualities: hot and cold, moist and dry. Earth is linked to water by the common quality of coldness, water to air by the quality of moisture, air to fire by heat, and fire to earth by dryness. Following a doctrine that can be traced back to Hippocratic physiology, the tetragram adds the four seasons of the year and the four humours of man to complete the image of cosmic harmonies that both inspired and retarded the further search for natural law'.

[54]   Berti, *Il principe dello studiolo*, p. 60.

[55]   Other workshops depicted are: 'laboratorio di polvere pirica', 'vetreria', 'oreficeria', 'fonderia dei bronzi', 'lanificio', 'pesca delle perle', 'miniera di oro', 'miniera di diamanti', 'raccolta dell'ambracane', etc.

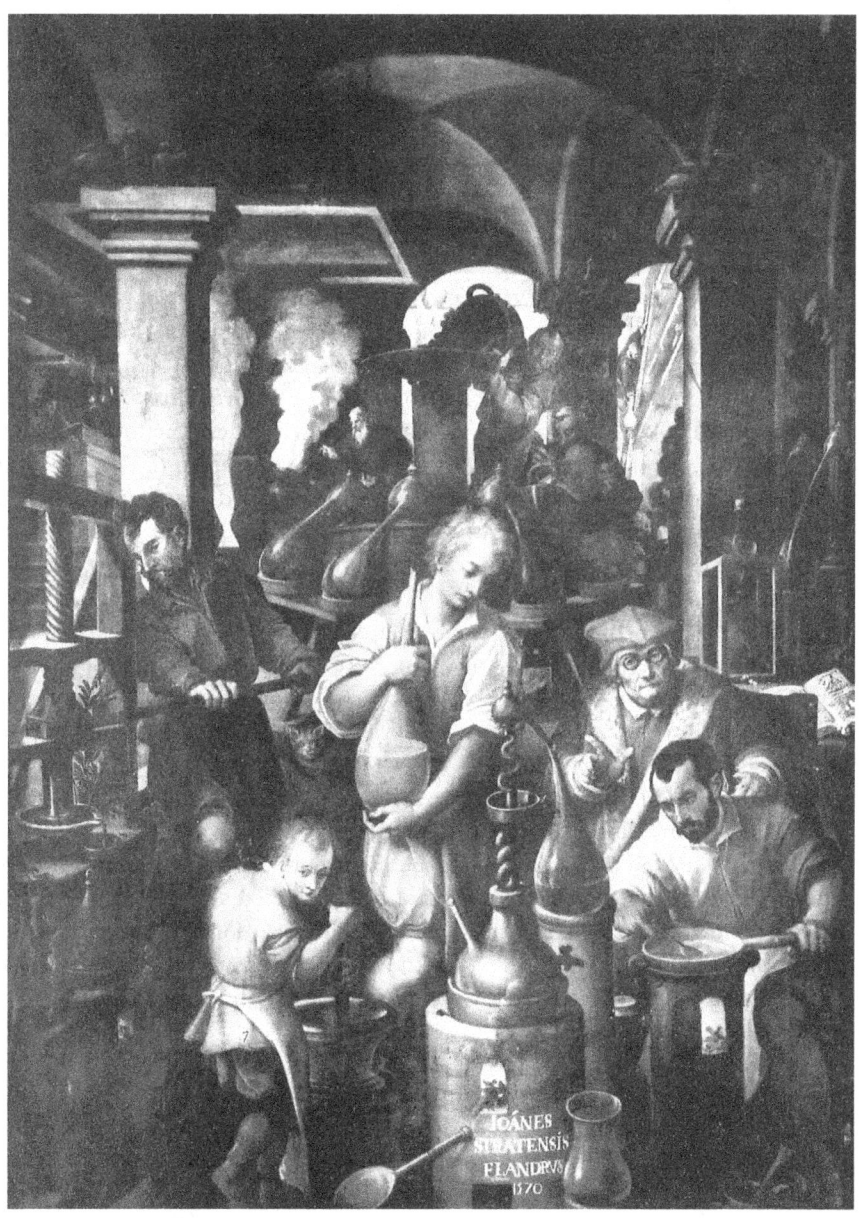

Figure 1.6   Giovanni Stradano, Francesco I working in the *fonderia*. Detail of 'the alchemist workshop', 1570. Florence, Palazzo Vecchio, wall of the *studiolo* of Francesco I

Francesco's *studiolo*, however, is much more than this. As Luciano Berti explains 'the *studiolo* that prince Francesco wanted was in fact the display or the museum, the precious casket where to gather the most refined products of the *fonderia*. And it also was the place where the various researches and products found a systematic conceptual unity, and were raised from the level of the workshop or laboratory to higher and more complex spheres.'[56] The central theme, art and nature, is rendered through the fantastic and symbolic transposition into visual images of the complex relationship between the universe, man, and man's work. In the vault of the *studiolo*, surrounding a representation of Nature and Prometheus (an allegory of the encounter between art and nature) the four Aristotelian elements – earth, fire, water and air – are depicted. Near them, however, the four qualities of hot, dry, cold and moist – are added; and in association with these the four humours ('complexions') of man: melancholy, bile, blood and phlegm, and the four seasons of the year. Borghini's '*invenzione*', in other words, contains the visual representation of the Hippocratic system (Figure 1.7). One of the pivots of the whole conceptual scheme is therefore Medicine, represented by its theoretical tenets.[57]

The *fonderia* in the Casino di San Marco was used intensively for a long time, since Francesco's natural son Don Antonio inherited both the Casino and a passion for medicine and pharmaceutical experiments. We can assume from the maps of the palace that Covoni includes in his book that a series of rooms without windows or direct access to the exterior were built to be the sites of the *fonderia* and the other workshops.[58]

Although in 1587, the year of Francesco's death, an inventory of the Casino di San Marco was drawn up, the items contained in the *fonderia* were not listed, probably because they were not considered worthy of note.[59] The *fonderia*, however, was taken into account in the inventory produced after the death of Don Antonio in 1621.[60] We know therefore that it was composed of three major rooms plus a small room by the garden and a part of the *loggia*.

---

[56]   Berti, *Il principe dello studiolo*, p. 61.

[57]   For the *studiolo* see also Lina Bolzoni, 'L'invenzione dello stanzino di Francesco I', *Le arti della memoria* (Florence, 1980); Marco Dezzi Bardeschi et al., *Lo stanzino del principe in Palazzo Vecchio* (Florence, 1980); Valentina Conticelli, '*Guardaroba di cose rare e preziose*': *Lo studiolo di Francesco I de' Medici. Arte, storia e significati* (Lugano, 2007).

[58]   Pierfilippo Covoni, *Don Antonio de'Medici al Casino di S. Marco* (Florence, 1892). See also Pierfilippo Covoni, *Il Casino di S. Marco costruito dal Buontalenti* (Florence, 1892).

[59]   ASF, Guardaroba Medicea, 36.

[60]   ASF, Guardaroba Medicea, 399. c. 3r: 'Inventario di tutto quello che si è ritrovato in diverse stanze nel Palazzo de il Casino del'Illustrissimo e Eccellentissimo Sig. Don Antonio Medici alla sua morte seguita il dì 2 di maggio 1621'.

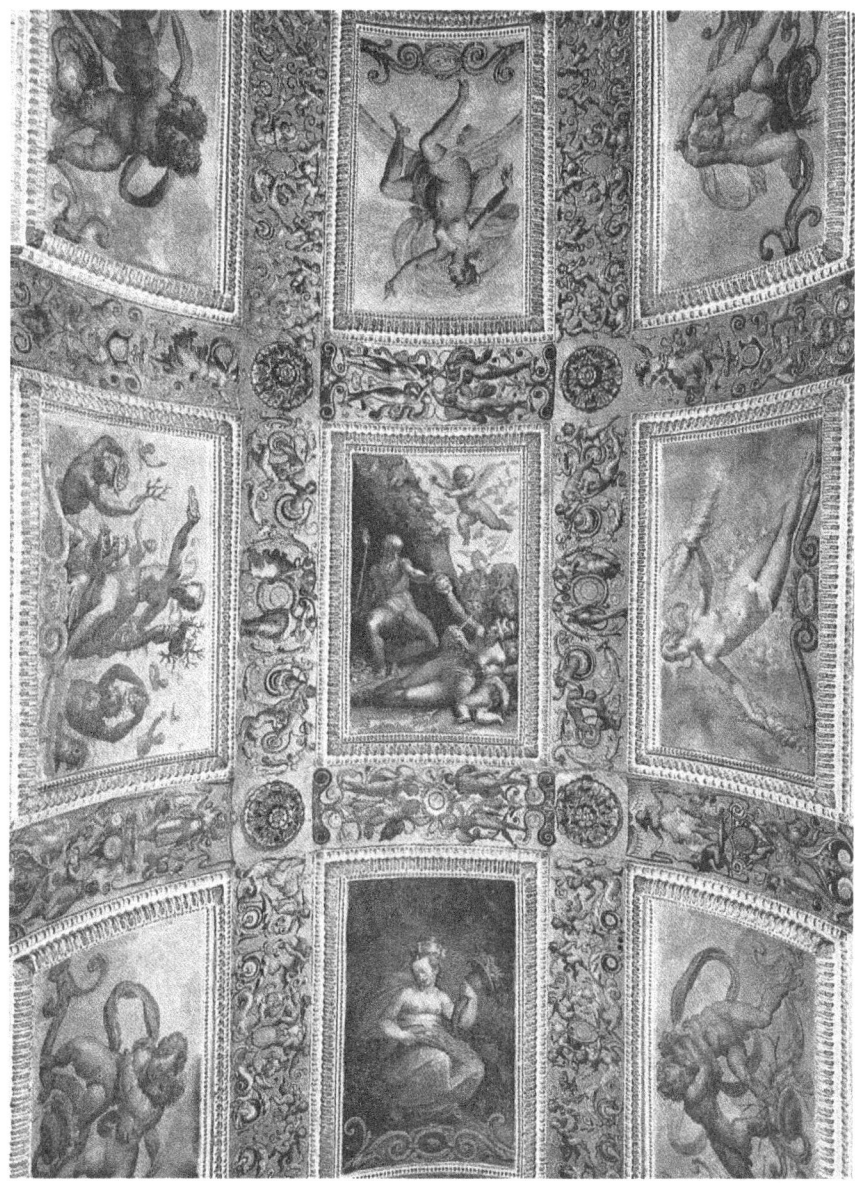

Figure 1.7   Ceiling of the *Studiolo* of Francesco I, Florence, Palazzo Vecchio

Before the description of the items of the *fonderia*, there is a complete list of the glass and porcelain containers (*alberelli, ampolle, vasi, scatole e scatolini, nasse*, etc.) and their medicinal contents, kept in eight cupboards in an adjacent room. The inventories of the Medici residences have been carefully examined especially by art historians, for the invaluable information about works of art they provide. The inventories of the books owned by the Medici are also often quoted and reported, as they are fundamental evidence of the cultural climate and circulation of ideas of the time. The description of the items contained in their laboratories has been neglected, probably because they were considered less interesting, although they are part of the same cultural context. In the case of Don Antonio in particular, the list of his books and the items of the *fonderia* are products of the same 'scientific' interest and field of enquiry. Don Antonio's books constitute a very specialized and up-to-date library, and are closely connected with the practical activities carried out in the laboratory. They all concern medical, '*spagiric*', and alchemical or chemical subjects. All the new ideas about chemical and Paracelsian medicine are present, along with the classics of herbal medicine.[61]

The inventory of the *fonderia* consists of 159 items (from c. 39v to c. 47v). Its rooms are crammed with all sorts of containers, tools and apparatus. The major equipment for distilling, such as furnaces, boilers, stills, etc. is located in the rooms attached to the garden.[62] Often the substances kept in various containers are recorded, and it is interesting to note that they are almost all mineral substances.[63] As is shown by the books of Don Antonio, he was much more interested in the new medical ideas of iatrochemistry than in traditional herbal medicine. In the second decade of the seventeenth century, plants had lost their absolute predominance. Vegetable substances, although present and still the basis of pharmacopoeia, are no longer material for experimentation in an avant-garde laboratory such as the one of Don Antonio de' Medici.[64]

The *fonderie* occupied a significant portion of the residences of the Medici and also of their thoughts. Although a number of people were employed in the *fonderia*, the grand dukes were personally engaged in the activities of the laboratory. They planned the medical recipes that were to be made, and they saw to the ordering of drugs, plants and minerals necessary to produce them. But what above all struck the

---

[61]   A partial list of the books of the inventory is reported in Filippo Luti, *Don Antonio de' Medici e i suoi tempi* (Florence, 2006), pp. 203–204.

[62]   'Inventario', cc.45v–47r.

[63]   Antimonio, cinabrio, litargirio, vetriolo, cristallo di montagnia, tartaro, allume di rocca, incenso, solfo, verderame, piombo, salnitro. The same can be said for the above-mentioned wardrobes of the *stanzino*, where only a few herbal substances are listed: balsamo occidentale (probably the West Indian balsam), aloe, contraerba, pignoli del Perù, bengui, agarico, mandragora.

[64]   For the penetration into Tuscany of Paracelsian ideas and iatrochemistry see Chapter 5, pp. 194–203.

imagination of contemporaries was the fact that they themselves spent a considerable amount of time in the laboratory, and worked there with 'their own hands'. Under the third grand duke Ferdinando, the pharmaceutical laboratory along with other workshops continued to be active. As has been seen, the *fonderia*, now located in the gallery at the Uffizi, was described as one of the wonders of Florence.

The supply of plants for the medicaments produced in the *fonderia* was obtained via various channels. As we can see from account books, they were sometimes purchased from apothecary shops. In the account books of the Speziale al Giglio of the period 1567–1568, for example, there are frequent orders from the grand-ducal laboratory, which were collected by the master of the *fonderia*.[65] At other times, mainly as far as the exotic herbs are concerned, they were purchased in Venice or directly shipped from Spain or Portugal. They were also ordered from herbalists (*erbolai* or *erboristi*) who collected them in the wild, as we can see from the following letter of 1601 requesting payment from the master of *fonderia* Niccolò Sisti to the *provveditore di guardaroba*:

> We will give, on behalf of Vostra Signoria, *lire* sixteen to the herbalists Francesco di Antonio Macherini and Marco di Simone for the payment of all the herbs and roots that go into the compound of 'acqua da pietra' and for all the herbs and other things that go into the 'olio da spasimo', and for all the herbs and other things that go into the compound of 'olio da ferite', provided from the above mentioned up to this day ...

And in another letter (1602) there is a list of various herbs and plants collected by Giovanni di Montereggi *erbolaio* and delivered to the *fonderia* at the Grand Duke Ferdinando's request, such as *acetosa, melissa, capraggine, corona pequinato*, and '49 pounds of absinth to make salt for the service of Madama Serenissima, as ordered by Mercuriale'.[66] This document provides evidence that at least some of the recipes ordered by the court physicians for the members of the family were directly produced in the *fonderia*.

The first three Medici grand dukes were all seen as medical advisers, and received frequent requests for medicines, recipes or rare medicinal substances from their courtiers or even foreign princes. Various letters provide evidence that they were considered to possess remedies for the most varied maladies. In a letter addressed to Cosimo a courtier asks him for 'some water distilled from asparagus which ... is a perfect thing for the urine', and a 'water for the eyes'.[67] In another letter (9 October 1572) Francesco Gonzaga, Count of Novellara, asks Francesco for 'a certain water that enhances beauty without doing any harm',

---

[65] See Chapter 6, pp. 204, 206.
[66] ASF, Guardaroba Medicea, 228 ins. 6, c. 582. Reported in ibid., pp. 477–8.
[67] ASF, MdP, 479, 62 (Medici Archive Project).

and in another (15 November 1575), Ercole Basso requests 'some of that most excellent secret for the stone in the kidneys'. Even the physician Baccio Baldini relies on the supply of the *fonderia* and asks Francesco (13 January 1583) for a 'bronze-coloured oil good for stomach-ache'.[68]

We have a first-hand record of some of the remedies produced in the grand-ducal laboratories from a small group of documents that have come down to us. One is the aforementioned short manuscript produced in Cosimo's *fonderia* (1556), which contains five recipes. One of these is the 'olio di scorpioni', also called 'oil of the Grand Duke', which contained, as well as the scorpions, a great number of vegetable ingredients (thirty-six ingredients in all), and became very popular at the time. The other recipes include an 'Elisir vitae probatissimo' prepared by distillation and containing seventy-four ingredients, 'olio da spasmo' 'matre balsamo'and 'olio da tutte le gomme seche'. These recipes were handed down in the Medici family and were also present (except for the latter) among the thirty-five 'secrets' produced by Antonio de' Medici at the Casino di San Marco.[69] These are Galenic recipes, based mainly on vegetable or animal substances. Of a very different kind are the recipes contained in another booklet, printed at the Casino di San Marco in 1604, which is all about chemical or 'spagyric' recipes, according to Paracelsian medicine, and to be discussed in Chapter 5, below.[70]

Plants and Gardens

The attention that the grand dukes devoted to the medical use of plants was only one aspect of their interest in the field of botany. Although the notes Cosimo wrote in the margins of Dioscorides's *Materia medica* show that he mainly concentrated on the curative faculties of plants, we have evidence that he had also absorbed Dioscorides' fundamental precept: the necessity of having direct knowledge of plants and of observing them in the various stages of their life. We will devote the next chapter to the influence on plant studies of the new teaching of *materia medica* at the University of Pisa and the establishment of a botanical garden. Here we will draw attention to the dukes' particular interest in plants for themselves, which was not less noteworthy than their commitment to medicine. The physician Baccio Baldini, in his biography of Cosimo describes his knowledge of plants thus:

---

[68]   ASF, MdP, 580, c. 79, p. 48; ASF, MdP, 679, c. 71, p. 113; ASF, MdP, 759, c. 66, p. 237.

[69]   BNCF, Magliab. XV, 140, *Segreti sperimentati dall'Ill.mo et Ecc.mo Sig. Principe D. Antonio de' Medici nella sua fonderia del Casino di S. Marco.*

[70]   *La fonderia dell'Ill.mo et ecc.mo Sig. Don Antonio Medici Principe di Capistrano – Nella quale si contiene tutta l'arte spagirica di Teofrasto Paracelso, & sue medicine. Et altri segreti bellissimi.* Stampato nel Palazzo del Casino di S. E: Illustrissima (Florence, 1604). See Chapter 5, pp. 199–200.

he knew an enormous quantity of plants, and the places where they hid themselves, where they would best flourish, where they would produce the most numerous and most flavourful fruit, the season in which they came into flower, and when they would come into fruit, and the virtues that many of them had to cure ills ...[71]

A passage of the aforementioned report of Ambassador Fedeli underlines Cosimo's interest in plants:

> He has the deepest knowledge especially of herbs and simples, and his gardens are full of them, and has them tended with particular care, and takes the greatest delight in having them planted, grown and experimented on, having at his disposal men highly skilled in that profession.[72]

Certainly Cosimo had a passion for plants, as is proven by the perseverance with which he planned and followed the works in the gardens of his villas and city residences. These gardens, above all those of his villa at Castello, and the Boboli garden behind the Pitti Palace, became famous mainly for their elaborate architectural design, their statues, grottoes, fountains and astonishing waterworks. While something of their structure and ornaments can still be seen today, as far as the planting is concerned, we can rely only on visual representation and written descriptions.

The renovation of the garden of the villa at Castello was one of the first things Cosimo embarked upon as early as 1537. The layout of the new garden was started by Tribolo and continued by Vasari, according to a project partly conceived by the humanist historian Benedetto Varchi.[73] Like the paintings in the Palazzo Vecchio, its magnificence and its scheme had the purpose of the glorification of the city of Florence and the Medici house. Some of the statues, for example, had to be arranged according to an elaborate plan reported by Vasari in his 'Vita di Niccolò detto il Tribolo': 'These [statues] had to indicate and show the greatness and bounty of the house of Medici and all the virtues of Duke Cosimo: that is to say Justice, Piety, Worth, Nobility, Knowledge and Liberality, which have always been in the house of Medici, and nowadays are all in our most excellent signor duca ...'[74] Only part of this project was completed, but the result, as we can see from Justus Utens' lunette, was magnificent (Figure 1.8).[75]

---

[71] Baldini, *Vita di Cosimo dei Medici*, p. 86.

[72] 'Relazione di Firenze di Messer Vincenzo Fedeli', p. 356.

[73] Giorgio Vasari, 'Vita di Niccolò detto il Tribolo', in *Le vite* (Novara, 1967), vol. 5, pp. 443–84. Azzi Vicentini (ed.), *L'arte dei giardini*.

[74] Ibid., pp. 469–72.

[75] Justus Utens' lunettes are kept in the Medicean Villa 'La Petraia'.

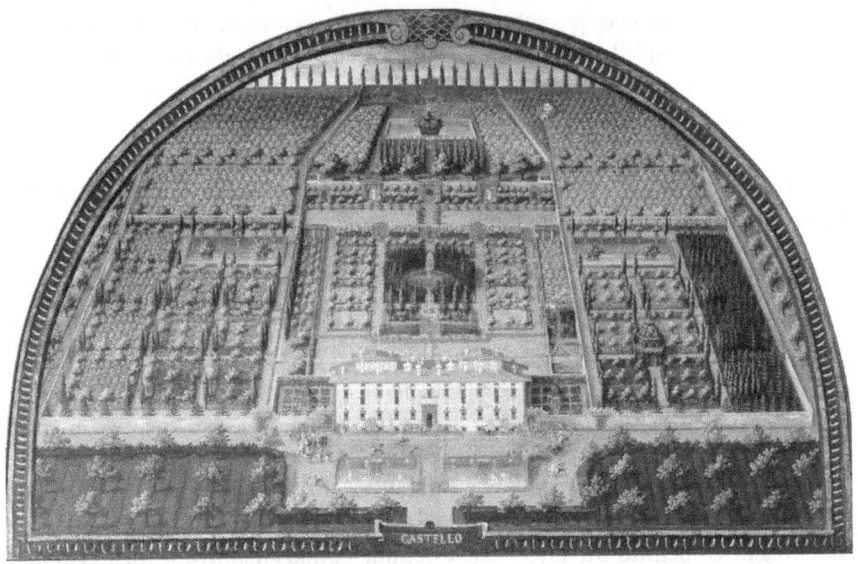

Figure 1.8   Justus Utens, Villa medicea a Castello 1599–1602, Florence,
              Poggio a Caiano

It is significant that the programme of sculpture of Castello included a fountain with a statue of Aesculapius, the god of medicine, in the herb garden. It would have underlined the vital role of the simples among which it was to be placed, and stressed the fact that the Medici were in charge of the health of the people and the state.[76] Aesculapius, in other words, had the same function in the garden as Cosmas and Damian had in the paintings, and was the traditional and pagan version of the physician saints. Another fountain with a statue of Aesculapius was later placed in the famous garden of Pratolino by the Grand Duke Francesco, as is described by Ulisse Aldrovandi who saw it in 1586 during one of his visits.[77]

Sometimes the vegetation was an integral part of the architectural framework, and Vasari, in his description of the garden, occasionally refers to it. He describes a large alley 'covered on its sides and above, in its height of ten "braccia", with a continuous vault of mulberry trees' and the labyrinth made of cypresses, laurels, myrtles and box, a garden of orange trees, and a '*salvatico*' of 'cypresses, firs, ilex, and other evergreens'. The garden represented a continuous interweaving of art and nature, as Claudio Tolomei put it in a letter of 1543 'now it seems a natural

---

[76]   Lazzaro, *The Italian Renaissance Garden*, p. 177 and p. 311, note 40.

[77]   'Descriptio brevis fontium Pratolini', Ulisse Aldrovandi 1586, in Barocchi and Bertelà, *Collezionismo mediceo*, p. 280.

artifice, now artificial nature.'[78] Many architectural elements were covered with vegetation, such as the walls that divided the garden into sections, the exterior of grottoes, and the trellises. On the other hand, trees and plants were often used as architectural elements themselves, as different forms of topiary, tall trees as obelisks, or trees and bushes forming the structure of a high labyrinth like the one at Castello. The alley of mulberry trees and the labyrinth in this garden are also described by the French writer and naturalist Pierre Belon (1517–1564), who adds interesting information about some plants that were then to be seen and that were an absolute rarity. These are the 'Indian figs', two 'real planes', trees recently imported, and some '*rhododendri*', which were actually oleanders, used in a garden for the first time.[79]

While the overall structure of the garden was the task of the architect, it is not always clear who was in charge of choosing the trees, plants and flowers. Some of them were the typical plants that we are used to seeing in Tuscany. Agostino Lapini, for example, in his *Florentine Journal* mentions them in relation to the laying out of the Boboli gardens: 'On Monday 12 May [1550] we started to level the ground in the garden at Pitti and provide it with sewers, to plant firs, cypresses, ilexes and bays'.[80] Although these are now among the most common of Tuscan plants, maybe they were not taken for granted in the sixteenth century, as Pierre Belon praises the Tuscans for selecting and growing evergreen species for their gardens.[81] The duke certainly played an important role in the planting, and we have a large number of letters that indicate that he often personally ordered the plants for his gardens and took great care to ensure that they would arrive at their destination in good condition. In a letter of 11 January 1565, he sent Andrea, the *fattore* in his villa at Castello, a long list of fruit trees, asking him to send cuttings to his garden in Pisa:

> Andrea, we need you to provide grafts of the fruit trees listed below and send them to Pisa well arranged, and divided with care into different bundles according to their type, wrapped up in straw, and on each bundle you will put a label indicating of which type they are ... Be careful to send all the below mentioned types, well arranged and paying attention not to make mistakes as to their qualities and quantities; do not send them all together but little by little, addressing them to ms. Zanobi Marignoli, making sure it does not rain ...[82]

---

[78]   Quoted in Lazzaro, *The Italian Renaissance Garden*, p. 61.

[79]   Pierre Belon, *Les Remonstrances sur le default du labour & culture des plantes & de la cognoissance d'icelles* (Paris, 1558); ch. 22, 'La grande beauté dont le jardin de Castello du Duc de Florence est orné', pp. 79v–80r.

[80]   *Diario fiorentino di Agostino Lapini: dal 252 al 1596, ora per la prima volta pubblicato da G.O. Corazzini* (Florence, 1900), p. 107.

[81]   Belon, *Les Remonstrances*, p. 80v.

[82]   Letter of 11 January 1565, ASF, MdP, 220, c. 72 (Medici Archive Project).

The location of the secret gardens or gardens of simples in the general scheme was certainly decided by the architect, but not the single herbs and essences. Cosimo was also very interested in these parts of the garden, as is shown in a letter of Vincenzo Ferrini to Pier Francesco Riccio, superintendent of some of the Medici villas, referring to 'a large number of herb plants that his Excellency wants to have planted at Castello'.[83] The duke was constantly kept informed about the gardens of his villas through letters from his superintendents. There is a long and very interesting report from Pier Francesco Riccio to Cosimo which describes the state of the plants and the works that were being done in the gardens of Boboli, Careggi, Poggio a Caiano and Castello. The language of such letters and the details included leave no doubt that Cosimo attached great importance to the planting, and followed its development. At least a few lines of it are worth quoting:

> [At Castello] the sweet orange trees have suffered a little and sometimes we fear some serious damage, but I hope that, in this weather, they will soon sprout new leaves. The leaves of the Indian figs could grow well, but even though they were well enclosed and covered, cold penetrated the covering. Andrea [da Castello] has pruned them to the ground and hopes they will recover. Two of them which were in ... are green and fresh.[84]

This letter refers to one of the new exotic plants that Pierre Belon tells of having seen at Castello: the so-called 'fico d'India', which was not the cactus that now bears that name (*Opuntia*), but the Indian Banyan tree (*Ficus Benghalensis*). Some decades later Agostino del Riccio informs us that this exotic tree could also be seen in the garden at villa Petraia and in the Rucellai and Salviati gardens.[85]

Love of plants, apart from their medical use, was inherited by Cosimo's sons Francesco and Ferdinando, and many documents provide evidence of this profound interest. We could begin by quoting the frivolous but significant account of Francesco looking at a flower, left by Agostino del Riccio: '... sometimes when he went into a beautiful garden, whether a roof garden or a natural garden, he would take a flower in his hand and gaze at that flower from all sides, observing every colour and beauty of it, to his great joy and delight'.[86] In 1582 Francesco planned a roof garden on the Loggia dei Lanzi, over the piazza della Signoria, where he was very keen on growing rare plants and flowers, as

---

[83]   Letter of 2 April 1547. ASF, MdP, 1173, c. 142.

[84]   Letter of 7 March 1551. ASF, MdP, 613, c. 21 (Medici Archive Project).

[85]   Agostino del Riccio, *Agricoltura sperimentale*, II, f. 429v. Quoted in Lazzaro, *The Italian Renaissance Garden*, p. 27.

[86]   Quoted in G. Targioni Tozzetti, *Notizie*, p. 243, from Agostino del Riccio, *Agricoltura sperimentale*, 'de' fior ranci', p. 874.

is indicated in a letter of 29 January 1583 from Simone Fortuna to the duke of Urbino:

> Walking with the Grand Duke in the new garden laid out on the high Loggia dei Pisani, I remembered the promise I had made to Your Highness of those rare seeds, as you had ordered. He let me have some seeds coming from the East Indies; he did not wish Your Highness to give them to anybody else, but use them as splendid ornament in your domestic gardens, and where shade and flowers are required, as he has shown me he had done using beautiful vases, many of which are made out of lead.[87]

The most relevant evidence of Francesco I and Ferdinando I's naturalistic interests is perhaps contained in the correspondence they exchanged with Ulisse Aldrovandi. In their correspondence, the centre of interest is natural science and their relationship is the relationship between scientists investigating nature. This letter of the Grand Duke Francesco to Aldrovandi is one among many which demonstrates his constant attempts to obtain rare plants for his gardens and the care with which he personally followed their growth:

> Many years ago, when my lord and master Grand Duke Cosimo was alive, one of those 'Guanabano' fruits was brought to us, and after taking some seeds, I had them put in a vase, and a plant came out and grew with leaves smaller than those of the orange tree, but larger than those of bay; but because it was not followed with the necessary care and perseverance, it was lost. Thus the seeds you have sent me are most cherished and I will have them planted and grown with the greatest care ... The beans I am sending have been collected from those I had seeded, and their flowers lasted almost until Christmas, but being in a place where they could not be covered, the extreme and extraordinary cold that came killed them ...[88]

Francesco's knowledge of plants is based on personal experience, and a few days later he even challenges Aldrovandi's botanical opinions: 'I do not think Guanabano is the Baba from India, and I presume I can show you the true Baba ...'. The exchange of plant material and information was a constant in their letters.

---

[87]   ASF, Urbino, Appendix 1, c. 468v, Barocchi and Bertelà, *Collezionismo Mediceo*, pp. 68–9, n. 235.

[88]   ASF, MdP, 269, folio 18 (Medici Archive Project).

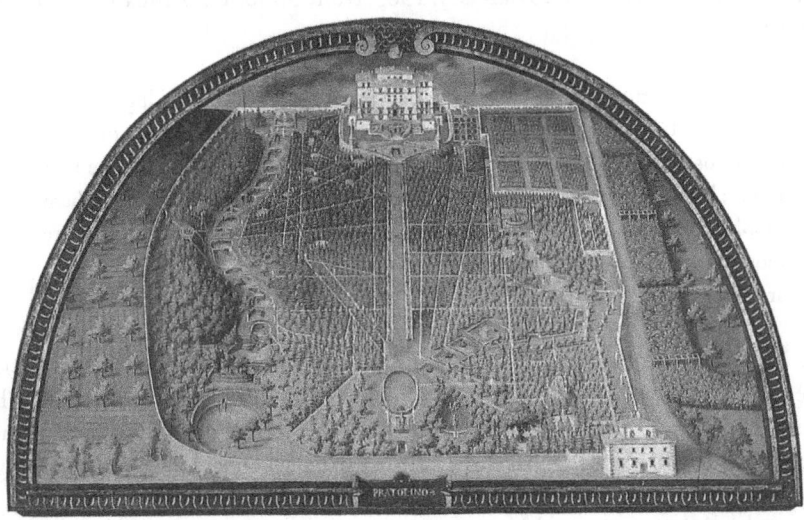

Figure 1.9   Justus Utens, Villa medicea di Pratolino, 1599–1602, Florence,
                Poggio a Caiano

Although Aldrovandi had sometimes favours to ask of Francesco, his esteem for the grand duke, whom he considered to be, like himself, a 'vero scrutatore della natura', seems genuine. His admiration for the garden of Pratolino is recorded in his notes, where he described the fountains and the rare plants he had seen there.[89] Pratolino, which Francesco had started in 1569, the same year of the *studiolo*, was regarded as one of the wonders of the time. As Luciano Berti points out, in the funeral rites following his death, the construction of Pratolino, represented in a picture by Ludovico Buti, was recalled as being one of his major achievements.[90] Although Pratolino was probably more famous for the fountains, statues, and incredibly sophisticated waterworks, a glance at Utens' lunette of Pratolino is sufficient to see the role played by vegetation (Figure 1.9).[91] Riguccio Galluzzi underlines the fact that

---

[89]   'Observata Pratolini Magni Duci', transcribed in Barocchi and Bertelà, *Collezionismo mediceo*, pp. 279–83.

[90]   Berti, *Il principe dello studiolo*, p. 91.

[91]   The most famous contemporary description of Pratolino is that of Francesco de' Vieri, 'Delle meravigliose opere di Pratolino e d'Amore' (Florence, 1586), reported in Barocchi and Bertelà, *Collezionismo mediceo*, pp. 284–302. The description is all based on a symbolical and

all the plants at Pratolino were the result of a careful choice: 'the wood plants, which had to be used as pure ornament of alleys and pleasure groves, were brought from distant lands, to add singularity to the delights prince Francesco was preparing for his villa of Pratolino.'[92]

Agostino del Riccio also adds: 'All vied with each other to present him [Francesco] with rare fruit trees and flowers, knowing that they were welcome; thus many plants were given to him; at the same time He had many plants brought from other Provinces, so that nowadays we all know them and our Florence and country gardens are full of them.' He mentions some of the rare plants imported by Francesco, such as some 'gelsomini pellegrini', the American aloe, and the Castagna cavallina (Horse chestnut). Aldrovandi too, in his list 'Observata Pratolini Magni Ducis', records a tree of 'Castanea equina', probably the first seen in Italy.[93]

Plants also constituted a constant interest for Francesco's brother Ferdinando. Two new grand villas, Artimino and the Ambrogiana were built under Ferdinando' s rule, and their gardens were laid out with great attention to planting. Ferdinando sent Giuseppe Casabona (Josef Goodenhuyse), the Flemish naturalist in charge of the *orto pisano*, on a trip to Crete in search of 'rare and singular plants for our gardens and for the use of medicine', as we read in a letter of 1591.[94]

In the course of the sixteenth century, the variety of species available increased enormously, as new plants continued to arrive from the New World, but also from Asia and the Levant. As far as flowers in particular are concerned, a radical change took place in the second half of the century. In a lecture published in the *Journal of the Royal Horticultural Society*, William Stern describes the 'revolutionary' discovery of the colourful Turkish gardens by the European ambassadors in Constantinople, which led to an unprecedented expansion of flowers in European gardens 'when ... importations of unpromising onion-like bulbs and knobbly tubers from Constantinople brought forth tulips, crown imperials, irises, hyacinths, anemones, turban ranuncoli, narcissi and lilies ...'.[95]

---

allegorical interpretation. Plants are very seldom mentioned, and only for their symbolical meaning. On de'Vieri's description see Suzanne Butters, 'Pressed Labor and Pratolino', p. 64 and pp. 78–87.

[92]   Berti, *Il principe dello studiolo*, pp. 203–206.

[93]   Barocchi and Bertelà, 'Observata Pratolini Magni Duci', *Collezionismo mediceo*, p. 278.

[94]   ASF, MdP, 280, folio 17 (Medici Archive Project).

[95]   William P. Stern, 'Master memorial lecture', *Journal of the Royal Horticultural Society*, (1965), p. 322.

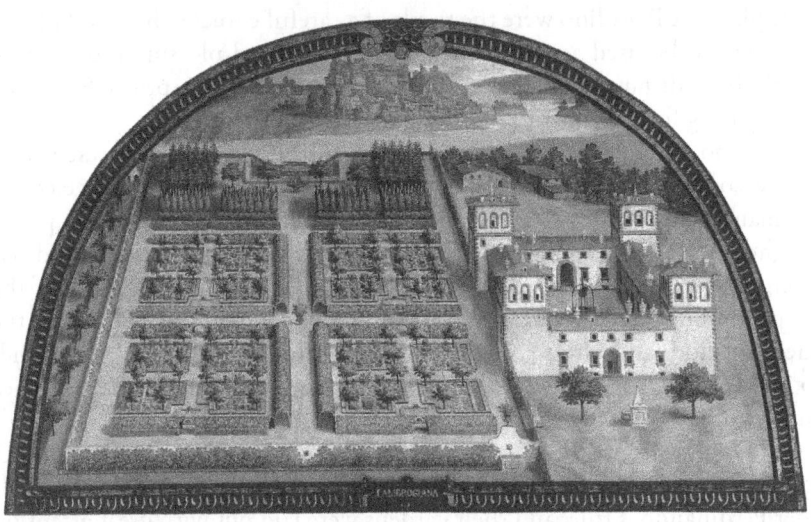

Figure 1.10   Justus Utens, Villa medicea l'Ambrogiana 1599–1602, Florence,
Poggio a Caiano

The absence of flowers in Tuscan gardens has often been discussed and commented upon. Among the lunettes representing the Medicean Villas, Justus Utens painted flowers only in the garden of the Ambrogiana (Figure 1.10). As this garden was laid out after 1587, we can assume that Utens represented here the new enthusiasm for flowers. He painted the beds, and placed flowers of a single variety in each of them; some, such as irises and tulips, although depicted with little attention to naturalistic details, are recognizable. The irises were not new, and the purple iris (*Iris germanica*) which was the symbol of Florence (the so-called Florence lily) could be there as a tribute to the grand duke. But certainly tulips, which began to be grown in Europe after 1593, cannot be interpreted in the same way. In Agostino del Riccio's *Agricoltura sperimentale*, there is an interesting chapter entitled 'on a king's garden' ('Del giardino di un re'). Among the various features that a king's garden should have, del Riccio includes a 'garden of flowers' where one should grow flowers that bloom in different times so that the king's garden could be attractive in each month of the year. In another section of his *Agricoltura sperimentale*, Agostino had in fact recorded the flowers that bloom in Tuscany in the different months. He also speaks of the difficulty of obtaining new bulbs such as 'milk' narcissi, white hyacinths, double peonies, tulips, Spain jonquils, double anemones, water elder, crown imperials, muscari, red lilies, etc., and he adds a list of towns where these bulbs can be obtained.[96]

Suzanne Butters's long description of the garden Duke Ferdinando laid out for his Roman villa on the Pincio provides further ample evidence of the interest and care he had for plants and flowers. He was actively engaged in choosing the plants for the new garden, and kept up a constant correspondence with his gardeners to be kept informed about their development.[97]

Conclusion

The wide-ranging cultural programme set up by Cosimo I, and developed by his sons, was aimed at creating the foundation of the new state. Patronage of letters and arts, with which the Medici family is usually still identified, was only part of that programme, which was broadened to include new 'scientific' aspects.

If the efforts to attract the most prominent European intellectuals to the re-founded University of Pisa are considered by historians as an outstanding element of Cosimo's cultural programme, the interest in medicine and natural science that the first three grand dukes cultivated, and the way in which their personal interests were channelled into the creation of their public image, has not been paid much attention. In a period when art and science were still closely linked, it is interesting to note how they were made to merge into the image of a religious and charitable prince, who was concerned both with the health of the state and with that of his subjects. The magnificent altarpieces and frescoes that suggested the identification of the Medici with the martyr physicians Cosmas and Damian; the sophisticated representation of medicine and the association of art and nature in Francesco's studiolo; the time spent and the work carried out in the laboratories to produce medicaments; the gift of these medicaments to the needy, courtiers and foreign princes; the study of plants for medicinal use and for the beauty of gardens; all these elements combined to build up a particular image of *magnificentia*, and at the same time offered objects for praise to contemporary biographers and foreign visitors. What emerges is, above all, Cosimo's ability to make them form part of a project aimed at multiplying the motives of internal prestige and international resonance.

It is difficult to gauge the influence of the personal interests of the grand dukes on the theory and practice of pharmacy and therapy, and on the study

---

[96]   Detlef Heikamp, 'Agostino del Riccio: Del giardino di un re', *Il giardino storico italiano*, in Giovanna Ragionieri (ed.), *Il giardino storico italiano* (Milan, 1981).

[97]   Butters, 'Ferdinand et le jardin du Pincio', *La villa Médicis*, vol. 2, pp. 392–401.

of plants. It is evident that the reform of the *Studio pisano* triggered a process that led to developments in medicine and plant study far beyond the initial support of Cosimo I. However, one can track some initiatives and behaviours of the grand dukes that are themselves novel and that offer material for reflection. Although one cannot know precisely how much manual work was actually carried out by them in their laboratories, the fact that they used 'their own hands', seems to have caused surprise ('something rare' in Ambassador Fedeli's words), but was never looked on contemptuously. That some manual skills were considered noble because they implied *scientia* and talent, was an acknowledged fact by the sixteenth century, as is proven by the general acceptance of painting and sculpture among the liberal arts. Medicine, in particular, had always combined the twofold aspect of theory and practice. We know, however, that physicians were held in higher esteem than apothecaries, who did not need a long university training to practise their profession. The *speziali* made 'with their own hands' the medicines doctors ordered, and were not allowed, at least in theory, to decide which medicine should be administered to a patient. The first editions of the *Ricettario fiorentino*, the Florentine pharmacopoeia, were made for apothecaries, but written by physicians. The edition of 1597, however, was drawn up by two doctors and two apothecaries appointed by Ferdinando I, and appeared with a long dedication in which the Medici were praised for their activities connected with pharmacy and therapy. It seems therefore that the personal involvement of the grand dukes in the production of medicaments had the result of diminishing the social gap between physicians and apothecaries. Furthermore, it is likely that their personal involvement also had a direct impact on the acceptance, in Italy, of Paracelsian pharmacy. Further research is needed on their use of the laboratory, which was not intended as a place where traditional medicaments were made, but was often aimed at improving them through new sophisticated apparatus, and at 'experimenting' on them.

As seen, the image of the prince-physician, along with its religious and social implications, was related to the idea of sacralization of power. This contributes to explain why commitment to medicine, and the work in the *fonderie* remained a prerogative of the grand dukes, and there is no evidence that it was imitated by their courtiers. On the contrary, enthusiasm for plants and gardens, and naturalistic interests in general, were shared by several members of the court. Agostino del Riccio in the 1590s, refers to some of them:

> I cannot praise enough those who have begun to adorn gardens in the manner they are today. The first was Grand Duke Cosimo, with his dear sons, Grand Duke Francesco, and Grand Duke Ferdinando, together with numerous others who have embarked in such a commendable undertaking, which would be too long to relate, such as the Salviati, Strozzi, Soderini, Gaddi, Acciaiuoli, Filicai,

Bartolini, Sommai, and a thousand more, whose names I will not mention, for the sake of brevity.[98]

Some of these 'signori' were plant connoisseurs such as Alamanno Salviati, whose garden was famous for the production of sweet 'zibibbo', a muscat grape, and many rare plants; or Alessandro Acciaiuoli, owner of the garden of Palazzo Corsini al Prato designed by Buontalenti, mentioned by Agostino del Riccio as the 'inventor' of roof-gardens. A well-known garden was that of the Serristori, parallel to the river Arno, as can be seen in Bonsignori's plan of 1584, mentioned by Benedetto Varchi as one of the most important gardens in Florence. Another famous garden was the so-called 'Paradise of the Gaddi', in the Via del Giglio, owned by the erudite collector and naturalist Niccolò Gaddi, 'man of confidence' to Francesco and then to Ferdinando.[99]

Love of gardens and the pleasure they provide were not a novelty. What was new was the importance now attached to gardens and their complexity, which, like the palace or villa they surrounded, became a symbol of aesthetic refinement and elegance. As far as plants are concerned, a new approach is reflected in the various documents we examined above. Plants were now sought after because they were beautiful or rare, and they began to acquire importance for reasons that had little to do with their utility. In addition, there was a new interest in their cultivation and their growth, from germination to maturity, was carefully observed and followed. The attention recommended by Dioscorides for simples was applied to all garden plants. Curiosity for new specimens and eagerness to grow them in the garden became an attitude shared by all the courtiers who could afford it.

---

[98]   Agostino del Riccio, *Agricoltura sperimentale*, vol. 2, ch. 15, p. 123, quoted in G. Targioni Tozzetti, *Notizie*, p. 285.

[99]   Cristina Acidini Luchinat, 'Niccolò Gaddi collezionista e dilettante', *Paragone*, 359–61 (1980), pp. 141–75.

Chapter 2
Medical Botany at the Re-founded University of Pisa

In the debate about intellectual innovation, Renaissance universities have traditionally been seen as the sites where knowledge was transmitted but not initiated. Universities, it was maintained, were traditional, if not retrograde institutions impermeable to change, where novel ideas were constantly held back. This general view has been partially challenged, and some exceptions acknowledged. As Charles Schmitt points out, there were cases in which 'perhaps both the intellectual level and the receptivity to new ideas found in the Renaissance university tradition was more progressive than is often admitted'.[1]

The emergence of natural history, and botany in particular, in sixteenth-century Italy are to be seen as an example of this receptivity to new ideas. The establishment of a chair of medical botany in Italian universities, a significant innovation in itself, brought about a series of new developments and practices which contributed to the gradual separation of botany from medicine and to the definition of a new disciplinary field. From this point of view, the University of Pisa, or the *Studio pisano*, as it is usually referred to, which reopened after a period of inactivity in 1543, seems to represent a privileged source of investigation.[2]

This chapter will focus on the study and teaching of *materia medica* at the faculty of 'Arts and Medicine' of the University of Pisa, in the period between circa 1540 and the end of the century. I will outline the role of the university in this particular context, both from the institutional and educational point of view. The importance attached to the university by Cosimo I, who considered it a central issue in his cultural policy, will also be underlined. The figure of Luca Ghini, who was the first lecturer of *materia medica* and founded the first botanical garden, and that of Andrea Cesalpino, who was his successor, and concentrated on the systematization of the vegetable kingdom, provide the focal points around which the features and methods of the new discipline took shape. Some observations regarding the use of terms need first to be made.

I sometimes use the term 'botany' to refer to the study of plants in general, or the adjective 'botanical' as it is clearer for us, although in the period under

---

[1]   Schmitt, 'Science in the Italian Universities in the Sixteenth and Early Seventeenth Centuries', p. 35.

[2]   Ibid., pp. 39–44. Siraisi, *Medicine and the Italian Universities*, pp. 331–4.

discussion the terms were not yet in use. I also occasionally use the term 'botanist' referring to a scholar, physician or apothecary particularly engaged in the study of plants.[3]

Plants were usually referred to by the term 'simples' (*simplices*) which directly associated them with their medicinal use. A 'simple' was, technically speaking, a drug made from one ingredient (as opposed to compound drugs made from many), which most of the time was a plant but could also be an animal or a mineral substance. As Karen Reeds suggests, the word's usage probably derived from the Latin title of Galen's treatise *De simplicium medicamentorum facultatibus*, or *De simplicibus*.[4] A professor appointed to lecture in medical botany was called *lector simplicium* and the lectureship *lectura de simplicibus* or *materia medica*; a botanical garden was called *orto* or *giardino dei semplici*. The study of plants, when seen as independent from medicine, was sometimes referred to as *res herbaria*.

I have used the words 'science' and 'scientific' in the sense we attribute to them today, only when they cannot be misunderstood. As is known, the term *scientia*, although in use, had a different meaning from that of the present day, sometimes changing according to the context, but certainly not corresponding to our concept of science.[5]

Cosimo I's Cultural Project and the University

When the young Cosimo I established his rule over the city of Florence and Tuscany, he set up a precise cultural policy programme for the new state.[6] As seen, his programme, along with the more traditional area of artistic patronage, included a series of initiatives in the 'scientific' field. Certainly the reopening of the *Studio pisano*, and particularly the reorganization of the faculty of medicine, played an important role in Cosimo's project, as is attested by his attempts to attract the most important physicians of the time. Although he undoubtedly achieved remarkable results, it is true that some eminent professors declined

---

3   The word botany (from the Greek *botane* meaning 'herb' or 'plant') and its derivatives began to be used towards the end of the seventeenth century and became usual in the eighteenth century. In his history of the *Studio pisano*, Fabbrucci uses the terms 'botanices cathedra', 'professor botanicarum rerum' and 'hortus botanicus'. Stefano Maria Fabbrucci, 'De Reliquis Insignibus Pisani Gymnasii Professoribus qui sub fausto Cosmi I Regimine floruerunt', in A. Calogierà (ed.), *Nuova Raccolta d'opuscoli scientifici e filologici*, vol. 6 (Venezia, 1709), pp. 59–61.

4   Reeds, 'Renaissance humanism and botany', p. 521, note 8.

5   Charles B. Schmitt, 'Recent Trends in the Study of Medieval and Renaissance Science', in Pietro Corsi and Paul Weindling (eds), *Information Sources in the History of Science and Medicine* (London, 1983), p. 223.

6   Galluzzi, 'Il mecenatismo mediceo e le scienze', pp. 189–215.

Cosimo's invitation and some others remained at Pisa only for a short time.[7] The prominent anatomist Vesalius, for example, spent only two months in Pisa in 1544, and the great German physician-botanist Leonhart Fuchs did not accept the duke's offer on the grounds, it seems, of religious reasons. Moreover, Pisa did not offer favourable living conditions at the time, as it was reduced to dire straits, and was plagued by an unhealthy environment. Although the reclamation of the marshes was one of Cosimo's achievements in the following years,[8] the physician Gabriele Falloppio in one of his works complains about the unhealthiness of the city where 'food, soil, air and water' were insalubrious.[9] Cosimo's attempt to make the *Studio pisano* the cornerstone on which the grand duchy's cultural prestige was founded certainly required a considerable effort both in terms of finance and commitment.[10]

The *Studio pisano* was founded in 1343, and from 1473, when Lorenzo de' Medici decided to move the state's university from Florence to Pisa, was considered the principal university of Tuscany.[11] During the early sixteenth century the *Studio* underwent a period of crisis due principally to the strife between Pisa and Florence, and had to cease its activity. It reopened on 1 November 1543 with a solemn ceremony and a memorable address by the eminent professor Francesco Robortello. The reopening assumed almost the character of a new foundation and it was seen as such by contemporaries. In fact, the warm support of duke Cosimo, the recruiting of new professors, and the drawing up of a set of new statutes made it seem an almost new institution.

A few observations on some general aspects of the actual organization of the University in the light of the statutes are worth noting.[12] The *Studio*, at

---

[7]   Siraisi, *Medicine and the Italian Universities*, p. 332.

[8]   Referring to the same fresco mentioned below (note 13), Vasari explains that he has placed a cornucopia in Pisa's hands 'that the prince makes flourish, since he has reclaimed and dried the marshes of that city, that caused pestiferous air ...' G. Vasari, *Ragionamenti sopra le invenzioni da lui dipinte*, in *Le vite*, ed. G. Milanesi (Rome, 1949), p. 215.

[9]   Quoted in Galluzzi, 'Il mecenatismo mediceo e le scienze', p. 195.

[10]   That Cosimo I attached great importance to the University is also attested by one of the frescoes of the pictorial celebration of the grand duke and his achievements painted by Vasari in the Palazzo Vecchio, where the duke was depicted with the allegorical figures of Pisa and the *studio*. See Vasari, *Ragionamenti*, p. 215. Lucia Tongiorgi Tomasi, 'L'Università e gli artisti', *Storia dell'Università di Pisa* (Pisa, 2000), pp. 666.

[11]   In 1472 the University of Florence had ceased its activity merging with Pisa. Only a few chairs were kept in Florence, but they were subordinate to the *Studio pisano* and the name of the professors and their salaries were included in the books (*rotuli*) of Pisa University; see Paul Grendler, *The Universities of the Italian Renaissance* (Baltimore, MD, and London, 2002), pp. 70–77, where the vicissitudes of the *Studio pisano* are summarized.

[12]   The Statutes have been transcribed in 'Gli Statuti di Cosimo I', *Storia dell'Università di Pisa*, pp. 572–645.

least formally, maintained its medieval characteristic of a union of students (*Universitas scholarium*). The students were divided into 'Nations' (*Nationes*) on the basis of their provenance. The foreigners (Transalpine or Ultramontane) were made up of three Nations (Germans, Spanish and French), while the Italians (Cisalpine or Citramontane) made up eleven Nations. Each Nation was led by a Counsellor while the head of the whole university was the rector. Both the counsellors and the rector were students, elected by their fellow students. Although the statutes stated that the rector was the supreme authority, second only to the duke, in fact his authority was only honorary.[13] The documents made clear that the running of the *Studio* was in fact carried out by two deputies, the *Auditore* and the *Provveditore*, closely connected with the government of the duchy. Important decisions therefore were taken under the dukes' surveillance. Besides, a series of norms aimed at maintaining strict control by the state were issued. Some laws issued under Cosimo I (1543), and then reinforced by his son Ferdinando I (1588), forbade the subjects of the Florentine state to attend a university outside Tuscany. Neither teachers nor students could leave the *Studio* for another university without obtaining the duke's permission; a degree obtained abroad was not recognized in the grand duchy.[14] The statutes, moreover, established that both professors and students before the final examination would have to swear allegiance to the state.[15] In 1564, a papal bull (*In Sacrosanta*) stipulated that they had to swear allegiance to the Catholic Church as well.[16]

Notwithstanding these protectionist rules, the *studio* was intended to be an international institution and an effort was made to attract foreign students. In fact, a considerable number of students came from abroad to study at Pisa.[17] The Medici took upon themselves also the maintenance of poor students. A document of 1542 established the founding of a college of students (*un Collegio di scolari*) in order to provide for those who 'oppressed by domestic poverty could not, without such help, show the excellence and the nobility of

---

[13] Danilo Marrara, 'L'età medicea 1543–1737', *Storia dell'Universita di Pisa*, Commissione Rettorale per la storia dell'Università di Pisa, vol. 1 (Pisa, 2000), pp. 89–97.

[14] Danilo Marrara, 'L'Università di Pisa come università statale nel granducato mediceo', *Rivista Giuridica della Scuola*, 8 (1965), pp. 11–12.

[15] 'Statuti', LIIII, p. 623 and LVIIII, p. 626.

[16] Marrara, 'Università di Pisa', p. 33.

[17] During the period between 1544 and 1609, of the 6,200 students who enrolled at Pisa more than half were from Tuscany and the majority of the rest from other parts of Italy. The students from outside Italy came from Germany (126), Spain (77), France (39), Portugal (30), Mallorca (26), Bavaria (26), Flanders (11), England (7), Poland (6), Tirol (3), Belgium (1) and Greece (1). P. Paganini, 'Statistica degli studenti pisani del secolo XVI', *Rivista critica della letteratura italiana*, 3 (1886–87), pp. 125–6.

their minds.'[18] A college (*Collegio Cosimo* or *della Sapienza*) to care for poor students was actually founded in 1543 under Cosimo's patronage, and another (*Collegio Fernando*) was established under the third grand duke's patronage.

Some aspects of the statutes that were more directly connected with the educational content of the curriculum are worth pointing out. There were three faculties in the *Studio pisano*: law (*utroque iure*, civil and canon law), medicine (*philosophia et medicina*), and theology (*theologia*).[19] The course of studies to get a degree in medicine lasted five years. During the first two years the students had to attend the courses of logic and philosophy (usually natural philosophy). They then progressed to medical studies proper. Only a very small number of students stopped at the first stage with a degree in philosophy; the majority went on to take a degree in medicine. Medical studies were divided into theoretical and practical medicine and surgery was taught as a separate subject. A new chair of medical botany (*lectura de simplicibus*) was established, as indicated in a single line of the new statutes: 'Those appointed to lecture on simples will read Dioscorides.'[20]

There are hardly any signs of innovation other than this in the 1543 statutes, which, surprisingly, remained in force until the end of the eighteenth century. The philosophical texts on which the medical curriculum were based did not change significantly from the ones prescribed in the preceding statutes of 1478. As far as the medical course was concerned, the texts were those of Galen and Hippocrates already indicated in the preceding statutes. The works of Avicenna, and Rasis, now considered 'barbarians' by some humanist scholars, were still included.

Nevertheless, as Nancy Siraisi observed, the *Studio pisano*, when reopened, actually 'offered notable opportunities for medical teaching, and a situation distinctly favourable to the most active and innovative areas of contemporary academic medical science'.[21] Cosimo's advisers Francesco Campana and Filippo del Migliore, who were in charge of the recruitment of professors, tried to attract to Pisa the most eminent scholars, and their efforts were not in vain. In fact, distinguished physicians such as Matteo Corti, Leonardo Giacchino, Giovanni Argenterio, Realdo Colombo, and Gabriele Falloppio accepted Cosimo's invitation to join the *Studio pisano*. Vesalius did not accept a permanent position, but he lectured on anatomy in 1544. The new lectureship on *materia medica*, after Leonhart Fuchs's refusal, was offered to the eminent physician-botanist Luca Ghini, who had taught the same subject at Bologna. The new teaching began in an intellectually stimulating atmosphere.

---

18 Fabbrucci, 'De Pisano Gymnasio sub Cosmo Primo Mediceo feliciter renovato', p. 7.
19 'Statuti', LIII, p. 622.
20 'Deputati ad lecturam de simplicibus legant Dioscoridem'. 'Statuti', XLIIII, p. 616.
21 Siraisi, *Medicine and the Italian Universities*, p. 331.

Luca Ghini and the New Teaching of *materia medica*

Although the acknowledgment of the necessity to introduce medical botany as an independent subject in the medical curriculum was per se a significant innovation, the new chair, established at Pisa and entrusted to Luca Ghini, brought about a series of developments that proved vital towards the definition of a new discipline.

Luca Ghini was born near Imola (Bologna) in *c.*1490. He studied philosophy and medicine at the University of Bologna where he took a degree in 1527, and was then appointed to teach practical medicine. As a professor at Bologna, Luca Ghini actively promoted the founding of a separate teaching of *materia medica*. In 1534, when the university offered him the post of lecturer on 'simples' he nevertheless refused it, on the grounds that the teaching was in conjunction with and ancillary to that of medicine, and that the salary was low.[22] It was only in 1539, that the *Studio bolognese* decided to yield to Ghini's request. It raised his salary, and assigned him a lectureship for which he would teach and 'demonstrate' medicinal simples, and interpret the books of Galen and other classical as well as modern medical authors.[23] This definition and description of the teaching is worth considering. Here simples are obviously still considered in connection with their medical utility, but the fact that they are mentioned in the first place is a novelty. The verb *monstrare*, to demonstrate, assumes an innovative meaning, as well as the reference to 'recent' authors.[24] Since the contract was drawn up after long negotiations between Ghini and the *Studio bolognese*, one can assume that the formulation had been worded by Ghini himself.

The texts usually prescribed in the faculties of medicine of Italian universities before a separate lectureship of *materia medica* was established suggest that most learned physicians, although entitled to prescribe medicines, had no control over the herbs and plants used to compose them. Although some of the classical authors mentioned in the curriculum had dealt with *materia medica* and the use of plant remedies, the sections of their texts containing these subjects were rarely read.[25] Even when they were read, the teaching was strictly based on the theoretical discussion of the texts. The only plants physicians happened to see were the ones, probably already dried, in the apothecaries' shops. As is known, the supply of plants (gathered or imported) and the production of medicines were undertaken by apothecaries, who were trained by apprenticeship. In order

---

[22]   Sabbatani, 'La cattedra dei semplici fondata a Bologna da Luca Ghini', pp. 13–53.

[23]   'Item d. M. Luca Ghino nominatim decreuerunt in quinquennium proximum simplicis medicinae tradendae et monstrandae munus, eamque ex Galeni et al.*i*orum medicorum veterum, et recentiorum libris in publicis scholis interpretandum.' Sabbatani, 'La cattedra dei semplici', p. 32.

[24]   Galassi, 'Luca Ghini', p. 194.

[25]   Reeds, *Botany in Medieval and Renaissance Universities*, pp. 44–54.

to get a licence to practise, they had to pass an examination set by the *Collegio degli Speziali*, but no written material had to be studied in order to obtain the licence. The physician and the apothecary, therefore, though closely associated in their professional life, and belonging, at least in Florence, to the same guild, were two very different figures. As far as medical botany was concerned, although there certainly were some exceptions, the theoretical and abstract knowledge of the physician often contrasted with the uneducated practice of the apothecary, leaving some doubts about the results of their collaboration. As will be seen, the innovations connected with a new way of studying plants, in conjunction with the humanistic approach to ancient texts, played a fundamental role in the renewal of pharmacology that took place in the second half of the sixteenth century. A common aim united humanists, naturalists, physicians and apothecaries.[26]

Although Ghini had at last obtained a lectureship of *materia medica* at Bologna, in 1544, when his five-year contract expired, he accepted Cosimo's invitation, and moved to Pisa. The reasons for his leaving Bologna were probably various. It seems that, as a result of the city's economic difficulties, professors' salaries were paid out late and irregularly. Ghini had to pay for his own botanical research and, above all, could not obtain permission to establish a botanical garden where he could pursue his study of plants and provide his students with plant demonstrations.[27] The situation in Pisa, where the project of a garden was welcomed by Duke Cosimo, was much more promising.

Edward Lee Greene's chapter about Ghini in his *Landmarks of Botanical History*, opens with a warning. Ghini, he says, 'has borne in tradition the reputation of having been foremost among Italian botanists of his time' and he adds 'I say in tradition because he published nothing and the fame that rests on tradition alone may not be quite secure.'[28] If one looks at how this reputation was built up, one sees that it was created in the first place by naturalists and scholars of his time, who had first-hand knowledge of Ghini's merits. One can rely on a vast number of opinions and comments about him that are found in letters or books written by Italian and European naturalists who were in a position to judge his talents. The list of contemporary scholars who expressed their praise for Ghini is impressive. Benedetto Varchi, Pietro Andrea Mattioli, and the exceptionally large group of his students (Ulisse Aldrovandi, Bartolomeo Maranta, Luigi Anguillara, Andrea Cesalpino, Francesco Calzolari, Raniero Solenandro, Gherardo Cibo), who, in their turn, played an important role in the development of plant study, all contributed to the building of his reputation. Scholars who expressed admiration for, or gratitude to, Ghini came from all over Europe, as is attested by the correspondence and writings of Turner, Fuchs, De

---

26   Palmer, 'Medical botany in northern Italy', pp. 149–57.
27   Galassi, 'Luca Ghini', p. 197.
28   Greene, *Landmarks*, p. 702.

Lobel, Tournefort and Gesner.[29] It is true, however, that, as he did not publish anything, his fame has progressively faded, and the reasons why he was held in such high esteem have often been forgotten. A small part of his writings, however, that has come down to us, mainly in manuscript form, provides some evidence of his understanding of medicine, and of *materia medica* in particular.

Luca Ghini's achievements are most of all to be seen in connection with what he created and put into practice. A freer approach to the classical texts together with direct observation of nature, led him to new ways of treating *res herbaria*. His name is above all tied to the new methods and techniques he found out or perfected and spread. The use of the botanical garden and of *herbaria* as didactic tools gave rise to a solid group of botanists who were the nucleus of a new community of naturalists.

Ghini's *Placiti* and Lectures

Even if Luca Ghini did not publish anything, some of his writings, kept in the library of Bologna University among Ulisse Aldrovandi's manuscripts, have come down to us. The first of them is the so-called *Placiti* (Opinions), written by Ghini at Mattioli's request. The second consists of a substantial number of Ghini's lectures on *materia medica* transcribed by Aldrovandi in his own handwriting, when he heard them in Pisa, probably in 1549 or 1550. Another series of lectures about syphilis (*De morbo gallico*), transcribed by a German student, was accidentally found in 1588 by Philip Schopf who had them printed in 1589 as an appendix to a medical text.[30] Another work sometimes quoted among Ghini's medical works is *Experimenta in praxi*. The only ascertained reference to this work is to be found in a list of the manuscripts extant in the library of the naturalist Georg Hieronymus Welsch, in the first page of his *Exotericarum Curationum et Observationum medicinalium Chiliades duae* (published in 1676).[31] However, in Welsch's work, which contains a substantial number (Sabbatani reports 1,400) of very brief summaries of the manuscripts in his library, no manuscript by Ghini is included.[32]

---

[29]   Galassi, 'Luca Ghini', pp. 198–9.

[30]   Luigi Sabbatani, *Morbi Gallici curandi ratio perbrevis: La cura del morbo gallico nelle lezioni di Luca Ghini* (Venice, 1921). See also Raffaello A. Bernabeo, 'Il "De morbo gallico" di Luca Ghini', *Museologia scientifica*, 8 (1991–92), p. 238.

[31]   Georg Hieronymus Welsch, *Georgii Hieronymi Velschii Exotericarum curationum et observationum medicinalium Chiliades duae* (Ulm, 1676). The book starts with 'Manuscripta e quibus duae curationum & observationum Medicinalium Chiliades subsequentes desumptae in bibliotheca Georgii Hieronymi Velschii'. In the first page: 'Lucae Chini [*sic*], *Experimenta in praxi*' is quoted.

[32]   Luigi Sabbatani, 'Di una supposta opera di Luca Ghini', *Archeion*, 5 (1924), pp. 37–40.

In 1551 Mattioli requested Ghini's opinion on a long 'list[33] of simples that he lacked, to include in his Dioscorides, because he did not know them.'[34] The list included more than eighty plants. In a letter written in 1558, Mattioli reveals that Ghini himself had written some books about plants, for which the illustrations had already been prepared. Why they were never published is hard to say, the only explanation we have, though improbable, is the one furnished by Mattioli himself:

> Although he had intended to publish certain volumes which he had written concerning plants, and had illustrated them with figures, after having read my commentaries, he wrote me not only a letter of congratulations upon my having anticipated him, and thus lightened his own labours, but he also sent me a very great number of plants, which I as duty bound have acknowledged as having been received from him when adorning my Dioscorides with the figures of them.[35]

It is likely that Ghini had already written about some of the plants requested by Mattioli, as he was able to grant Mattioli's wish in a very short time and in November of the same year he sent him his opinions, on the majority of the plants listed. The *Placiti* were transcribed and printed in a long article by G.B. De Toni in 1907.[36] Only a few sections have been reproduced and translated into Italian by Fabio Garbari[37] and in English by Edward Lee Greene.[38]

A passage of the *Placiti* ('De Thalictron')[39] has sometimes been quoted as an example of Ghini's independent attitude toward Dioscorides's authority:[40]

> There was a certain old man of Bologna, in his day first among the herbarists of the time, who used to say that the very etymology of the name Dioscorides shows what kind of a man he was; that Greek name always sounded to him like *Deus Discordiae*. And really what the good old man said in jest and to provoke a laugh is not far from being true. Dioscorides did indeed transmit so great a number of

---

[33]   Biblioteca universitaria di Bologna (BUB), MS Aldrovandi 98, vol. 2, c. 53v–55r, 'Catalogo delli Semplici che mi manchano da mettere nel Dioscoride perché non li conosco'.

[34]   BUB, MS Aldrovandi 98, vol. 2, 33r-53r, 'Clarissimi atque Excellentiss. Lucae Ghini in celebri Pisana Academia materiae medicae professoris doctissimi. De quibusdam simplicibus placita ad Andream Mathiolum senensem celeberrimum medicum conscripta, idibus Octobris an. LI – Pisis'.

[35]   Quoted and translated by Greene, *Landmarks*, p. 801.

[36]   Luca Ghini, *Placiti*, in Gian Battista De Toni, 'I Placiti di Luca Ghini', *Memorie del Reale Veneto Istituto di Scienze Lettere e Arti*, 27 vols (Venice, 1902–1907), vol. 8, pp. 3–49.

[37]   Fabio Garbari, 'Luca Ghini a Pisa, cardine della cultura botanica del XVI secolo', *Museologia Scientifica*, 8 (1991– 92), pp. 230–33.

[38]   Greene, *Landmarks*, pp. 715–22.

[39]   Thalictrum, an herbaceous perennial plant of the family Ranunculaceae.

[40]   Garbari, 'Giardino dei semplici', pp. 31–2.

succinct, short, shabby and imperfect plant descriptions that, through such brief hints as he has given it may be impossible to arrive at a determination of the plants; hence concerning many of them we have such a variety of opinions, such seemingly opposite judgments about so many plants as renders it doubtful whether they can be recognized if ever found, and among this number is Thalictron ...[41]

Edward Lee Greene draws our attention on another point of the *Placiti*, concerning Horminum:[42]

It does not signify anything that Dioscorides failed to make mention on all these (under Horminum), for he did the same thing in the case of many other genera. Not in all of them which he undertook to describe did he give an enumeration of the species; and I think that you yourself, good Sir, have observed many more species of Cynosorchis than Dioscorides enumerates, more kinds of Tithymalus, more in Ranunculus, Polygonatum, Aconitum, daughters of Asphodelus, of which last I have in the garden three species over and above that described by Dioscorides ...'[43]

The Florentine humanist Benedetto Varchi, who had heard Ghini's lectures in Bologna, points out his ability for original thought as a rare quality:

And though the custom of modern philosophers is always to believe what is written in the classical authors and most of all in Aristotle, without proving anything, sometimes it is no less a sure thing to do otherwise and to depend on *esperienza*; I found some others who share this opinion, especially Luca Ghini, most distinguished physician and herbalist ...[44]

The passage is interesting also because it underlines the necessity of personal observation (*esperienza*) as opposed to dogmatic belief. A critical approach to the texts of the ancient writers of *materia medica* was not new and can already be found among the humanists of the preceding generation. The physician Nicola Leoniceno (1428–1524), who was professor at Bologna University for a long period, and who probably was one of Ghini's masters, had written a book the title of which was very significant: *De Plinii ac plurium aliorum in medicina erroribus* (1492). Ermolao Barbaro (1454–1493) had written a much more ponderous book on the same subject, *Castigationes plinianae*, in which he claimed to have corrected over five thousand mistakes in Pliny's *Historia Naturalis*. Edward Lee Greene, commenting

---

[41]   Greene, *Landmarks*, p. 718.
[42]   Horminum pyrenaicum (dragonmouth), of the family Lamiaceae.
[43]   Greene, *Landmarks*, p. 720. Quoted also by Giovanni Cristofolini, 'Luca Ghini a Bologna: la nascita della scienza moderna', *Museologia Scientifica*, 8 (1991–92), pp. 207–21.
[44]   Quoted from Varchi's *Questione dell'Alchimia* by Galassi, 'Luca Ghini', p. 195.

on Leoniceno's and Barbaro's works on Pliny, points out that some historians have objected to the fact that they were not botanists, and that a philological work had nothing to do with plant study. He very convincingly challenges their objection, demonstrating that Leoniceno and Barbaro would never have been able to write their works without a thorough knowledge of plants, and that their familiarity with them is apparent on every page and in every paragraph of their works.[45] The classical authors were assuming a new role; they did not represent the *summa* of knowledge anymore, but the indispensable platform on which one could begin the great work of checking, reorganization and integration. Not enough attention has been paid to the fact that when plants are involved, philological accuracy was not enough to regain a full understanding of the original texts.[46] While philology applied to literary and philosophical texts required comparison with the original written texts, philology applied to natural history texts often required comparison with nature. There was no way to review a botanical text other than that of direct observation of the plants from life.

If it is true that a reading of the *Placiti* reveals a freer and more critical approach to the authors from antiquity, it also confirms that the starting point was always Dioscorides. Ghini's constant research is aimed almost exclusively at finding in nature the plants that Dioscorides included in his *Materia medica*. One could object that this is obvious, as the *Placiti* were about Dioscorides' plants unknown to Mattioli. But the quest for plants to which Ghini is referring goes back a very long way. From what he says it is clear that he has been looking for those plants for years, and that his method of research was closely dependent on Dioscorides' words.[47] And this is one of the reasons why he laments that Dioscorides' descriptions lack clarity, and that often only a few species of certain plants are mentioned. This was not contrary to 'experientia', as his method was to look for plants in the field, checking personally if their attributes corresponded to what Dioscorides wrote, proceeding on the basis of trial and error, looking at them in the various stages of their growth, smelling and tasting them. He does not confine himself to finding them; he reproduces them, grows them, and records them in his *herbarium* or in pictures.

The reading of the *Placiti* reveals a series of other interesting aspects. First of all, the passages quoted above provide a very clear example of the confusion of nomenclature and the difficulty of interpretation that reigned in the field of medical botany. Second, one can see how complicated and aleatory was the retrieval of information and material concerning unknown plants. Several

---

[45]   Greene, *Landmarks*, pp. 560–61. Although the errors found in Pliny were attributed mainly to nomenclature difficulties and the negligence of copyists, and their criticism was mainly philological, these works, especially Leoniceno's, introduced a new attitude towards the classical authors. Fuchs's first book 'on the medics' errors' was published in 1530.

[46]   On this point see Reeds, 'Renaissance humanism and botany', p. 527.

[47]   See for example, 'De Crocodilio', Ghini, *Placiti*, p. 24.

Placiti contain stories of monks, merchants, seamen, soldiers, cardinals and many others who provided information about a plant or some kind of plant material. The section on 'Balsam', for example, refers first to a Greek monk, then to a Florentine merchant, and further on, to a superintendent of grand ducal triremes.[48] In the section on 'Aspalatho 1°' Ghini declares that he had no idea what that plant was until he received a piece of wood that was considered to be aspalatho by a Florentine tradesman. He believed that it was asphalato, although he had to confess that it was not bitter in taste (as Dioscorides had written).[49] It was very bitter, however, after it was ground. So he sent part of it to the *speziale* Baldassare Pepoli (his and Mattioli's friend) for the preparation of theriac, and sent a small portion to Mattioli.[50] Another identification, that of papyrus, is proposed by Ghini to Mattioli almost as a riddle. There are ships, he says, that bring sugar from Madeira, St. Thomas and Brazil to the port of Leghorn. Sugar is wrapped in different kinds of leaves, some of which are said to be papyrus. He will send three different leaves, so that Mattioli can judge himself which of these could be the right one. He is going to add a small sheet of papyrus written (he thinks) in Arabic letters which was given to him by a merchant from Pisa who maintained it had been found in the chest of a corpse, sold as a mummy.[51]

The *Placiti* are also a demonstration of the activity connected with the botanical garden, which is often mentioned, always referred to as '*hortus illustrissimi Ducis nostri*'.[52] Some of the plants unknown to Mattioli were already grown in the botanical garden, which means that Ghini always tried, when he was given seeds or suitable plant material, to see if they would take root in the Tuscan soil and climate and to grow them in order to follow their growth and show them to his students.

The attention of historians of botany has focused exclusively on the *Placiti*, overlooking the fact that we have at our disposal the transcription, by Ulisse

---

[48] 'Retulit mihi Monachus quidam graecus'; 'Eadem narravit mihi mercator quidam Florentinus ex Capponum familia'; 'Matheus Pratensis qui iam in Illustrssimi Florentinorum ducis triremibus scribam agit'. Ghini, *Placiti*, pp. 17–18.

[49] Ghini, *Placiti*, p. 18. Another rather vague identification of asphalato by the physician Luigi Anguillara is reported by Paula Findlen, *Possessing Nature: Museums, Collecting and Scientific Culture in Early Modern Italy* (Berkeley, CA, 1994), p. 205: 'Finding myself at the house of the most excellent physician messer Ioseppe Cincio in Rome in 1545 ... I came across a piece of wood on a table in his *studio* that smelled like a rose but without any bitterness, from which I quickly determined that it was asphalato and communicated this with many.' From Anguillara, *Semplici*, pp. 37–8.

[50] De Toni ('I Placiti di Luca Ghini', p. 18, note 3), cites the long letter sent by Mattioli to the apothecary Baldassare Pepoli concerning the preparation of theriaca, where aspalatho is mentioned.

[51] Mattioli, *Discorsi* 1573, p. 135.

[52] See for example 'De hormino', Ghini, *Placiti*, p. 29.

Aldrovandi, of a substantial number of the lectures Ghini gave at Pisa.[53] De Toni, alone, paid some attention to them and noted down a list of the titles of the first section. The only information with which he provides us in relation to the content, however, is two or three comments concerning some particular plants. Other scholars who dealt with Ghini either did not take them into consideration at all, or else seem to have confused them with the *Placiti*, assuming that they were one and the same.[54]

The lectures are very different from the *Placiti* for a series of reasons. They were academic lectures, addressed to students and not to an eminent colleague, and therefore the tone is much more professorial, even if there are sometimes some references to Ghini's personal experiences and a few digressions. Although the statutes of the *Studio pisano* prescribed that they had to be based on Dioscorides, there is a great display of erudition, and all the classical writers of *materia medica*, together with more recent and contemporary authors, are often mentioned in the customary humanistic manner. Unlike Dioscorides, moreover, the plants are arranged in alphabetical order, and their '*temperamentum*' (in terms of hot/cold, dry/humid and relative degrees) is often included, more in a Galenic than in a Dioscoridean style. It has to be remembered that Luca Ghini was not new to the task of 'reader of simples' and that, while in Pisa the new statutes prescribed only Dioscorides's *Materia medica* as the subject of the course, at Bologna University Galen and recent authors were also included. It is very likely that the content of the lectures Ghini held at Pisa was very similar to that of those held at Bologna. It is worth noting, however, that the lectures do not follow a regular pattern. Sometimes an entire lesson is dedicated to a single plant, at other times two or more plants are grouped together. Some of the lessons, moreover, are much longer than others.

Besides the content, there are other aspects worth considering. For example, it would be interesting to investigate not only *what* was taught, but also *how* it was taught, and what exactly happened during a lecture. Unfortunately there are no descriptions of how a lecture was held, or what went on in the classroom. However, one can assemble some information from different sources, and try to imagine what a lecture on simples at Pisa, in those years, might have been like.

The statutes stated that public lectures which were always held in Latin in the halls (*scholae*) of the university had to last one hour, 'even if the students were noisy'. Professors who left their desks before the hour was up, had their salaries reduced by way of a fine.[55] Although there is no specific reference to the lectures of

---

[53] BUB, MS Aldrovandi 98, vol. 2, 69v-148r, 'Ex lectionibus D.L. Ghini in Academia Pisana legentis collecta'. The lectures are 86 numbered from 1 to 103. Lectures 10, 14, 67, 69, 70, 72, 75, 76, 78, 80, 85, 86, 87, 91, 92, 94, 95 are missing.

[54] Garbari, Tongiorgi Tomasi and Tosi, *Giardino dei semplici*, p. 31.

[55] 'Statuti', XLIII, p. 614.

materia medica, one can assume that they followed this general rule. It is not clear, however, what exactly happened during the hour's lecture. We know that while the authorities laid down that the lectures should be oral (*libero vocis decursu*), the usual practice consisted in the dictation of notes. Fabroni, in his *Historiae Academiae Pisanae*, reports a list of sixteen amendments to the statutes, issued in 1583 by the *Auditore* Concini, the last of which concerned the matter of note-dictating. It explicitly warned professors not to dictate notes and established that defaulters should be fined according to the decision of the rector.[56] The notes were particularly useful to students, because the texts on which the lectures were based were usually very large, very costly and seldom available. The students, therefore, were firmly against the veto on dictation and many lecturers tried to comply with their wishes without breaching the embargo they were under. They did so simply by speaking very slowly.[57] The issue of the oral character of lectures was long debated among contemporary academics. There is an account of this ongoing debate written in a later period (1612) where the *Auditore* Antonio Curini proposed a solution consisting of speaking for forty minutes, and dictating a summary of the lecture for the remaining twenty minutes.[58] Given the extant transcription of Ghini's lectures by Aldrovandi, which were prior to the amendment of 1583, one can assume that Ghini used to dictate notes to his students.

A detail, however, is worth pointing out. In *Lectio* 32 'De Bedeguar', Ghini, commenting on that plant, refers to the fact that he is showing a specimen to the students: 'the plant I am showing you ...'.[59] Ghini therefore used dried plants in the lecture hall, probably those he did not have at his disposal in the botanical garden. Bedeguar, a kind of thistle also called 'white thorn', in fact, is not included on the list of plants grown there. It is very likely that Ghini's lectures consisted of reading, commenting, probably dictating notes, sometimes showing dried specimens, and at other times proceeding to the *ostensio* in the garden of simples annexed to the *Studio*.[60] If part of the lecture was spent in the demonstration of dried specimens or live plants in the garden, it explains why some of the lectures in Aldrovandi's manuscripts were longer than others

---

[56] Angelo Fabroni, *Historia academiae pisanae*, 3 vols (Pisa: 1791–95; reprint, Bologna: Forni editore, 1971), vol. 2, p. 3.

[57] Giuseppe Ongaro and Elda Martellozzo Forin, 'Girolamo Mercuriale e lo studio di Padova', *Girolamo Mercuriale – Medicina e cultura nell'Europa del Cinquecento*, in A. Arcangeli and V. Nutton (eds), *Girolamo Mercuriale: Medicina e cultura nell'Europa del Cinquecento* (Florence, 2008), p. 41.

[58] Marrara, 'L'età medicea' 1543–1737', p. 163.

[59] 'Hanc plantam quam vobis ostendo ...' Ghini, *Placiti*, p. 7.

[60] Luca Ghini (as well as his successor Andrea Cesalpino) was both professor of *materia medica* and curator-demonstrator in the garden. In other universities, for example at Padua, the positions were sometimes held by two different persons. See Grendler, *The Universities*, pp. 348–50.

and they did not follow a standard pattern. First-hand observation, by then, had probably become a fundamental part of the teaching of *materia medica*. From a didactic point of view this was certainly a crucial innovation which involved a substantial change in the understanding of *res herbaria*.

The only work by Luca Ghini which was published in the sixteenth century seems to be his *De morbo gallico*, a short treatise on syphilis, which appeared as an appendix to Johann Marquard's *Practica theorica empirica morborum interiorum* (1592).[61] This treatise is based on a number of Ghini's lectures, and is interesting above all because it provides us with some information on Ghini's attitude toward the use of new American medicinal plants for the treatment of what was commonly believed to be a new American disease. I will examine this work in detail in Chapter 4.

Andrea Cesalpino

In 1555, after Luca Ghini had left Pisa, Andrea Cesalpino (1519–1603) took his place both as lecturer of simples and director of the botanical garden. In about 1569 he left the teaching of *materia medica* for that of practical medicine. After fourteen years, in 1592, when the famous physician Mercuriale was invited by the grand duke to the *Studio pisano*, Cesalpino left Pisa for Rome. He was probably vexed by the fact that Mercuriale was appointed to teach the same subject, but with the higher position of *professore sovraordinario* (Cesalpino was *professore ordinario*) and with a higher salary. In Rome he was appointed physician to Pope Clement VIII, and he taught medicine at the Sapienza University as *professore sovraordinario* with a salary of 1,000 *scudi*, the same offered to Mercuriale in Pisa. He died in Rome in 1603, aged 84.

As far as the various practices of natural observation and data recording were concerned, Cesalpino seems to have followed his master's teachings. He took care of the botanical garden and supervised, with Luigi Leoni, the works for its move to a new location in 1563. Aldrovandi in his manuscripts reports a series of lists of plants[62] seen in Pisa's garden of simples during Cesalpino's tenure as director that testify to the increase of species grown, some of them coming from the New World.[63] In his dedication to the Grand Duke Francesco I of his

---

[61]   These lectures were transcribed in Luigi Sabbatani with a long introductory comment, in *Lucae Ghini Morbi gallici curandi ratio perbrevis*. See Chapter 4, pp. 159–61.

[62]   Andrea Ubrizsy Savoia, 'Le piante pisane nei manoscritti di Aldrovandi', *Museologia Scientifica*, 9 (1992), pp. 363–80.

[63]   It seems that in the 1570s the garden underwent a period of decay. In a letter to Aldrovandi of 1571, when Cesalpino had left the teaching of *materia medica* and the garden was under Leoni's superintendence, the apothecary from Lucca Giovan Battista Fulcheri

work *De plantis*, Cesalpino refers to his botanical expeditions.[64] From the same source and from a letter to Bishop Tornabuoni, we know that he produced two herbaria, one of which has come down to us. However, Cesalpino paid much more attention than Ghini to the theoretical and philosophical side of natural history. He was a keen botanist and an eminent physician, but he was also a *subtilissimus philosophus*, as declared on the title page of his *De plantis*.[65] In a period when Platonic philosophy was recognized in the university curriculum, and the *Studio pisano* established the first lectureship in that subject,[66] Cesalpino was a convinced Aristotelian. Famous, among philosophers, was his controversial debate with the first professor of Platonic philosophy Francesco Verino. Charles Schmitt, commenting on the lack of new ideas at the University of Pisa in the field of philosophy, considers him to be the most original thinker of the Pisan circle.[67] It is certainly this philosophical attitude that allowed him to consider the *res herbaria* from a novel viewpoint and to take a decisive step in the emergence of botany as a new and independent discipline. He was, according to historians, the inventor of systematic botany.[68]

Unlike Ghini, Cesalpino's reputation is supported by a large number of publications which cover different fields, such as philosophy, medicine, botany, mineralogy and even history. Historians, especially in recent years, have usually only examined one of his works or a particular subject area, and very rarely has Cesalpino's personality been examined in its entirety.[69] Almost all the authors who have written about him have underlined his philosophical, or better, his peripatetic approach. His philosophical works were usually regarded as an original interpretation of Aristotelianism; his Aristotelianism, however, was often considered, especially by historians of botany, to be a serious hindrance to original thinking. Cesalpino not only wrote philosophical works where he expounded and commented on Aristotle, such as the *Peripateticarum quaestionum libri quinque* (1571), but also all his other works were filtered

---

wrote: 'if that garden in the future is not more diligently taken care of, it will become a kitchen garden'. Quoted by Garbari, Tongiorgi Tomasi and Tosi, *Giardino dei Semplici*, p. 24.

   [64]   Andrea Cesalpino, *De plantis Libri XVI* (Florence, 1583).

   [65]   Cesalpino, *De plantis*, 'Dedication'.

   [66]   Charles B. Schmitt, 'The Faculty of Arts at Pisa at the time of Galileo', *Physis*, 14 (1972), pp. 263–7.

   [67]   Ibid., pp. 264–5.

   [68]   Greene, *Landmarks*, p. 808.

   [69]   Lynn Thorndike devotes an entire chapter to Cesalpino, in which he examines his various works: *A History of Magic and Experimental Science* (New York, 1923–58), 8 vols; vol. 6, ch. 40, 'Cesalpino's View of Nature', pp. 325–38.

through a philosophical vision. This vision was not only a characteristic of his writings, but was, very often, the *sine qua non* of his writings.[70]

Historians of medicine have considered his medical works and, above all, have discussed his theory of the circulation of blood, which, some have argued, preceded that of Harvey. Cesalpino's medical works, however, cover a much larger area. Pharmacology constitutes the object of his *De Medicamentorum Facultatibus*, in which he expounds at length the theory at the basis of the use of medicinal herbs and minerals, and which includes a section on distillation.[71]

His *Daemonum investigatio* should also be numbered among his medical works, although it is usually ascribed to the rather vague category of 'demonology'.[72] It is interesting to consider it, as it adds important information about Cesalpino's intellectual personality, and at the same time provides a good example of the use of natural herbal remedies in a 'supernatural' case on the part of a university physician. The occasion of the work is explained by Cesalpino in the first page of the treatise. An assembly of theologians, philosophers and physicians was held at the *Studio pisano* to discuss the cases of demonic possessions which had occurred to some nuns in the Monastery of S. Anna in Pisa. The purpose of the assembly was 'to judge from a careful examination of the symptoms whether disease stems from natural causes or whether there lurks another supernatural cause which does not respond to medical treatment but which only divine aid can remove'.[73] Cesalpino, as the title suggests, deals with the question from a medical point of view; his approach, however, is strictly philosophical. The views of Aristotle and Hippocrates are drawn together with the principles of Catholic religion to support his belief that demons exist and that possessions are caused by supernatural forces. Demons, which are not always evil spirits, are the *trait d'union* between God and Nature. Therefore, although incorporeal, they can operate on natural events and cause diseases. According to this view, disease seems to be at the same time 'demonic' and natural, as the demons are nothing but means mediating between divinity and man.

A short chapter at the end of the treatise is devoted to the treatment of demonic possessions. Cesalpino has no doubts about the efficacy of medical treatment and of the use of natural remedies;[74] he lists the herbal remedies indicated by

---

[70] Andrea Cesalpino, Andreae Caesalpini Aretini *Peripateticarum quaestionum libri quinque* (Venice, 1571).

[71] Andrea Cesalpino, *Andreae Caesalpini Aretini De medicamentorum Facultatibus, Liber Secundus* (Venice: Giunta, 1593), chapters XVIII–XIX, pp. 286–90.

[72] Andrea Cesalpino, *Daemonum investigatio peripatetica in qua investigatur locus Hippocratis si quid divinum in morbis habetur* (Florence, 1580).

[73] Mark E. Clark and Kirk M. Summers, 'Hippocratic medicine and Aristotelian science in the *Daemonum investigatio peripatetica* of Andrea Cesalpino', *Bulletin of the History of Medicine*, 69(4) (1995), p. 528.

[74] Cesalpino, *Daemonum investigatio*, ch. 24, p. 168.

Hippocrates, Dioscorides, Homer, Galen and Pliny. Some of the herbs are used as *amuleta* and can be useful to protect soul and body from malignant influence, such as *betonica* (according to Dioscorides and Antonio Musa Bresavola). His medical advice is to use natural medicaments like *aromata* and *suffumigia* which, by their volatile and penetrating properties, can enter more deeply into the body, reach the evil spirits, and, permeating through them, alter or expel them.[75] He mentions a series of herbs that can serve the purpose, and adds that Theriaca and Mitridatum, which are very effective against poisons, can be very useful in the case of demonic possessions, especially when diluted in an alcoholic liquid such as *aqua vitae*.[76]

This book has been a source of unease for historians who considered Cesalpino's achievements in medicine and natural history as steps of an imaginary stairway to scientific progress. The few authors who have written about the whole literary production of Cesalpino consider his acceptance of demonic influence as a drawback on his way to science and try to find justifications for it.[77] Francesco Fiorentino, referring to the *Daemonum investigatio* says that 'Here Cesalpino takes a step backwards, and returns to sorceries, witchcrafts, and similar vulgar prejudices.' And further on: 'He was credulous enough not to resist the vulgar fables of his time ...' and concludes that 'this booklet is his Achilles's heel'.[78] Lynn Thorndike, who in his *History of Magic* also devoted a whole chapter to Cesalpino, considering a great part of his works, was not far off this line of thought as he judged negatively the fact that Cesalpino wrote 'credulously on witchcraft' despite his being 'the most distinguished Italian scientist' and believes that 'his entitling his deluded mixture of theology and gross superstition a Peripatetic investigation must be regarded as a blot upon the escutcheon of Aristotelism'.[79]

Cesalpino's Herbarium (1563): A First Attempt at Classification

Herbaria, i.e. collections of dried plant specimens, a practice which had recently come into use, were used as a means to record and preserve the plants gathered in the wild, to exchange data and information with fellow naturalists, or as a

---

75 As far as demonic possessions are concerned, this is a very traditional medical advice. Already Mondino dei Liuzzi (*c.*1270–1326) had suggested using the fumes of some burnt herbs to expel evil spirits. Galassi, 'Luca Ghini', p. 192.

76 Rue, clary sage, fennel, peony root (also good for epilepsy), balsam, alkermes and all the substances that are scented such as amber, musk, cinnamon, nard, aloe wood.

77 See Francesco Fiorentino 'Vita ed opere di A. Cesalpino', *Studi e ritratti della Rinascenza* (Bari, 1911), pp. 325–38; Ugo Viviani, *Vita e opere di Andrea Cesalpino* (Arezzo, 1922).

78 Fiorentino, *Studi e Ritratti*, pp. 214–16.

79 Thorndike, *History of Magic*, chapter XL, 'Cesalpino's View of Nature', pp. 325–38, p. 338.

didactic tool.[80] Cesalpino probably used them for all these reasons, but he was also interested in a different use. A herbarium was the only way to have at one's disposal all the plants at the same time, irrespective of the place or time of their growth and vegetation, and thus enabled comparison. Comparing specimens was precisely what Cesalpino intended to do in order to find what he was most interested in, a new criterion of classification. The taxonomic principles he finally evolved were expounded at length and in detail in the first book of his work *De plantis* (1583). His herbarium, however, is significant as it shows that Cesalpino was concerned in the problem of plant classification twenty years before the publication of *De plantis*, and provides a direct insight into the process that lead to it. The dedicatory letter to Tornabuoni reveals Cesalpino's intention, and the theory underlying his methodology. Surprisingly, the whole letter is centred exclusively on taxonomy, which shows that this was the main function he attributed to his herbarium, even if it is very unlikely that the same interest was shared by the recipient Bishop Alfonso Tornabuoni who had simply asked for 'a gathering of simples glued on sheets in order to recognize them'.[81]

Cesalpino goes straight to the subject, avoiding any preamble, and explains why a classification was necessary: 'Although the number of plants keeps growing almost constantly, and such a number cannot be comprehended by the human intellect, by gathering many of them according to their similarity, and so reducing them to a small number, we can easily have knowledge of them as is appropriate'.[82] The arrangement of plants in a number of genera (groups), Cesalpino observes, had already been attempted by Theophrastus (*c.*371–*c.*287 BC), who did a good job, but neglected medicinal plants ('circa l'herbe medicinali se ne passò leggiermente'), and by Dioscorides who, on the contrary, dealt only with medicinal plants. He believes that the correct procedure is that of Theophrastus who considered the differences in the appearance of each plant, and according to their 'parts', gathered together those which belonged to the same stock (*schiatta*).

Theophrastus and Dioscorides represent two very different approaches to plants. As the titles of their works suggest, Theophrastus, in his *Historia plantarum* deals with plants in general, quoting particular plants in order to make clear his point of view; Dioscorides in his *Materia medica*, on the contrary, is interested only in medicinal plants, and devotes a chapter to each of them (circa 600), pointing out their medical properties. Theophrastus

---

[80] See Chapter 3, pp. 96–7.

[81] Andrea Cesalpino, 'Al R.mo Monsignore il S.or Alfonso vescovo de Tornabuoni', p. 3. The dedicatory letter is published in Théodore Caruel, *Illustratio in hortum siccum Andreae Caesalpini: Rudimentum ex plantis libro Agglutinatis vigere scio in testimonium eorum, quae in hoc volumine a me dicuntur* (Florence, 1858).

[82] Ibid., p. 1.

observes plants so as to be able to define the vegetable kingdom. Dioscorides observes and describes each single plant that can be useful to man so that it can be recognized and used according to his prescriptions.

As to systematization, Theophrastus needs a general frame into which to arrange his material. He divides vegetables into four categories 'which are the fundamental and essential categories which comprehend, it seems, the totality or the majority of vegetables: trees, bushes, shrubs, herbs.'[83] He gives a definition of each of the four categories, but points out that they are not absolute; some plants, according to their features, could be ascribed to one or other category. 'These definitions must be accepted with all due reservation and must be viewed as schematic formulas.'[84] There could be other criteria, he adds, therefore 'it is not necessary to follow rigorously the definition and our division must be considered a simple scheme'.[85] Theophrastus's classification is very general and very simple; it is based on plant morphology and is very easily understood.[86] For someone used to dealing with sixteenth-century herbals, which are usually written by physicians, with an almost exclusive attention to medicinal plants and their properties, the impact of Theophrastus is unexpected. Theophrastus's works on plants, completely unknown before the beginning of the fifteenth century, had been translated into Latin in 1483 and went through many editions in the first half of the sixteenth century.[87] Although Theophrastus was not unknown to sixteenth-century scholars, as his name is often quoted in the herbals of the time, his works did not attract the attention that might have been expected, and were never included in the syllabus of the universities. The explanation usually provided is that a general, philosophical approach did not interest the naturalists of the time, who were almost always medical men. This is surprising, however, as the education of physicians was very much

---

[83]   Suzanne Amigues, *Théophraste, Recherche sur les plantes. A l'origine de la botanique* (Paris, 2010), p. 9.

[84]   Ibid.

[85]   Ibid., p. 10.

[86]   As Suzanne Amigues points out 'this classification of vegetables according to their biological form is still in use in some scientific works of high level such as Flore forestière françoise (1989–2008), published by the Institut pour le Développement Forestier.' Ibid., p. 9, n. 12.

[87]   Aristotle's views on natural history were known from other works such as *De anima, Parva naturalia*, etc. and above all the books on animals where he draws a parallel, often discussed in the literature of the time, between animals and plants. The book *De plantis*, usually referred to as Pseudo Aristotelian, now attributed to Nicolaus from Damascus (first century AD) had been considered part of the Corpus aristotelicus during the Middle Age, and played a considerable role in spreading a peripatetic approach to the vegetable realm. Roger Bacon and Albertus Magnus wrote commentaries to *De plantis*. In the sixteenth century Giulio Cesare Scaligero wrote commentaries to this book and to the two books of Theophrastus. See Reeds, *Botany in Medieval and Renaissance Universities*, pp. 7–9.

centred on natural philosophy, and we know of controversies between medical men on questions that were purely philosophical (for example, the discussion about plant illustration). Although the curriculum of the faculties of medicine included a substantial philosophical training, philosophers and naturalists were seen as representatives of contrasting ways of understanding knowledge.

Undoubtedly it was Dioscorides's *Materia medica*, and not Theophrastus's books on plants, that came to constitute *the* model to which all sixteenth-century herbals conformed. The scope and aims of their works were different, and it should be noted that even the small section Theophrastus devoted to medicinal plants (usually published as chapter IX of *Historia Plantarum*) has been proved not to be originally part of this work.[88] Dioscorides in the preface to his *De materia medica* addresses physicians and advises them to observe plants in all the stages of their life as a function of their medical use; Theophrastus, in the first book of his *Historia plantarum*, observes plant morphology to find the differences and affinities that allow him to organize the study of plants in general.

Cesalpino himself points out that it is very rare to find a physician-naturalist who is at the same time a philosopher, and that is why, although Theophrastus had 'indicated the way', the problem of classification was never seriously taken into account. No one seems to have followed in his steps because 'among naturalists, very few have combined this profession with the study of philosophy ...'.[89] To embark on a reorganization of the vegetable kingdom both the general vision of the philosopher and the attention to particulars of the naturalist were necessary. Cesalpino is aware that only a botanist with a philosophical vision, as he rightly considers himself to be, can commit himself to such an undertaking. He will look for the similarities and dissimilarities that will allow him to divide plants into groups, and will proceed by trial and error. And this is when the herbarium comes into play; to begin with he sets out before him all the plants he has collected, and groups them 'roughly for this first time' ('*per questa prima volta grossamente*') dividing them into different sections.

This use of the herbarium on the part of Cesalpino is the perfect example of the methodological shift brought about by the new techniques of plant recording. As was pointed out, the removal of plants from their habitat for

---

[88] Amigues, *Théophraste*, 'Introduction', pp. X–XI.

[89] Cesalpino, Dedicatory letter, p. 2. Julius Caesar Scaliger, in the preface of his commentary to *De plantis pseudo-aristotelicus*, lamented the negligence of the ancients and of contemporaries and recognized that a new order was necessary to put an end to the chaos of botany. However, he did not propose a new way of classification. Also Girolamo Cardano devoted a section to plants in both his encyclopaedias (*De subtilitate* and *De varietate rerum*), where he dealt with philosophical issues and plant products. He speaks of the *differentiae* of plants briefly, admitting that they are too many and too complicated to be dealt with.

examining them, lead to a new method of studying plants which is at the root of scientific botany. After the re-discovery of first-hand observation 'in the field', plants were detached from their natural environment and gathered in botanical gardens, collections, and *herbaria* which became the new sites and tools of research. This became possible 'by decontextualizing nature, by curiously tearing out water lilies from water so that they could be dried, measured, printed, and compared with other living forms detached from local ecology and most of the senses'.[90]

Cesalpino then proceeds to explain briefly the criteria according to which he is going to group the plants. The centre of his reasoning is what Aristotle defines as the vegetative soul,[91] which is the principle that accounts for the faculties of nutrition and reproduction. He does not attach great importance to the organs of nutrition, as roots do not present sufficient differences, he observes, to provide a basis for taxonomy.[92] He concentrates instead on the modes and instruments of reproduction; comparing their incredible variety, one can find the similarities that allow the grouping of plants in genera and in families.[93] It is not sufficient to compare the 'parts' of the plants, such as 'flowers, seeds, roots, stems and other parts', one has to start from the true essence of plants. He will not go into philosophical and technical matters – Cesalpino continues – but will confine himself to indicating some groups into which he has divided the specimens. The first group is constituted of trees and shrubs; the second of those plants which have their seeds exposed, without any cover; the third by the plants whose seeds are contained in 'vases'. The last group is that of the plants that do not seem to have seeds.

---

[90] On this aspect, see Scott Atran, *Cognitive Foundations of Natural History: Towards an Anthropology of Science* (Cambridge, 1990) p. 134; Brian W. Ogilvie, *The Science of Describing: Natural History in Renaissance Europe* (Chicago, IL, and London, 2006), pp. 221–2.

[91] Cesalpino, Dedicatory letter, p. 4. The concept of vegetative soul is drawn directly from Aristotle. It is present in *De plantis of Pseudo-Aristotle*, but Theophrastus never refers to it directly. See Luciana Repici, *Uomini capovolti, le piante nel pensiero dei Greci* (Rome and Bari, 2000), pp. 200–11.

[92] 'Havendo adunque la natura variato quanto ha possuto, d'intorno alle radici non posseva molto variare'. Cesalpino, Dedicatory letter, p. 4.

[93] 'Adunque da e modi vari del produrre e semi, o quello che ha proportione con e semi genitali, & dalla simiglianza di quelli ho rintracciato e generi & le spetie delle piante, conciosiache quelli più propinquamente mi dinotano la virtù dell'anima, per la quale tutte hanno l'esser' loro.' Ibid., p. 5.

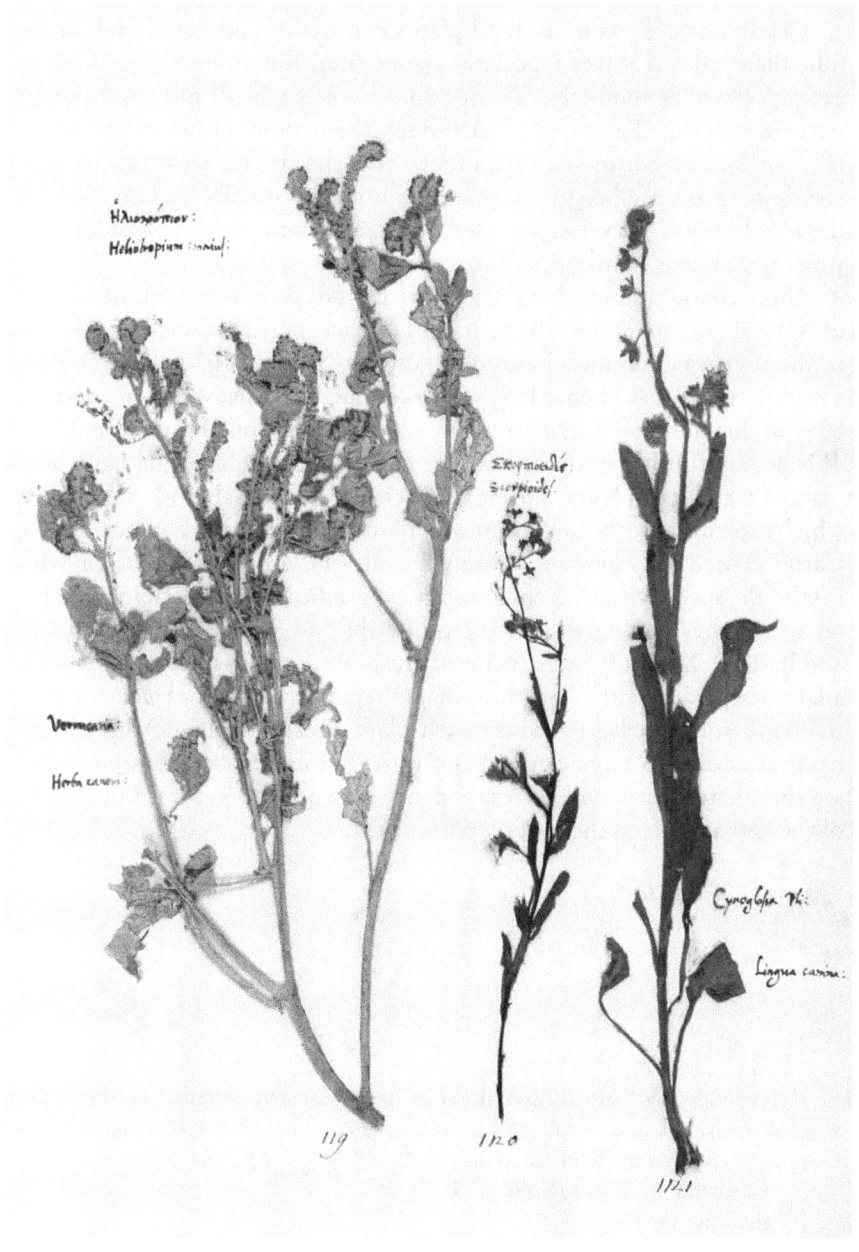

Figure 2.1　One page (f.120) of Cesalpino's herbarium, 1563. Sezione botanica, Florence, Museo di storia naturale dell'Università

Cesalpino's collection of dried plants consists of 266 folios, and on each folio there are two or three specimens (sometimes four or five). Each folio and each specimen is numbered. The specimens are 768 in all and correspond to circa 760 species (Figure 2.1).[94] Although the number of plants included in *De plantis* twenty years later are about 1300, the criteria according to which Cesalpino proceeded to group them did not substantially change. The same theory, although not yet expounded in detail as in the first book of his major work, was already in his mind.[95]

The herbarium, after a long series of vicissitudes is now kept in the Museum of Natural History of the University of Florence. In 1717 it was examined and studied by the Florentine botanist Pier Antonio Micheli (1679–1737), who left a manuscript (BOT-Mich. MS9) with a commentary, that was then continued by Giovanni Targioni Tozzetti in 1737–38 and by his son Ottaviano in 1796.[96] This manuscript is constituted of 276 folios and includes a catalogue of the plants ('Catalogus plantarum Horti Sicci Andreae Cesalpini') and a *notizia* which explains how the herbarium was found.[97] In 1858 the botanist Teodoro Caruel carried out a new and thorough study of Cesalpino's herbarium which lists all the specimens, with their numbers as indicated by Cesalpino, the page on which they are glued, and the transcription of names (in Latin, Greek and Italian). The study of Caruel is of great interest because he carries out his analysis in parallel with Cesalpino's major botanical work *De plantis*, recording the book and the chapter where each plant is contained, and the scientific name according to Linnaean nomenclature.[98] From his accurate study we can see that there is an actual correspondence between the 'genera' and 'families' of the herbarium and those of *De plantis*.

---

[94]   Guido Moggi, 'L'erbario di Andrea Cesalpino', *Gli erbari aretini da Andrea Cesalpino ai giorni nostri*, in Chiara Nepi and Enrico Gusmeroli (eds), *Gli erbari aretini da Andrea Cesalpino ai giorni nostri* (Florence, 2008), pp. 12–13.

[95]   Cesalpino, Dedicatory letter, p. 14.

[96]   Ibid., pp. 14–16.

[97]   The manuscript is described by Stefania Ragazzini in *I manoscritti di Pier Antonio Micheli conservati nella Biblioteca Botanica dell'Università di Firenze* (Florence, 1993), pp. 17–20.

[98]   Théodore Caruel, *Theodori Caruelii Illustratio in hortum siccum Andreae Caesalpini: Rudimentum ex plantis libro Agglutinatis vigere scio in testimonium eorum, quae in hoc volumine a me dicuntur* (Florence, 1858).

Cesalpino's *De plantis*

Twenty years later, when *De plantis* came out (1583), we can see how Cesalpino's principles of classification had been developed and refined.[99] In the dedication of his work to Grand Duke Francesco, some topics dealt with in the letter to Tornabuoni are repeated or specified. It is clear that the *raison d'être* of the book is the new organization of the vegetable kingdom. If the decline and chaos of medical botany was a customary topic in the literature dealing with plants of the time, here the focus has shifted. Usually the authors lamented the state of the discipline in relation to the irresponsible use of medicinal herbs, which were often substituted with wrong, even poisonous ones. The solution envisaged was therefore medical, and consisted in the retrieval of the true plants listed by ancient authors, above all Dioscorides. Even when the issue of how to arrange the sequence of plants in a book was discussed, it was always dealt with as a side issue, something which was not relevant. In Cesalpino's work systematization is the central point, and for that reason plants are seen in their own right. In other words, *De plantis* is not a medical book. A phrase, towards the end of the dedication, removes all doubts: 'I have considered it superfluous to add the medical properties [of plants]; in fact these have been expounded by many authors, and above all, at great length by Dioscorides and Galen.'[100]

In the dedicatory letter to Francesco I, Cesalpino sets out very clearly the reasons why he has embarked on this work. The first argument is, as in his letter to Tornabuoni, the impossibility of dealing with the vastness of the vegetable kingdom without a serious philosophical reflection. Here, however, he states more exactly 'that the number of species is continually increasing not because Nature produces new forms, but because new forms are revealed to us every day'.[101] A great deal of work has been done to recover the study of plants of the ancients;[102] Luca Ghini in the *academia pisana*, Mattioli, and other prominent scholars have produced exhaustive commentaries to Dioscorides (one of

---

[99] Andrea Cesalpino, *De plantis Libri XVI* (Florence, 1583). On Cesalpino's taxonomy, see: Julius Sachs, *History of Botany (1530–1860)* (Oxford, 1860), pp. 37–58; A.G. Morton, *History of Botanical Science* (London and New York, 1981), pp. 128–44; C.E.B. Bremekamp, 'A re-examination of Cesalpino's classification', *Acta Botanica Neerlandica*, 1 (1953), pp. 580–93; Atran, *Cognitive Foundations of Natural History*, pp. 138–58; Greene, *Landmarks of Botanical History*, Part II, pp. 807–83; Ernst Mayr, *The Growth of Botanical Thought: Diversity, Evolution, and Inheritance* (Cambridge, MA, and London, 1982), pp. 158–62; Ogilvie, *The Science of Describing*, pp. 223–6.

[100] 'Facultates quoque addere superfluum duxi: cum enim hae apud multos authores praecipuè Dioscoridem & Galenum admodum copiosè legantur.', Cesalpino, *De plantis*, p. VI.

[101] Ibid., p. II.

[102] Cesalpino mentions 'Ruellius, Hermolaus, Brasavolus'. Ibid., p. III.

them Anguillara);[103] exotic plants, both from the East and West Indies have been listed and described in two books, by Garcia da Horta and Monardes.[104] Notwithstanding these efforts, botany is in a deplorable state. Comparing it to an unruly army, he continues:

> I recognise just this to be the condition of things in the botanical world today, where the vastness and intricacy of the disorder appal the mind, give rise to countless and inextricable errors, and are the source of endless controversies; for if the genus is not known, no description of a plant, however accurately it may have been transmitted, will enable one to identify it with certainty, and such descriptions are apt to mislead; for if the genera are confused all is confusion, necessarily.[105]

No knowledge can exist, he adds, which ignores this general rule: 'All science consists in the gathering together of things that are alike, and in the distinguishing and separating of the unlike.'[106]

Once again Cesalpino stresses that among the *antiqui* the only author who turned his attention to the problem of classification was Theophrastus, 'who showed the way'.[107] Dioscorides ordered plants according to their medical properties, and this, he points out, is a most 'unnatural' order. The most fallacious, however, was the alphabetical order, which is the furthest from nature. He then states the reasons why a classification according to nature is the most appropriate. It is based on natural *differentiae*, which are easier to recognize, and are not subject to changes in environmental conditions; it is the best way to help the memory, as the immense number of plants can be grouped in orderly and much less numerous genera. The natural way of classification is also profitable for medicine, as the plants belonging to the same group, very often have similar faculties; moreover, according to this system, plant description will be easier, shorter and more precise because, once the features of a genus are expounded, there is no need to repeat them for all the species belonging to that genus. Pictures are no longer required, as the *differentiae* between species are better conveyed by words.

Also the new plants which arrived from distant lands had to find a place in Cesalpino's taxonomy. It had to be 'predictive', that is to say it had also to work

---

[103] Ibid.

[104] Ibid., p. IV.

[105] Ibid., p. II, as translated and quoted by Greene, *Landmarks*, p. 816.

[106] 'Cum igitur scientia omnis in similium collectione & dissimilium distinctione consistit', Cesalpino, *De plantis*, p. IV.

[107] Ibid.

for plants of which no one knew the existence.[108] This was possible because his system was based exclusively on plant morphology. In the dedicatory epistle of *De plantis* he justifies himself in advance if some of the 'new' plants were not placed in the right order. This was not to be ascribed to a deficiency of the system, he explains, but to the fact that often only parts of the exotic plants (roots, wood, dried leaves, etc.) were shipped from abroad, and an examination of the whole plant was not possible.

Cesalpino devoted all the first book of *De plantis* (XIV chapters) to the explanation of the criteria at the basis of his taxonomy. The first eleven chapters of the first book describe the parts that constitute the plants. The vegetative soul, which is the pillar that supports his theory, is mentioned in the very first line of the text: 'The nature of plants has only that sort of soul through which they are fed, grow and generate their like ...'. Unlike animals, that are more complex organisms and therefore need a more elaborated system, plants need only 'nutriment for the conservation of the individual and the seed for the perpetuation of the species'.[109] Two concepts, already touched on, seem to emerge more clearly: that of the species as a fixed form and that of the seed as the depository of the true essence (*substantia*) of the species.[110] The plant has two organs (*partes*) necessary to perform these fundamental functions: one is the root, through which the plant draws its nourishment; the other is the stalk (for herbs) or trunk (for trees) that carries the fruit for the propagation of the species. As we will see further, these fundamental parts provide the basis on which the grouping of plants is determined.

The parallel with animals, which vouches for the Aristotelian foundation of his reasoning, is always present and leads the development of the exposition. Aristotle had located the animals' soul in their heart (*cor*). But where is the 'animae principatus' in a plant? Cesalpino looks for the best place to locate the 'cor'in plants and finds it in the point of conjunction between the root and the shoot.[111] He then proceeds to expound the function of nutrition with the parts

---

[108] See Kristian Jensen, 'Description, Division, Definition: Caesalpinus and the Study of Plants as an Independent Discipline', in Marianne Pade (ed.), *Renaissance Readings of the Corpus Aristotelicum: Proceedings from the Conference held in Copenhagen, 23–25 April 1998* (Copenhagen, 2001), p. 201.

[109] Cesalpino, *De plantis*, p. 1.

[110] Atran maintains that the idea of the immutability of the species was conceived by Cesalpino and was not an Aristotelian concept. According to Atran, for Aristotle the species was dependable on a series of factors that Cesalpino would define 'accidental'. Atran, *Cognitive Foundations*, pp. 138–9.

[111] 'radix germini coniungitur, locus videatur cordi plantarum oportunissimus', Cesalpino, *De plantis*, p. 3. Julius Sachs, who devoted an important part of his *History of Botany* to Cesalpino, criticized this point, attaching some importance to it. Bremekamp comments on Sachs's point of view demonstrating that the concept of 'cor' was used

that provide for the absorption and the distribution of nourishment; the modes of propagation (*generatio*) and the parts involved among which are the seed, the flower, the fruit. He also devotes a chapter to minor 'parts' such as tendrils, thorns and hair.

The last three chapters of the first book are those in which Cesalpino sets out the principles of his classification and its theoretical justification. In chapter XI he explains the traditional (Theophrastus's) general division of tree, bush, shrub and herb (*Arbor, Frutex, Suffrutex and Herba*), defining first tree and bush. He then discusses the various definitions of herb enunciated by his predecessors, challenging their criteria and expounding the reasons why they cannot provide a valid principle of classification. In the next chapter (XII) he repeats the principle according to which the characters at the basis of a classification should be found in the 'parts' of the plant that perform the two primary functions of nutrition and growth, and the generation of the like. Root and shoot account for nutrition, while 'fruit and the parts that contribute to the making of the fruit' ('fructus & partes ad fructificatione facientes') account for propagation.

He condenses (chapter XIII) the four Theophrastian classes of tree, bush, shrub and herb into two classes, including the bushes in the class of trees, and joining the herbs with the shrubs. In the letter to Tornabuoni of 1563 he had not considered the root a significant organ for plant classification, dismissing it as not presenting sufficient variety. Here he finds a role for the root as the part that indicates if a plant belongs to the tree or the herb class. If the root is hard and woody, the plant is a tree, if it is soft, it is a herb.[112]

The first general division is therefore based on the first fundamental function of the plant, i.e. nutrition. This division, however, must be subdivided into smaller groups, according to the second fundamental function of the plant, that of reproduction. The parts of functional importance that must be taken into account are therefore the fruits and the seeds, and anyway those that constitute the organs of fructification ('modo fructificandi').[113] One has to discard (chapter XIV) all those aspects (*differentiae*) that are only 'accidental' and do not represent the essence (*substantia*) of the plant. Cesalpino has a very clear idea of the characters that are to be counted as *accidentia*: they are those which are not the plants' own and are not perpetuated through the seed, but might change according to the environment, climate, manner of cultivation and perception, such as size, colour, odour, taste, or medicinal properties. Only the 'natural' differences were substantial, that is to say those related to the plant essence, all the others were accidents. In order to define more precisely which are

---

by Cesalpino very seldom in his classification, exerting an insignificant influence on it. Bremekamp, 'A re-examination of Cesalpino's classification', p. 582.

[112] Cesalpino, *De plantis*, p. 27.

[113] Ibid., p. 28.

the *differentiae* that must be considered in a plant's organs, Cesalpino restricts them only to three: the number, the position and the aspect.

The remaining fifteen books of *De plantis* deal with the description of about 1,500 individual plants arranged in thirty-two groups.

The principles by which Cesalpino decides to group the different classes and genera are diligently justified through observation and logical reasoning. The general criteria summarily expounded in his letter to Tornabuoni twenty years before are here discussed, explained, and supported by a rational justification. It has been pointed out that there were other naturalists who tried to put some order in botany, but no one, before Cesalpino, felt the need to define criteria or to justify them.[114]

It is clear that close observation of plant morphology was one of the distinctive features of his method. His observation is sometimes supported by arguments very similar to what we would now call 'experimental method'. For example, when he investigates how plants draw water from the soil, this is how he proceeds. It cannot be the kind of force that a magnet exerts on iron, he argues, since in magnetism what is larger attracts what is smaller, and therefore it would be the soil's water that attracts the plant and not vice versa. Nor can a plant absorb moisture through a force like that exerted by a vacuum, as the earth also contains air and, as is demonstrated by cupping glasses applied to the ground, air would prevail, and the plants would absorb air instead of water. But there are substances, like linen, sponges, and powders that are more inclined to absorb water than air. Hence the nutritive function, he concludes, must be carried out through parts that have this kind of property.[115]

It is not surprising that *De plantis* was not much appreciated by contemporary scholars.[116] Caspar Bauhin refers to *De plantis* in one of his letters and defines it 'learned but most obscure' ('doctus sed obscurissimus'), and declares that he had much trouble in understanding it and doubted that students would be able to do so.[117] His contemporaries expected a new book of the kind they were familiar with. It was not obscure just because Cesalpino's classification was difficult to grasp, but also because they did not find the information they had been used to look for in a 'herbal', which was taken for granted to be a medical book. Cesalpino, in fact, consistent with what he had expounded in the dedication, did not mention the medicinal properties of plants, with the only exception of

---

[114] Ogilvie, *The Science of Describing*, p. 221.

[115] Cesalpino, *De plantis*, pp. 3–4.

[116] Cesalpino did not provide schemes or *tabulae* to make his system more easily understood. Schemes of Cesalpino's classification were drawn up by Ray in *Methodus nova*, 1682 (pp. 161–6); Linnaeus (*Classes plantarum*, 1738); Sachs (*History of Botany*); Bremekamp ('A re-examination of Cesalpino's classification', pp. 591–3). Bremekamp's schemes are also reported (by the editor) in Greene, *Landmarks*, pp. 812–14.

[117] Reeds, *Botany in Medieval and Renaissance Universities*, p. 19.

some plants of recent importation, the use of which was still controversial.[118] As it was a book on plants, and not on the medical virtues of plants, it was not considered useful by contemporary physicians, and therefore not often taken into account. The enormous success of Mattioli's *Discorsi* provides evidence of what contemporaries expected from a book on plants.

The most frequent remark made by botanical historians, and other authors who dealt with the subject, is that Cesalpino's classification is theoretical and artificial.[119] Although not all of these writers (I have considered mainly Sachs, Bremekamp, Atran and Mayr) based their analyses on the same premises, their conclusions converge, as they all point out that Cesalpino's principles of classification were chosen by philosophical reflection to justify groups that already existed. When Cesalpino describes, in his letter to Tornabuoni, how he first set out all the plants of his herbarium under his eyes to group them according

---

[118] The entry on Guaiacum, the new drug *par excellence*, for example, contains some medical information. Cesalpino, *De plantis*, pp. 105–107.

[119] Julius Sachs criticizes him on the grounds that he had trodden a 'dangerous path and one which led succeeding botanists astray ... since the natural system can never be laid down upon a priori principles of division.' Sachs, *History of Botany*, pp. 40–41. Bremekamp explains that 'The artificial nature of the arguments by means of which Cesalpino tried to make the choice of his characters acceptable, makes it probable that these characters were not ... chosen on account of a preconceived notion, but that they must have been brought to light by the analysis of natural groups, i.e. of groups of plants that are similar in habit.' Referring to the concluding chapters of the first book of *De plantis* he maintains that 'The arguments which according to this exposition lead to the choice of his characters, were merely arguments by which he tried to justify the choice after the latter had been made, and by which any other choice could have been justified as well.' Bremekamp, 'A re-examination of Cesalpino's classification', pp. 584–5. Bremekamp tries to reconstruct the procedure according to which Cesalpino determined his classification. Scott Atran, commenting on Bremekamp's analysis, points out that there was no need to imagine a particular procedure, since the groups were already part of what he calls folk biology: 'The families and sections of natural families that Cesalpino did produce were, to a significant extent, already known to local folk and herbalists of the time: '*Graminae, Leguminosae, Liliaceae, Labiatae, Verbenaceae, Umbelliferae, Cruciferae, Ranunculaceae, Cucurbitaceae, Euphorbiaceae, Compositae, Rosaceae, Caryophillaceae and Primulaceae.*'According to Atran, it was more likely that Cesalpino 'attempted by trial and error' to find the characters of fructification organs that would *preserve* these groupings. Atran, *Cognitive Foundations*, pp. 151–8. Ernst Mayr also points out the 'artificiality' of Cesalpino's system. He states that it is evident that Cesalpino 'could not have arrived at his groupings merely by applying logical division' and that he evidently started out with certain 'natural groups' that he already had in mind: 'Cesalpino, thus, followed a two steps procedure. He first sorted his plants by inspection into more or less natural groups and then searched for suitable key characters that would permit him to arrange these groups in accordance with the principles of logical division.' However, he concludes, 'the 32 groups of plants recognized by him are, on the whole, remarkably "natural"'. Mayr, *The Growth of Botanical Thought*, pp. 160–61.

to their differences and affinities, he would already have had in mind some groups known by him intuitively or by tradition. All naturalists saw natural groups of plants as having an affinity to one another. Affinity, however, was recognized and accepted intuitively, and no effort had been made to understand or define it rationally. These natural groups, Julius Sachs explains, 'present themselves to the unprejudiced eye as naturally as do the groups of mammals, birds, reptiles, fishes and worms in the animal kingdom'.[120] But Cesalpino based his attempt at classification on the philosophical definition of a plant and its nature. At the beginning of his book he states that nutrition and reproduction are the two functions of a plant. The organs of nutrition and reproduction, therefore, are the *partes* on which to base the divisions and subdivisions of the vegetable kingdom. While not rejecting the 'natural' groups, he attempted to explain rationally the affinities and differences that were recognizable in the 'natural' groups.[121]

This issue of artificiality is the most recurrent criticism of Cesalpino's system. It is, however, intertwined with a series of different opinions on its general significance to the history of botany. Julius Sachs (1890) regards Cesalpino as 'the first who converted observation into real scientific research.' 'He endeavoured to express with clearness and on principle' that which the German fathers of botany had felt indistinctly, 'that there is an actual connection of relationship among plants expressed in their organization as a whole.'[122] Morton regards Cesalpino's Aristotelism as an inevitable negative influence on his thought, but then he argues that 'the outmoded aspects of Cesalpino's thought' are 'completely thrown into the shade by the remarkable conceptual advances he made in spheres of botany so important for the future'.[123] He even criticizes Sachs' lack of sympathy and understanding of Aristotle, and his failure to appreciate Cesalpino's 'creative assimilation of knowledge' inherited from Greek science, and to realize his great capacity for empirical observation.[124] Agnes Arber, in her book on herbals, is the most negative of all, and devotes to Cesalpino just a few very brief sections. She finds him too abstruse and obscure, a step backwards from Albertus Magnus's achievements. The artificiality of his system is once again the principal criticism, but she does not justify her opinion on the basis of an analysis of Cesalpino's work.[125] Edward Lee Greene, on the contrary, praises him highly, analyses at

---

120   Sachs, *History of Botany*, pp. 3–4.
121   Ogilvie, *The Science of Describing*, pp. 223–5.
122   Sachs, *History of Botany*, pp. 40–41.
123   Morton, *History of Botanical Science*, p. 130.
124   Ibid., note 44, pp. 157–8.
125   Arber, *Herbals*, pp. 116–17, p. 136, pp. 152–3. Scott Atran reports a quotation from Agnes Arber on Cesalpino and discusses it as an example of ill-founded assertion. Atran, *Cognitive Foundations*, pp. 151–2.

length his method of classification, and agrees with Linnaeus in considering his work the first example of systematic botany.[126]

Historians usually agree on the fact that Cesalpino was the first to point out clearly that systematic botany implied the investigation of natural relations of plants to each other, and that usefulness and medical properties were 'accidental' and not belonging to the true essence of the plant.

Oddly, Cesalpino's *De plantis*, at a distance of many centuries, was not only the first book inspired by Theophrastus, but in common with Theophrastus's *Historia plantarum*, was paid little attention by their successors. However, Cesalpino's philosophical reflection on the vegetable kingdom, in conjunction with the importance he attached to observation, and his consideration that a collection of all plants was not something to strive for, constituted a new way to approach the natural world. While contemporary naturalists concentrated their efforts on collecting as many natural specimens as they could, believing that once the task was completed, all the secrets of nature would be revealed and the 'book of nature' read at last, Cesalpino's attitude showed an alternative path.

Cesalpino went beyond first-hand investigation of plants and concentrated his efforts on developing a system of classification based on rational principles. As Brian Ogilvie points out 'most Renaissance naturalists did not see any need to go beyond common sense when they organized their histories of plants. From the perspective of later centuries, Cesalpino was ahead of his time; from his contemporaries' point of view, he was imagining problems that did not exist.'[127] Exclusive attention to plant morphology and the method of logical division based on similarity and dissimilarity of characters, remained the basis of all successive taxonomies, up to Linnaeus and beyond.[128]

Conclusion

Universities, unlike courts, were institutional places where precise functions were performed, on the basis of a set of fixed rules. While the figure of a courtier is elusive and not easily definable, that of a university professor was unambiguously defined by his role. The intellectual endeavours and achievements of Luca Ghini and Andrea Cesalpino were made possible and sustained by their roles as *lectores simplicium* within the university. As we will see in the next chapter, the methods that allowed a new way of studying plants were at the same time fundamental teaching tools. The chair of *materia medica* certainly represented an innovation within the context of the university, and from which a completely new way

---

[126]   Greene, *Landmarks*, pp. 808–31.
[127]   Ogilvie, *The Science of Describing*, pp. 225–6.
[128]   Mayr, *The Growth of Biological Thought*, p. 161.

of viewing natural history rapidly took root. Its novelty is attested also by the fact that it was not met with unanimous approval and was often considered as a lesser subject. Knowledge of simples had too long been left in the hands of wise women and apothecaries and it still occupied a low place among university professors. Even after medical botany was recognized as part of the curriculum of the faculty of medicine, it was hardly considered on the same level as other teaching. In the *Studio pisano*, for example, it did not reach the level of 'ordinary' teaching, and remained 'extra-ordinary' throughout Ghini and Cesalpino's tenures (only Aldrovandi in Bologna had succeeded, by his authority, in rendering it *ordinario*).

This view about the teaching of *materia medica*, is well expressed in a letter of Falloppio to Aldrovandi of 23 January 1561. Here Falloppio blames Aldrovandi for his decision to leave philosophy for the teaching of medical botany.[129]

> You are throwing yourself into something which has already achieved its apex, and cannot go further. There is nothing left but to have some illustrations printed, and make a comment on Theophrastus's *De Causis plantarum* ... I really do not know whose spell you have come under. I hear that you are now teaching the history of animals of Aristotle, and that of metals, and I do not know what else. I praise everything, but think of these lectures held in public, and compare them with lectures about *Parva Naturalia*, *De generatione et corruptione*, *De anima*, *Meteorologica* and the like, which contain so many philosophical speculations. When you reach the apex of the former you will be an excellent herbalist, while of the latter you will be an excellent philosopher, and your soul will be elevated by speculations, while in the former it will be abased by observation.[130]

The teaching of natural history was scorned by Falloppio as a subject unworthy of a great mind, as it only involved observation, and not philosophical speculation. Within the traditional hierarchy, theory was always regarded as superior to practice. It was a deep-rooted belief, as Falloppio himself was a great connoisseur of simples and, as an anatomist, he could not be suspected of considering 'practice' inessential. It was the subject itself which was considered of little account, even though Aristotle had dealt with it. Falloppio certainly knew that both Galen and Avicenna, the authors who were considered fundamental in the study of medicine at the university, had devoted substantial parts of their work to simples and pharmacology. However, these sections of

---

[129] This is the description of the teaching in the university roll of 1560–61: 'Legat philosophiam naturalem ordinariam, de fossilibus, plantis et animalibus'. Grendler, *The Universities*, p. 350.

[130] *Epistolario di Gabriele Falloppia*, ed. Pericle Di Pietro (Ferrara, 1970), p. 56. The letter is also quoted by Fiorentino, *Studi e ritratti della Rinascenza*, p. 202.

the great medical writers were considered only ancillary, and not central, to their literary production.[131]

The letter of Falloppio is also significant in that it confirms that observation had become the basis of the study of simples. Observation, however, as a new way of acquiring knowledge of the natural world required new habits and methods which allowed its practice and the preservation of the results obtained. These will be the subject of the next chapter.

---

[131] Avicenna, for example, had devoted the second book of his *Canon* to simples, and the fifth to the medicinal preparations. If we examine the rolls (*rotuli*) of the faculty of medicine at Pisa in the second half of the sixteenth century, we see that, although Galen and Avicenna were almost always present among the prescribed texts, the parts of their works concerning medicinal plants and the way to use them are never mentioned.

Chapter 3
New Ways of Studying Plants

The first university courses entirely devoted to the study of plants were established in the faculties of medicine. Physicians, according to the ancient medical writers, were required to have a thorough knowledge of the simples they were using in their prescriptions. To know a plant, Dioscorides had explained, meant to see it sprout from the soil and follow all the stages of its growth. All its parts, seeds, roots, leaves, stems, bark, flowers and so on, had to be taken into account. It was evident that the course of medical botany held in a lecture hall, once again based on a book, even if dealing exclusively with plants, could not provide all the information the future physicians were supposed to acquire. Luca Ghini, who had promoted the new teaching of *materia medica*, first at Bologna and then at Pisa, was well aware of what a *lector simplicium* would need to convey these kinds of notion. They were the same as he, as an observer of natural things, needed for his study of, and research on plants. First of all a place where one could grow plants and watch them develop day by day; observation, however, was of little use if it could not be recorded and conveyed. To this end, a series of techniques were devised, the initiation and dissemination of which was often attributed to Luca Ghini and his group of pupils. This chapter examines the scientific activities and procedures that were established, perfected, and spread in the second half of the sixteenth century, and became the common ground on which naturalists began to base the observation of the natural world, the recording of natural data, and its communication.

Gardens of Simples

A garden where plants could be seeded, transplanted and propagated, and where their development could be examined and monitored in detail was one of Ghini's fundamental requirements, and one of the reasons why he left the University of Bologna where he could not obtain funds to establish it. The fact that Duke Cosimo was willing to support his project was probably what convinced Ghini to accept his invitation to lecture on simples at Pisa.[1]

---

[1]   Fabio Garbari and Lucia Tongiorgi Tomasi, 'Le origini dell'orto dei semplici: dall'Orto dell'Arsenale all'Orto Novo di via Santa Maria', in Garbari, Tongiorgi Tomasi

Medicinal herbs had always been grown in monastic gardens, and gardens of simples were also often established near hospitals. There is evidence that there was a garden of simples in Pisa next to the *Ospedale nuovo* near the Cathedral.[2] Marcello Virgilio Adriani, in his commentary on Dioscorides' translation (1518), in the chapter on Eupatorium, refers in passing to the garden of the Hospital of Santa Maria Nuova in Florence: 'I have seen in the gardens of the larger hospital of our city a plant growing, which, by exhibiting all the marks attributed to Eupatorium by Dioscorides, should prove to be that.'[3] We also know that 'secret gardens', that is to say small enclosed plots of ground for aromatic and medicinal herbs, were to be found in most private gardens, and that some apothecaries used to have gardens of their own in which to grow simples.[4]

The garden of simples founded in 1544 in Pisa by Luca Ghini under the duke's patronage however, had a different and novel function. It was an institution of the University, established in connection with the new chair of *materia medica*. The plants and herbs of the new garden, therefore, were not only to be used to prepare drugs and remedies. The relationship with medicine was still fundamental, but the educational and 'experimental' approach appeared to be pre-eminent. The didactic use of the garden was certainly one of Ghini's interests. In a letter sent from Bologna on 2 February 1545 to Francesco Riccio, the duke's secretary, he gives an account of his excursions to the Apennines in search of plants for the botanical garden at Pisa; he states that the garden is intended to be useful for students ('d'utile alli scolari').[5] As previously mentioned, the professor appointed to lecture on simples spent part of his lectures in the garden, showing students the plants referred to when commenting on Dioscorides. The importance of this practice for the future generation of naturalists cannot be underestimated. It soon became the usual teaching method, and other botanical gardens attached to universities were established in Italian university towns. One of Ghini's students, Luigi Anguillara, founded a botanical garden in Padua in 1545, the same year as the foundation of the *orto pisano*; Ghini himself laid out another garden of

---

and Tosi, *Giardino dei semplici*, pp. 15–26. Giovanni Calvi, *Commentarium inserviturum Historiae Pisani Vireti Botanici Academici* (Pisa, 1777).

   [2]   Garbari, Tongiorgi Tomasi and Tosi, *Giardino dei semplici*, p. 28.

   [3]   Greene, *Landmarks*, p. 574.

   [4]   We know, for example, that the *speziale* Stefano Rosselli (1523–1597) had a garden near his Villa di Quarata at Antella, where he had gathered a great quantity of plants collected during his excursions in Tuscany or ordered from distant lands. Guglielmo Volpi, 'Intorno all'origine del Giardino dei semplici di Firenze', *Archivio storico italiano*, 9(1) (1922), p. 87.

   [5]   Garbari, Tongiorgi Tomasi and Tosi, *Giardino dei Semplici*, p. 277.

simples in Florence.[6] Bologna's garden was founded by Ulisse Aldrovandi in 1568. Soon after, other European towns and universities created their own physic gardens.[7]

The garden of simples at Pisa was organized from the outset as a place where 'esperienza' could be undertaken. An impressive number of specimens were planted in the garden, most of them collected by Ghini himself and his assistants, or sent by colleagues and correspondents. A list of the plants extant in the garden is recorded in one of Aldrovandi's manuscripts.[8] As one can see from the title above the *catalogus* 'the number of plants at this time [between 1549 and 1553] was 620', more or less the number of plants that appear in Dioscorides' *Materia medica*. The list includes only a part of them ('only the most beautiful and rare'), that is to say about 340.[9] Most of them were useful from the pharmaceutical point of view, although some seem to have been chosen for purposes other than their practical use. What is worth noting is the fact that this list is considered to be the first list of plant seeds (index seminum) in the history of botany.[10] Since the seeds were available to botanists, it placed the garden, its director, and the *Studio pisano* at the centre of a web of correspondence, exchanges and requests. In subsequent lists, always concerning the first *orto pisano*, Aldrovandi notes the appearance of the first American plants, a 'pianta maxima' (sunflower), and a 'pomus amoris' or 'tumatulum pomum' (tomato).[11]

---

[6]   See below, pp. 92–3. Volpi, 'Intorno all'origine del Giardino dei semplici di Firenze', pp. 81–90. P. Luzzi and F. Fabbri, 'I tre giardini botanici di Firenze', *I giardini dei semplici e gli orti botanici della Toscana* (Perugia, 1993).

[7]   Leiden, 1587; Basel, 1588; Montpellier, 1597; Oxford, 1621; Paris, Jardin du roi, 1626; London, Chelsea Physic Garden, 1673.

[8]   BUB, MS Aldrovandi 136, vol. 14, 'Catalogus omnium plantarum quae erant in horto publico studiorum tempore Luca Gini qui publice profitebatur lectionem simplicium, et horti studiorum praefectus erat. Numerus autem eo tempore plantarum erat 620. Hic tamen describam ex hillo horto pulchriora simplicia et rariora, in quibusdam vero eius opinio apparebit.'

[9]   The list is transcribed and discussed in G.B. De Toni, 'Spigolature Aldrovandiane: Le piante dell'antico Orto Botanico di Pisa ai tempi di Luca Ghini', *Annali di Botanica*, *Annali di Botanica*, 5(3) (1907), pp. 421–40.

[10]   Fabio Garbari, in AA.VV., *Livorno e Pisa: due città e un territorio nella politica dei Medici* (Pisa, 1980), p. 527. The first Index seminum to be printed was that of the botanical garden of Padua in 1591.

[11]   Andrea Ubrizsy Savoia meticulously reports the lists of plants from the botanical garden and Pisa countryside that are included in Aldrovandi's manuscripts in 'Le piante pisane', pp. 363–80.

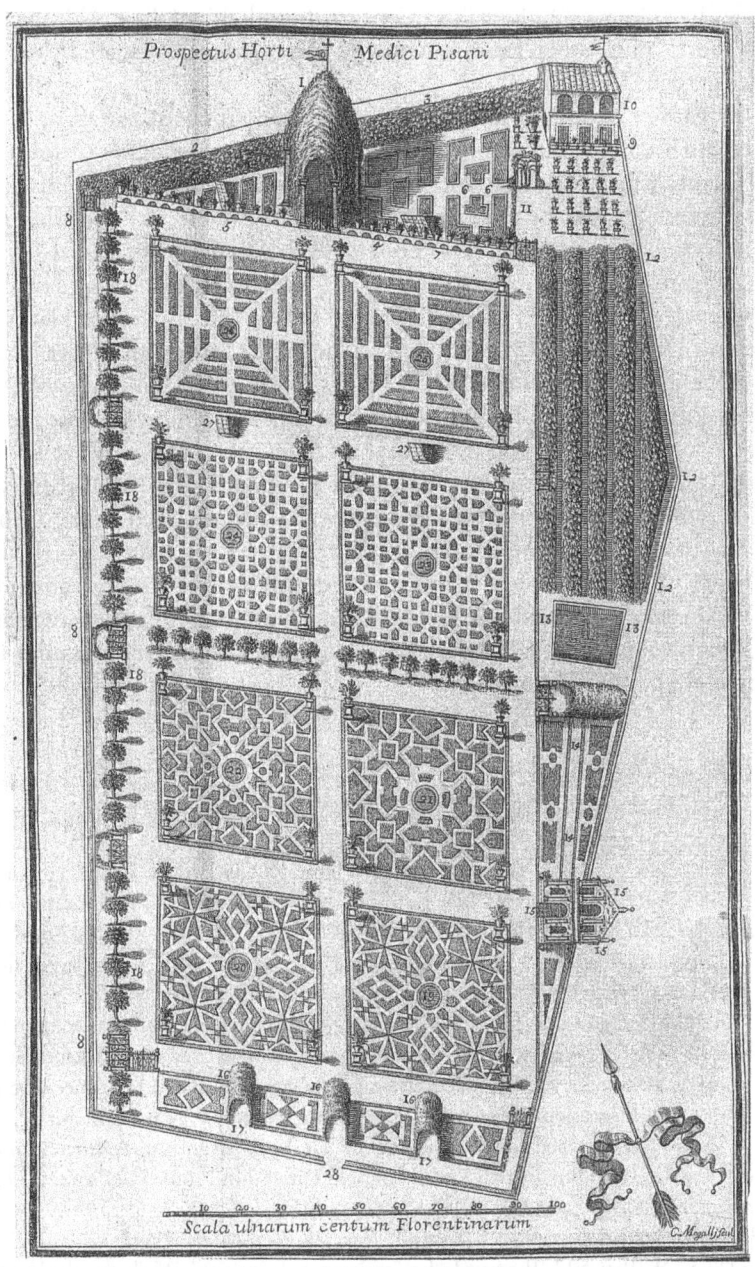

Figure 3.1   The garden of simples at Pisa. From Michelangelo Tilli, *Catalogus plantarum horti Pisani*, 1723. Florence, Biblioteca Nazionale Centrale

The garden was moved twice in the second half of the sixteenth century. In 1563, when Cesalpino was in charge, it was moved to make space for the needs of the adjacent Arsenal. This second garden was smaller than the first, and was set up in less favourable ground, as it was distant from the university, and was close to the walls of the city which shaded it for a great part of the day. Probably for these reasons, Grand Duke Ferdinando moved it again, and a third garden was laid out where it remains today (Figure 3.1). At the entrance we can still see the memorial tablet of 1595, where it is underlined that the garden was intended for students who wanted to study the nature and faculties of plants, but was also open for all those who were willing to visit it.

Aldrovandi's manuscripts provide us with other lists of the plants he had seen, or had requested from the *orto pisano* and the country around Pisa. Thus we have an idea of the development and increase of specimens grown in the garden under the tenure of Andrea Cesalpino and later of the *semplicista* Giuseppe Casabona or Benincasa (the Flemish Josef Goodenhuyse), who became prefect of the *orto pisano* when it was moved for the second time, after 1591. A vast number of plants were taken from Pisa to be grown in the botanical garden that Aldrovandi had, in the meantime, founded in Bologna (1568). Between 1569 and 1583 Aldrovandi requested 128 species that were not yet present in the *catalogus* at the time of Ghini.[12]

While we have a plan of the third *orto pisano*, we do not have any precise information about the layout of the first and the second Pisan botanical gardens. From the so-called 'Scorzi map', which is the oldest map of the city that has come down to us, we can guess that they were roughly square.[13] Actually a square divided into four sections, subsequently subdivided into several smaller beds, seems to have become the model of the botanical gardens that were laid out in the second half of the century.[14] The closest example that can be provided is certainly the second Tuscan botanical garden that was founded very shortly after that of Pisa, the Florentine *giardino dei semplici*, or *giardino delle stalle*, as it was often called.[15] The garden was set out on a piece of land Cosimo had leased from

---

[12] Ubrizsy Savoia, 'Le piante pisane', p. 373.

[13] In the 'Scorzi map' (end of the seventeenth/beginning of the eighteenth century) the three botanical gardens are designed, although they never coexisted. See Tongiorgi Tomasi, 'Le origini del Giardino dei Semplici', in Garbari, Tongiorgi Tomasi and Tosi, *Giardino dei semplici*, note 2, p. 25; Emilio Tolaini, *Forma Pisarum. Storia urbanistica della città di Pisa. Problemi e ricerche* (Pisa, 1979), pp. 213–16. In the third botanical garden the square model was doubled, as the ground was in the shape of a long rectangle.

[14] See for example, Andrea Ubrizsy Savoia, 'The botanical garden of Padua in Guilandino's day', in Alessandro Minelli (ed.), *The Botanical Garden of Padua 1545–1995* (Venice, 1995), pp. 173–95.

[15] Volpi, 'Intorno all'origine del Giardino dei semplici di Firenze', pp. 81–90. Luzzi and Fabbri, 'I tre giardini botanici di Firenze'; Leopoldo Del Migliore, *Firenze città nobilissima illustrata* (Florence, 1684; Repr. Facsimile Bologna, 1968), pp. 238–9.

the nuns of San Domenico in 1545, near the Convent of San Marco, in that area of the city where the Medici had already built a menagerie and stables. It was designed by Tribolo (Niccolò Pericoli), the architect who, in those same years, was also in charge of the works in the garden at Castello. The duke, who had already established a *giardino dei semplici* in Pisa, intended to have another one in Florence. Leopoldo Del Migliore (1684) describes the layout of the garden:

> Then the beauty of this garden, associated with the above mentioned utility, consists of the partition of the ground, ingeniously made according to various mathematical Figures; the same figures necessary to separate and distinguish from each other the qualities of simples, as reported by Serlio ... It [this garden] is separated and divided into four parts by means of alleys or paths covered with a vault of bay, which form a cross, as they run in straight lines from the four corners of the square in which the garden is contained.[16]

The reason the duke wanted to have another botanical garden set out in Florence was to allow the Florentine students who had moved to Pisa, where the faculty of medicine was now established, to study plants during their vacations. It should also be noted that the hospital of Santa Maria Nuova served as a medical school for the training of future Tuscan physicians, and therefore it was likely that a number of students spent part of their time in Florence.[17]

Given the great importance Duke Cosimo attributed to plants, both from the medicinal and the aesthetic point of view, there was also another reason that could have induced him to found a garden of simples in Florence. As was written in the tablet outside the *orto pisano*, a garden of simples was a place that not only students, but also all the citizens who wanted to, could visit and enjoy. Although many courtiers had laid out splendid private gardens, which also contained sections of medicinal herbs, the city did not have a public space where citizens could walk, converse, observe plants, and admire the beauties of nature. A public garden was perhaps seen by Cosimo as an important addition to the image of beauty and grandeur that Florence had to acquire, no less important than palaces and churches. The preparation of the *giardino delle stalle*, as Del Migliore relates, was entrusted to the most skilled men, and above all to Luca Ghini.[18] While Tribolo was in charge of the design, Luca Ghini, shortly after the layout of the *orto pisano*, was entrusted with the planting of the new Florentine garden. This garden was greatly expanded under Grand Duke

---

16 Del Migliore, *Firenze città nobilissima*, p. 238.

17 G. Cellai, L. Fantoni and P. Luzzi, 'Intorno all'origine del giardino dei semplici di Firenze: Il Monastero di S. Domenico in Cafaggio', *Atti e memorie dell'Accademia toscana di Scienze e Lettere la Colombaria* (Florence, 2009), pp. 80–97.

18 Del Migliore, *Firenze città nobilissima*, pp. 238–9.

Francesco and his *semplicista*, the Fleming Casabona.[19] The botanist Giuseppe Casabona was introduced to the Medici by Niccolò Gaddi, a prominent figure in the political and intellectual circles of the city, who was also a keen connoisseur of plants and simples. His garden in via del Melarancio, the so-called 'Paradiso dei Gaddi', was praised as one of the most beautiful gardens of Florence, and was also known to include a section where medicinal plants were grown.[20] Casabona, invited by Gaddi as a guest, quickly acquired a great reputation for his botanical knowledge, and was soon welcomed to court by Grand Duke Francesco, who conferred on him the title of *semplicista*. In this capacity he supervised the garden of the Casino di San Marco, the *giardino delle stalle* in Florence, and also the third botanical garden in Pisa.

The botanical garden played a significant role also from another point of view. Cosimo's effort to give the university a dominant position within his cultural project gained considerable advantage from the *orto pisano*. It served as an important vehicle of renown and consensus for the grand duchy. It is known from books, letters and journals that the garden was visited and praised not only by Italian, but also by many foreign visitors throughout the sixteenth century. The naturalists Pierre Belon, Charles de l'Ecluse (Clusius), Matthias de Lobel and Pierre Pena, to name but a few, visited it and wrote about it praising the garden as well as the grand duke's liberality. The fact that plants in this garden could be seen that could not be seen elsewhere is repeated over and over again. Mattioli reported that in the garden one could find 'many rare plants that were never seen in Italy up to that moment' and praises the 'most excellent Cosmo Duke of Florence'.[21] The French botanist Pierre Belon refers to the garden in his *De neglecta cultura stirpium* where he mentioned the men of *scientia* and the rare plants that are gathered there to the advantage of those who want to study them. He adds his praise for the grand duke: 'I think one should not omit to say that this eminent prince, besides all his other virtues, has seen fit to promote science with such great enthusiasm that he did not spare any expense'.[22] As Galluzzi points out, the symbolic importance of possessing all the plants of the known world would have been stressed by scholars and visitors of the time. It was interpreted as a sign of power and it certainly contributed to build up Medicean prestige.[23]

The attempt to concentrate in a small space all the plants found in nature was paralleled by another initiative. A collection of natural objects was started and exhibited in a room annexed to the garden, the so-called *Galleria*. The purpose

---

[19] Calvi, *Commentarium inserviturum*, pp. 71–84.

[20] Acidini, 'Niccolò Gaddi', pp. 141–75, 359–61.

[21] Galluzzi, 'Il mecenatismo mediceo', p. 196.

[22] Pierre Belon, *De neglecta cultura stirpium* (Antwerp, 1589), p. 64. Reported in Garbari, Tongiorgi Tomasi and Tosi, *Giardino dei semplici*, 'Appendix 1', p. 282.

[23] Galluzzi, 'Il mecenatismo mediceo', p. 196.

was primarily scientific and didactic, as is attested by the fact that it was, at least at the beginning, a collection of *naturalia* as opposed to *artificialia* and that it was, like the garden, connected to the *Studio*. This collection, started under Cosimo I, was enlarged under Francesco I, and especially under Ferdinando I by the new director of the garden, the Franciscan friar Francesco Malocchi.[24] There is an interesting letter of 1 July 1599 to Aldrovandi in which Malocchi asks advice about the rarest things, both plants and natural objects, that can be found in the Genoese Riviera, as the grand duke had asked him to carry out research in that region.[25] Then, among Aldrovandi's manuscripts, one can actually find the list of the things Malocchi collected in Liguria, between the 15 July and 2 September 1599, for the *Galleria* and the botanical garden. As far as 'natural things and materials' (*'robe e materie naturali'*) are concerned, there are the most disparate objects, the main part of which are minerals and marine material, such as 'extravagant' shells, corals and pearls. As to plants, there is a list of almost 200 of them, some of which were probably planted in the garden, and others dried and kept in a herbarium.[26]

The importance of this kind of collection, 'whose purpose was to bring all of nature into one space',[27] for the development of natural history, has been recently extensively studied.[28] It is important to note that although the *lectura de simplicibus* was primarily focused on plants, there is evidence that it was not the only subject dealt with by professors of *materia medica*. We know, for example, that Luca Ghini gave a series of lectures on minerals, as Benedetto Varchi informs us,[29] and that he collected and exchanged natural objects with his correspondents. Pharmacology had always dealt with other substances, both animal and mineral, as well as with simples and the new interest in the natural world gave birth to a new group of collectors. Collecting, Lorraine Daston and Katherine Park observe, was no more an activity of patricians and princes, but of scholars and medical men as well: 'Unlike princely collectors, who continued to prize precious materials and elaborate workmanship, physicians and apothecaries collected mainly *naturalia*, which reflected their own interests

---

[24]   Fabio Garbari, 'I "Prefetti" del giardino, dalle origini', in Garbari, Tongiorgi Tomasi and Tosi, *Giardino dei semplici*, pp. 46–7.

[25]   BUB, MS Aldrovandi 136, vol. 28, cc. 60v – 61v. Quoted in Tosi, *Aldrovandi e la Toscana*, p. 430.

[26]   BUB, MS Aldrovandi 136, vol. 30, cc. 98r–105v. The list is reported in Garbari, Tongiorgi Tomasi and Tosi, *Giardino dei Semplici*, Appendix 1, pp. 284–9.

[27]   Findlen, *Possessing Nature*, p. 1.

[28]   See for example Giuseppe Olmi, *L'inventario del mondo: catalogazione della natura e luoghi del sapere nella prima età moderna* (Bologna, 1992) and Findlen, *Possessing Nature*.

[29]   Galassi, 'Luca Ghini', p. 195. He refers to *Questione dell'Alchimia*.

in therapeutics and were also relatively affordable.'[30] In this period some private collections of this kind were begun, such as the 'museums' of the apothecaries Ferrante Imperato in Naples, and Francesco Calzolari in Verona, and above all of Ulisse Aldrovandi in Bologna. Aldrovandi's description of his collection gives an idea of his immense effort to retrieve and collect the entirety of natural objects, including those from distant lands. Among the enormous number of the items amassed, he lists his dried and painted plants:

> Today in my microcosm, you can see more than 18,000 different things, among which 7000 plants in fifteen volumes, dried and pasted, 3000 of which I had painted as if alive. The rest – animals terrestrials, aerial and aquatic and other subterranean things such as earths, petrified sap, stones, marbles, rocks, and metals – amount to as many pieces again. I have had paintings made of a further 5000 natural objects – such as plants, various sorts of animals and stones – some of which have been made into woodcuts. These can be seen in fourteen cupboards, which I call the Pinacotheca. I also have sixty-six armoires, divided into 4500 pigeonholes, where there are 7000 things from beneath the earth, together with various fruits, gums, and other very beautiful things from the Indies, marked with their names, so that they can be found.[31]

It is not by chance that at Pisa the collection of *naturalia* was attached to the botanical garden and was under the supervision of the garden's director. Botany, among the various branches of natural history was the first to emerge and take form. It was, as Schmitt points out, 'the growth point from which a number of other natural history subjects developed.'[32] The museum of *naturalia*, like the botanical garden, was perceived as a necessary step towards the reform of *materia medica* and the advancement of medical knowledge. Apothecaries were the first to collect *naturalia* as they were the objects of their profession; Ferrante Imperato, for example, declared that his museum was 'full of an infinite number of rare things for the apothecary's profession.'[33] Physicians, through the new lectureship of *materia medica* established in the universities, were now equally involved in the investigation of natural objects. As Paula Findlen observes 'natural history had become part of the 'expertise' required to become a physician', thus physicians 'increasingly collected natural specimens to fit their image as observers of nature and practitioners of *materia medica*.'[34]

---

[30] Lorraine Daston and Katharine Park, *Wonders and the Order of Nature 1150–1750* (New York, 1998), p. 149.

[31] Quoted by Daston and Park, *Wonders*, p. 154.

[32] Schmitt, 'Science in the Italian Universities', p. 40.

[33] Findlen, *Possessing Nature*, pp. 245–6. All ch. 6 'Museums of Medicine' of Findlen, *Possessing Nature*, deals with this topic.

[34] Ibid., pp. 246–7.

With reference to the botanical garden, another aspect is worth pointing out. It is the insistence on the beauty of trees, herbs and flowers. The garden of simples was useful, but was also considered beautiful and pleasant. Plants were no more seen, not even by physicians, only as pharmaceutical elements; they began to be considered for themselves. In the letter to Cosimo's secretary that has already been quoted, Luca Ghini himself refers to 'many and very beautiful plants' (*molte e bellissime piante*). Some years later Agostino del Riccio in his *Agricoltura sperimentale*, praising the third grand duke Ferdinando, describes the botanical garden as a 'beautiful and fair garden full of simples and plants of great virtues' where the 'honorable students and Doctors go to argue about those plants and at the same time see their beauty'.[35]

The beauty of plants is now referred to again and again also where one would not expect it. One line of the title of the botanical garden plants' list mentioned above, as it appears in Aldrovandi's manuscript, is significant: 'I will describe here the most rare and beautiful (*rariora et pulchriora*) simples of that garden'.[36] Although the plants are referred to as 'simples', which is the term used for medicinal plants, their beauty is underlined. There is an item on the list which testifies that plants were now studied not only for pharmaceutical reasons. This item reads: 'Many unknown plants, nevertheless beautiful.'[37] It is evident that these plants had not been gathered and transplanted because they were useful but in order to be studied in their own right.

Herbaria

Aldrovandi's manuscripts provided evidence that Ghini, along with the written text of the *Placiti*, sent Mattioli sixty-nine dried plants with labels (*epigrammata*), all of which are listed. As De Toni notes, if Ghini could send such a substantial number of plants in such a short time, it was clear that he was already in possession of the dried specimens. In one of his *Placiti*, 'De Horminio', he stated that he was going to send two plants 'dried and glued to sheets of paper' ('essiccate e attaccate col glutine alle carte').[38] In a letter to Ulisse Aldrovandi of 16 October 1553, Ghini wrote that he was sending him some dried plants ('erbe secche') adding that he had collected at least 600.[39] From a series of letters of pupils and colleagues who thank him or comment on his generosity it is known that he often sent them dried specimens and even prepared small herbals for

---

[35]   Agostino del Riccio, *Agricoltura sperimentale*.The section containing this passage is reported in Garbari, Tongiorgi Tomasi and Tosi, *Giardino dei semplici*, 'Appendix 1', pp. 278–9.

[36]   BUB, MS Aldrovandi 136, vol. XIV, 'Catalogus omnium plantarum'.

[37]   Ibid.

[38]   'De Hormino', Ghini's *Placiti*, p. 29.

[39]   The letter is published in Tosi, *Ulisse Aldrovandi e la Toscana*, p. 48.

students who were embarking on botanical studies. Francesco Calzolari, the eminent apothecary of Verona who was one of Ghini's pupils, mentioned in a letter of 1555 to Aldrovandi 'a book of simples well dried that is more than anything else dear to me', sent to him by Luca Ghini.[40]

The dried specimens mentioned above, so often used by Ghini, were the result of a novel method of preserving plants for future study and research. The plants were collected and pressed, usually between cloths, and then glued to sheets of paper and labelled. As Edward Lee Green points out, naturalists of the previous generation, when walking in the country, 'took ancient texts with them, in manuscript or in memory', looked at the plants and left them there.[41] There is not sufficient evidence to attribute the invention of this new method to Ghini, but certainly he was the first to employ it extensively, to exchange specimens with colleagues and correspondents and to use it for his demonstrations in the lecture hall. He certainly taught it to his pupils as is attested by a series of *horti sicci*, as herbaria were often called, that have come down to us. One of them is a small herbarium of 202 specimens of plants collected in the garden of simples at Pisa, now kept in Florence. It is anonymous, but universally attributed to a priest from Lucca, Michele Merini, one of Ghini's pupils. Much more substantial are the ones by Andrea Cesalpino, Ulisse Aldrovandi and those attributed to the naturalist Gherardo Cibo.[42]

Andrea Cesalpino, as we have seen, is known to have produced two herbals. While the one he gave to Cosimo I is now lost, the other one, dedicated to Bishop Alfonso Tornabuoni, is still extant and is kept in the Museo di storia naturale at the University of Florence. It consists of 768 specimens and is a useful reference for botanical historians as it exemplifies his criteria of classification.[43] Aldrovandi's *hortus siccus*, kept in Bologna, is a gigantic work of more than 4.000 specimens collected in sixteen volumes, ordered alphabetically. Lucia Tongiorgi Tomasi draws attention to a group of five herbaria now at the Biblioteca Angelica in Rome, that have been attributed to Gherardo Cibo, a naturalist and a painter who can be counted among Ghini's pupils.[44] In a period when nomenclature and description were such imperfect tools, the possibility of collecting and having to hand specimens of real plants was an invaluable means of recording and exchanging information.

---

[40] See De Toni, *Placiti*, pp. 12–13.

[41] Greene, *Landmarks*, p. 709.

[42] Lucia Tongiorgi Tomasi, 'Dall'essenza vegetale agglutinata all'immagine a stampa', *Muselogia Scientifica*, 8 (1991–92), p. 278; 'Gherardo Cibo: visions of landscape and the botanical sciences in a sixteenth-century artist', *Journal of Garden History*, 9 (1989), pp. 199–216.

[43] Tongiorgi Tomasi, 'Dall'essenza vegetale agglutinata', pp. 278–9. I have dealt at length with Cesalpino's herbarium, in Chapter 2, pp. 70–76.

[44] Tongiorgi Tomasi, 'Dall'essenza vegetale agglutinata', pp. 281–3.

Field Trips

Another practice that became more and more common among botanists was that of excursions made specifically to observe and collect plants for the purposes of study and research. With regard to Italy in particular, long journeys to distant lands were seldom undertaken. We know that Aldrovandi, at a mature age, had entertained a project to visit the New World, but he was never able to put it into practice.[45] As far as the study of plants is concerned, the most 'exotic' trip was maybe that of the Venetian Prospero Alpino (1553–1616) who, as physician to the new Venetian consul to Cairo, in 1580 accompanied him to Egypt and described some fifty species used in Egyptian medicine in his book *De plantis Aegypty*.[46]

The specific reasons for these field trips were various. Certainly the humanistic re-discovery of texts from antiquity and the critical attitude that led to the retrieval and identification of simples mentioned in them were at the root of most expeditions of this period. Theophrastus, Pliny and Dioscorides' interest in the plants around the Mediterranean determined the geographical scope of Italian naturalists. Dioscorides' *Materia medica*, which was considered the fundamental text on simples, played an important role. The attempt to identify all the plants Dioscorides had described was supported by the need for pharmaceutical reform. Many simples used in medicinal recipes were not those to which Dioscorides had referred, with apothecaries often substituting certain items with others which could well have been harmful or even poisonous. The search for plants originally mentioned by Dioscorides, therefore, in the light of the recovery of the real ancient remedies, was of paramount importance.[47]

A famous account of a botanical expedition is that of Francesco Calzolari, one of Luca Ghini's students and a learned apothecary and collector in Verona. His *Viaggio di Monte Baldo*, contains a passionate description of beautiful landscapes and an accurate list of all the plants found on this mountain near Verona.[48] In his dedication to the physician-botanist Prospero Borgarucci, he sets out his aim to clear up the mistakes caused by the ignorance of simples, which put in jeopardy the reputation of doctors and apothecaries, and the lives of patients. He refers to Pietro Andrea Mattioli as the one who, more than anybody else, had clarified and perfected *materia medica*, and claimed that 'no other work more perfect, more exquisite, or more precious than his [Mattioli's] can be.'[49] The naturalists and friends who are reported to have joined him during his excursions are, among others, Luca Ghini, Ulisse Aldrovandi and Luigi Anguillara.

---

45   Ulisse Aldrovandi, 'Discorso naturale', in Sandra Tugnoli Pattaro, *Metodo e sistema delle scienze nel pensiero di Ulisse Aldrovandi* (Bologna, 1981), pp. 173–232.

46   Minelli, *The Botanical Garden of Padua*, p. 65.

47   Palmer, 'Medical botany in northern Italy', p. 151.

48   Francesco Calzolari, *Il viaggio di Monte Baldo* (Venice, 1566).

49   Ibid., p. 3.

In fact, the *Commentarii in libros sex Pedacii Dioscorides Anazerbei, de materia medica* of the Sienese physician Pietro Andrea Mattioli played a fundamental role in this search for Dioscoridean plants, and, as Richard Palmer points out, it furnished the focus that the botanical movement needed.[50] The book, first published in Italian in 1544 without illustrations and with a modest apparatus of comments, went into numerous editions both in Italian and Latin, acquiring each time new characteristics, extending with the number of plants described and the accompanying commentary increasing over time. It became a phenomenal publishing success; in 1568 Mattioli himself declared that 30,000 copies had been sold from the first ten editions alone.[51] Mattioli used to supplement the research for his *Discorsi*, as his commentaries were usually called, by frequent requests for information and material from other colleagues. He was known to be very vindictive and even to retaliate against those who dared to criticize him, and to be full of praise for those who were willing to cooperate. Although Mattioli was very careful to keep all the success for himself, his way of proceeding through a succession of contacts and different contributions, resulted in a sort of cohesive web of relations among contemporary naturalists. Paula Findlen sees the *Discorsi* as one of the centres around which a natural history community began to form.[52]

It is not known exactly what criterion Luca Ghini followed in his field trips to gather plants for Pisa's botanical garden. As the *lectura de simplicibus* was based on Dioscorides, it is likely that he tried to collect the greatest possible number of simples included in *De materia medica* in order to be able to show them to his students. The list of plants of 1548 considered above, however, suggests that this was not the only criterion he adopted. He was one of the first to use excursions for a didactic purpose, demonstrating plants to his students in the field. This habit became a common practice, continued by his students, as is noted in a passage of Aldrovandi's autobiography referring to the year 1557, when he lectured in Bologna: 'Having obtained a license from the Senate, in May he [Aldrovandi] went forth with many students, first seeing all the valleys from Padusa as far as Ravenna, in which he observed the major part of the plants [described] by the ancients as well as many which they did not describe. Then he left Ravenna for Rimini, from Rimini to Avernia, where St. Francis lived, and there he found many plants not described by the ancients ...'[53] In two other sections of his autobiography concerning field trips, Aldrovandi recounts that he used to gather plants to dry them for his herbaria.[54]

---

50   Palmer, 'Medical botany in northern Italy', p. 152.

51   Arber, *Herbals*, pp. 81–2.

52   Paula Findlen, 'The Formation of a Scientific Community: Natural History in Sixteenth-Century Italy', in Anthony Grafton and Nancy Siraisi (eds), *Natural Particulars: Nature and the Disciplines in Renaissance Europe* (Cambridge, MA, 1999), pp. 369–400.

53   Quoted by Schmitt, 'Science in the Italian Universities', p. 41.

54   'La vita d'Ulisse Aldrovandi cominciando dalla sua natività sin' a l'età di 64 anni vivendo ancora', transcribed in *Il teatro della natura di Ulisse Aldrovandi*, ed. R. Simili

A passage in *Botanologicon*, a dialogue written as early as 1534 by the German humanist and botanist Euricius Cordus (1553–1535), provides some interesting information about his way of identifying plants. Cordus is addressing four fellow medical students at Erfurt:

> Whenever it pleases you let us go forth. I will not keep you back; nevertheless I, just as if none of you were here, shall follow my usual practice of taking along a little book or two. I take the greatest delight in these sallyings into the country, where I can have before me fresh and growing those herbs which I have read about at home, and may compare them with the pictures of others which I carry in memory; also taking such note of their names and reputed virtues, as I may gather from such old women whom I meet upon the way. By the use of all these means I am the better able to arrive at a sound conclusion, or at least a more probable opinion, about the identity of a thing ...[55]

Therefore the 'probable' identification was made by comparing the plants described in the 'books' he took along, with the 'fresh and growing herbs' he encountered. The information contained in the books, it is worth noting, had to be supported by oral tradition as it was provided by 'old women' he met.[56] Claudia Swan reports the fact that 'field guide' editions were available at the time. An example from some years later is a small format edition of Fuchs's *De historia stirpium*, with reduced versions of the original woodcuts. In the title it is clearly expressed that the 'contracted' format (*in exiguam angustioremque formam contractae*) was intended for walkers or travellers (*deambulantes vel peregrinantes*) interested in identifying the plants *in situ*.[57]

In the background of his plant illustrations the botanist and artist Gherardo Cibo (1512–1600) depicts naturalists in the act of studying and collecting plants in the wild. In the illustration of hellebore, he represented the customary way of using books to compare the description of a plant with the natural specimen. In the foreground the plant is drawn in detail, and in the background two botanists are depicted while observing a plant 'on the field', one reading from an open volume, the other holding the plant in his hands (Figures 3.2 and 3.3).[58]

(Bologna, 2001), p. 141.

[55] Euricius Cordus, *Botanologicon* (Cologne, 1534), pp. 26–7, as translated by Greene, *Landmarks*, pp. 366–7. Quoted also in Swan, 'The Role of the "Libri Picturati"', p. 189.

[56] This issue is discussed below, p. 120.

[57] Swan, 'The Role of the "Libri Picturati"', p. 191.

[58] See Findlen, *Possessing Nature*, p. 168. L. Tongiorgi Tomasi 'Gherardo Cibo: Visions of landscape', pp. 199–216.

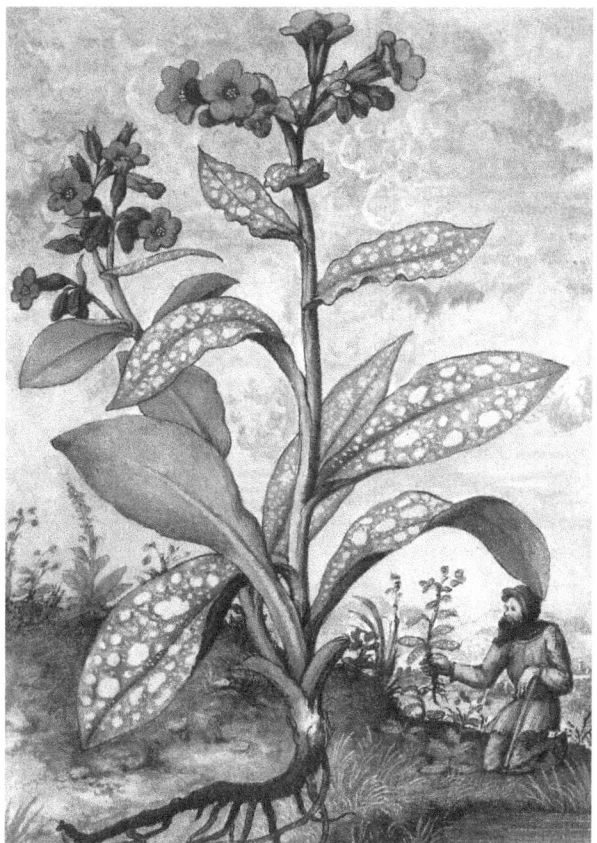

Figure 3.2   Gherardo Cibo, 'Pulmonaria'. In the background a botanist
              picking up the plant. British Library, MS Add. 22332

Cordus, unlike Aldrovandi, did not mention the means by which he
used to record his observations. The herbaria were not yet in use at the
time. Cordus's son Valerio, who was instructed by his father, was renowned
for the innovative method of his long and accurate descriptions. In fact, the
improvement of plant description, which was very poor at the time and of little
help in identifying specimens, never seriously concerned Italian naturalists.
Although Ghini, found fault with Dioscorides' insufficient and often obscure
descriptions, he did not seem to make any serious attempt to improve this
shortfall. Ghini, and Aldrovandi after him, always relied on the visual aids of
dried and painted plants.

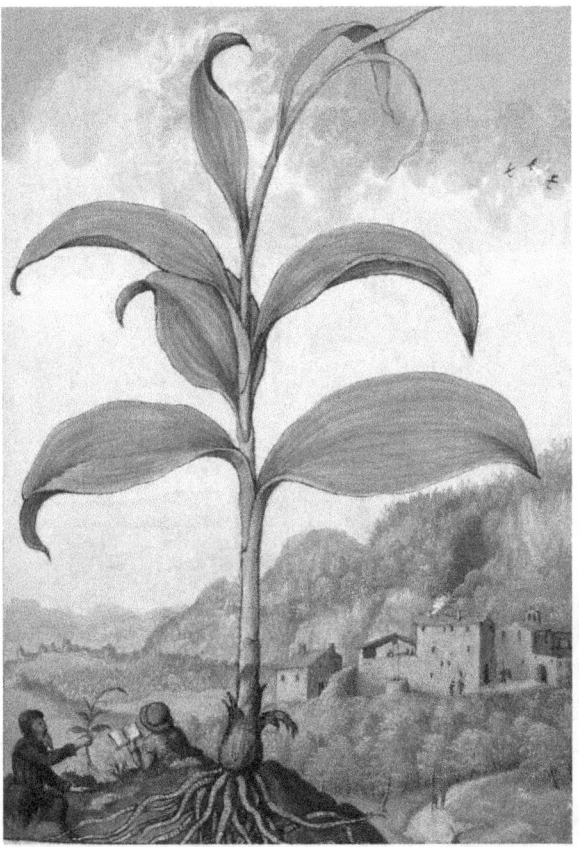

Figure 3.3   Gherardo Cibo, 'Elleboro biancho'. In the background botanists
               looking at the plant and at a herbal. British Library, MS
               Add. 22332

Botanical Illustration

The great strides taken in botanical drawing that took place after the 1540s
originated from the wish to record plant observation and possess at least a
representation of all available specimens. The emergence of printing was not in
itself sufficient to change the stylized representations of old herbals, and up to the
1530s no significant improvement had taken place. Illustrations, which should have
been an aid to plant identification and in support of their descriptions, had become
completely useless. The drawings were never made from life, but copied from other
drawings, which in turn were copies of copies, and had acquired features that made
them as far from the originals as they were from nature (Figures 3.4 and 3.5).

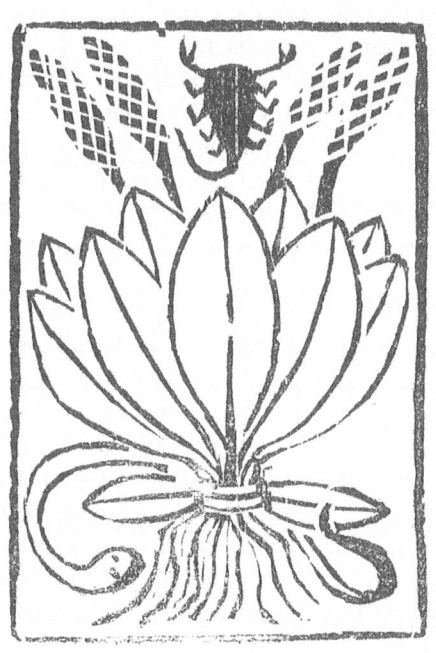

Figure 3.4   'Herba Plantago', f .11v, *Herbarium Apulei*, the first printed
herbal (1481). Milan: Edizioni Il Polifilo, 1979, vol. 1

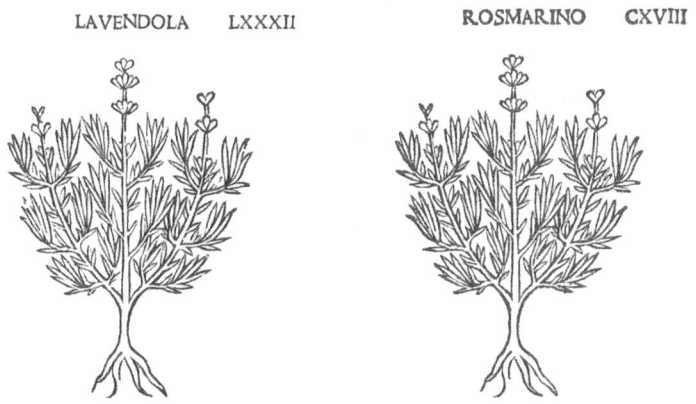

Figure 3.5   *Herbolario volgare*, the first printed herbal in Italian (1522).
The same wood-cut is used for rosemary and lavender. Milan:
Edizioni Il Polifilo, 1979, vol. 2

Plant description, on the other hand, was scant and inadequate, and offered little help as far as identification was concerned.

How plants could be recognized is hard to say. Agnes Arber suggests 'that a knowledge of the actual plants was, in practice, transmitted by word of mouth and that the herbals were only used as reference books, to ascertain the reputed qualities of herbs, with whose appearance the reader was already quite familiar'.[59] The gathering of simples was not the physician's task anyway, and the apprentice apothecary, as previously mentioned, learned from peasants and old women.

It is debatable whether the return to represent nature from life originated with the 'herbalists' or with the 'artists'.[60] It has been suggested that there were two parallel paths, one pertaining to art, the other to science, both stemming from and testifying to a transformation in attitudes towards the natural world. Some rare examples of early fifteenth-century Italian manuscript herbals, that contained naturalistic representations of plants are recorded in the history of botanical illustration.[61] Yet the ability to reproduce nature in a realistic manner, so that viewers might be deceived, according to the classic formula of imitation of nature, is a common assumption of the Renaissance theory of art. And certainly art had already achieved the capacity to 'imitate nature' through the representation of realistic detail, before scientific illustrations made a regular appearance in herbals.[62]

Cosimo's *Scrittoio*

At the time, anyway, art and science were not separate and contrasting fields. Art, as ability to imitate nature, could be useful to represent plants in the herbals. This function of art is pointed out by the humanist historian Benedetto Varchi (1503–1565) in his *Lezzione nella quale si disputa della maggioranza delle arti* (1546), where he parallels the woodcuts of Vesalius's anatomy and Fuchs's book of plants to Bacchiacca's paintings in the Florentine *scrittoio* of Cosimo I, in the Palazzo Vecchio: 'It [painting] is also of great utility in the sciences, as is seen in the book of Anatomy by Vesalius ... in the book of Plants by Fuchsio and even

---

[59] Arber, *Herbals*, p. 119.

[60] Pacht, 'Early Italian Nature Studies and the Early Calendar Landscape', pp. 25–31.

[61] Blunt, *The Art of Botanical Illustration*, pp. 25–30; Wilfrid Blunt and Sandra Raphael, *The Illustrated Herbal* (London, n. d.), pp. 68–81.

[62] The link between naturalism in the visual arts and the birth of modern science has been variously discussed by historians of science, philosophers of science, and art historians. See for example, Baldasso, 'The role of visual representation in the scientific revolution: A historiographic inquiry', pp. 69–88; Baroncini, 'Note sull'illustrazione scientifica', pp. 527–43. I discuss further this issue in my Conclusion, pp. 268–9.

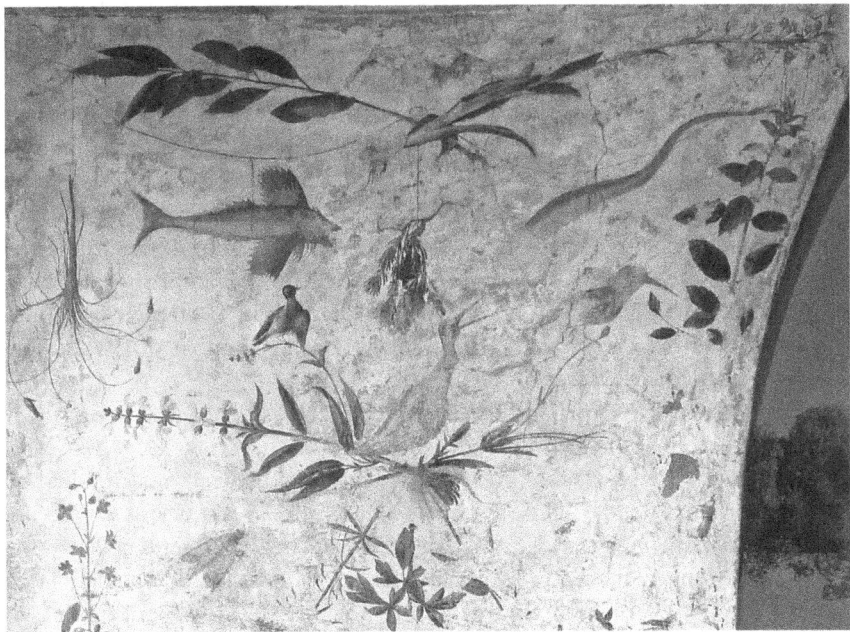

Figure 3.6   Bacchiacca, plants on a wall of the *Scrittoio del Duca* (*c.*1545). Florence, Palazzo Vecchio

better, and with a higher degree of naturalism, in those [paintings] by Francesco Bacchiacca, painted for the Most Illustrious Duke of Florence, as may still be seen in His Excellency's study.'[63]

The naturalistic frescoes painted by Bacchiacca (Francesco Ubertini) around 1545 for the *scrittoio* of Cosimo I in the Palazzo Vecchio are a very rare example of botanical illustration used in an unusual context (Figure 3.6). Sadly, only parts of them have survived, but what remains has been recently restored.[64] Naturalistic paintings of leaves, flowers, fruits and vegetables were not a novelty at the time, but they usually were in the form of decorative

[63]   Benedetto Varchi, *Lezzione nella quale si disputa della maggioranza delle arti e qual sia la più nobile, la scultura o la pittura* (1546). In *Trattati d'arte del Cinquecento fra Manierismo e Controriforma*, 3 vols (Bari, 1960), vol. 1, p. 39. The passage is quoted and translated in Tongiorgi Tomasi, *The Flowering of Florence*, p. 35. See also Olmi, *L'inventario del mondo*, p. 21. Also Vasari praises Bacchiacca's paintings 'fece a sua eccellenza uno scrittoio tutto pieno di uccelli di diverse maniere e d'erbe rare, che tutto condusse a olio divinamente.' Vasari, *Le vite*, vol. 6, p. 314.

[64]   The *scrittoio* of Cosimo I is in the *mezzanino* between the first and the second floors. It is not open to visitors.

wreaths, garlands, or festoons. Sometimes the choice of fruits, and above all vegetables, was surprising, as in the case of the onions, carrots, pumpkins, courgettes, eggplants, turnips, artichokes and cucumbers painted by Giovanni da Udine in the festoons that complemented the frescoes by Raphael in the Loggia of Psyche at the Farnesina in Rome, which seem to eschew the usual allegorical and symbolical function.[65] Giovanni da Udine himself worked in Florence with Vasari, and among the painters of his circle there were some other masters of this genre, such as the Tuscan Cristofano Gherardi whose biography is included in the *Vite*.[66] Although the flowers and fruits contained in their festoons were 'liberated', as Nicole Dacos puts it, 'from their symbolical meaning' and 'secularized', their function was primarily that of a frame, and they were never the subject of the painting.[67]

The plants painted by Bacchiacca in the Palazzo Vecchio are of a completely different sort. First of all they *are* the subject of the painting; second, they are single plants depicted as floating in space, rendered in a very realistic manner (some of them with their roots), more as botanical illustrations or pictures in a herbal than in a floral arrangement. The plants represented, moreover, seem to have been chosen more among Tuscan wild or medicinal plants than among the usual ornamental or symbolic flowers.[68] Finally, to underline the fact that they are playing the leading role in the painting, they are, in their turn, framed by a floral wreath. In her article about the plants depicted in the *scrittoio*, Maria Adele Signorini, noting that some of the plants seem painted from life and some others from dried specimens, conjectures that the latter might have been copied from Ghini's own herbarium.

This is the period when Luca Ghini, appointed reader of *materia medica* at the *Studio pisano*, started the botanical garden in Pisa, and was very active in gathering herbs for the garden, for his herbaria, or to have them painted. Being personal physician to the grand duke, he had occasion to discuss about plants with him, a subject they both had very much at heart. Plant pictures had become one of the most frequently used ways of recording plants and of acquiring knowledge of unknown species, and were commonly exchanged between naturalists. We know that Cosimo used to have animals and plants depicted by his court painters, and being constantly in contact

---

　　65　　Nicole Dacos, 'Alle fonti della natura morta italiana, Giovanni da Udine e le nature morte nei festoni', in *La natura morta in Italia* (Milan, 1989) pp. 55–68.

　　66　　Vasari, *Vite*, 'Vita di Cristofano Gherardi detto Doceno dal Borgo San Sepolcro, pittore', pp. 105–35; 'Vita di Giovanni da Udine, pittore', pp. 395–410.

　　67　　Dacos, 'Alle fonti della natura morta', pp. 67–8.

　　68　　An interesting article reporting all the plants still visible in Cosimo's scrittoio is that of Maria Adele Signorini, 'Sulle piante dipinte dal Bachiacca nello scrittoio di Cosimo I a Palazzo Vecchio', *Mitteilungen des Kunsthistorischen Institutes in Florenz*, 37(2/3) (1993), pp. 396–407.

with Aldrovandi, Ghini and occasionally with other naturalists, had frequent opportunities to exchange natural objects and pictures with them.[69] As far as printed herbals are concerned, however, plant illustrations from life had appeared for the first time only in the German books (of which we will speak below) of Brunfels, and above all of Fuchs, and constituted a novelty. And undoubtedly it was a novelty to represent plants in that way on the walls of a room. The peculiarity of the composition, and the fact that the fresco was commissioned by Cosimo for his study, suggest that it was realized according to a precise idea of the duke himself. The choice of plants, and their lay out, so similar to the new realistic depictions of plants and to the new illustrations of printed herbals, can be seen as further evidence of the naturalistic interests of the duke.

Luca Ghini is known to have made constant use of botanical drawings. Evidence that he had plants painted from life is provided by the Flemish Matthias de Lobel and the French Pierre Pena who reported that Ghini used to have both dried and painted plants 'In cartas ipse conderet et affabre pingendas curaret'. The same thing is confirmed by Giovanni Targioni Tozzetti in 1754 and Giovanni Calvi in 1777.[70] We also have evidence that Ghini sent a series of his botanical illustrations to Leonhart Fuchs, who included them in his unpublished *Erbario figurato*.[71] Although we do not know who was the painter from whom Ghini commissioned the pictures of his plants, we know that they were of a very high quality, since Fuchs, having managed to see one of these plants from life, declared that it was not necessary to reproduce it, as Ghini's picture was already perfectly accurate.[72] In a letter of 1558, Mattioli reports that Ghini had already prepared the illustrations for a work on plants that he was writing, and that he intended to publish.[73]

---

[69]   Bacchiacca was often asked to paint natural objects. See for example, two letters, one of 1550 in which Bacchiacca is asked to paint a recently hunted bird: 'un uccello tutto bianco con ali nigre, piedi et gambe lunghe et becco longo', and another one in 1551 in which it is said that a bird will be sent from Cosimo in Pisa to Florence to be depicted by Bacchiacca (Medici Archive Project).

[70]   Lucia Tongiorgi Tomasi, 'Dall'essenza vegetale agglutinata', p. 283.

[71]   S. Seybold, 'Luca Ghini, Leonhard Rauwolf und Leonhart Fuchs. Uber die Erkunft der Aquarelle im Wiener Krauterbuchmanuskrpt von Fuchs', *Jahreshefte der Gesellschaft für die Naturkunde in Wurttemberg* (Stuttgart, 1990), 145, pp. 239–326. Garbari, 'Luca Ghini a Pisa', pp. 227–8.

[72]   Signorini, 'Le piante dipinte nello scrittoio', p. 397.

[73]   See Chapter 2, p. 61.

Brunfels and Fuchs

It was not until Brunfels's *Herbarum vivae icones* (1530–36) and, most of all, Fuchs's *Historia stirpium* (1542) were published, that naturalistic botanical drawings were available to a wide public and recognized as a means of recording nature.[74]

Although dried plants could be prepared by the naturalist himself, it was obvious that many plants, such as succulents, or parts of them, and most fruit, could not be preserved in an *hortus siccus*. In addition, the colour of dried leaves and flowers was not permanent, and it had to be specified in a note. Illustrations did not have these drawbacks, but presented another series of problems. First of all, they required a much more sophisticated skill. Botanists had to hire painters and work in close collaboration with them. Printing presented some additional problems. Woodcuts, which was the technique most used at the time, needed further specialized craftsmanship; the drawing had to be copied and then carved into woodblocks. In a picture such as a botanical illustration, where detail is essential, it is evident that great ability and accuracy were indispensable. Moreover, while in the original watercolour or gouache colours could be accurately reproduced, they could not be printed. Colour, if desired, had to be added by hand on each copy.[75] For all these reasons, scientific illustrations were a very difficult and expensive undertaking.

De Historia Stirpium's outstanding results were also due to the cooperation between the author and his artists. In the introduction Fuchs refers to the great care devoted by him and his artists in portraying the plants described in the book. Their successful collaboration is underlined in the book's frontispiece, where Fuchs had the painter, the delineator and the engraver portrayed (Figure 3.7). Fuchs's illustrations had great success, as was testified by their European fame. The woodblocks were used again and again, and the illustrations copied in numerous herbals. The case of Otto Brunfels's *Plantarum Vivae Eicones* was different. Here the beautiful 'vivae eicones', as the title suggests, are the *raison d'être* of the book, and the artist, not the botanist, was the real author. Thus Brunfels's text took second place to Weiditz's illustrations and not viceversa. Also the peculiar style of the pictures was Weiditz's choice. As Claus Nissen puts it: 'The artist too was responsible for an all too objective approach: it was not the botanist who called for the exact reproduction of chance damage and other accidental features of plant specimen. For the latter invariably visualizes a picture of the species, an ideal never completely matched by reality.'[76]

---

[74]   Otto von Brunfels, *Herbarum vivae icones, ad naturam imitationem, summa cum diligentia et artificio effigiatae* (Strasbourg, 3 vols, 1530, 1532, 1536); Leonhart Fuchs, *De historia stirpium commentarii insignes* (Basel, 1542). On Brunfels and Fuchs's herbals, see Blunt, *Art of Botanical Illustration*, pp. 45–56; Zucchi, 'Brunfels e Fuchs', pp. 411–65.

[75]   On this point, see Agnes Arber, 'The Colouring of Sixteenth Century Herbals', *Nature*, 145 (1940), p. 803.

[76]   Nissen, *Herbals of Five Centuries*, p. 38.

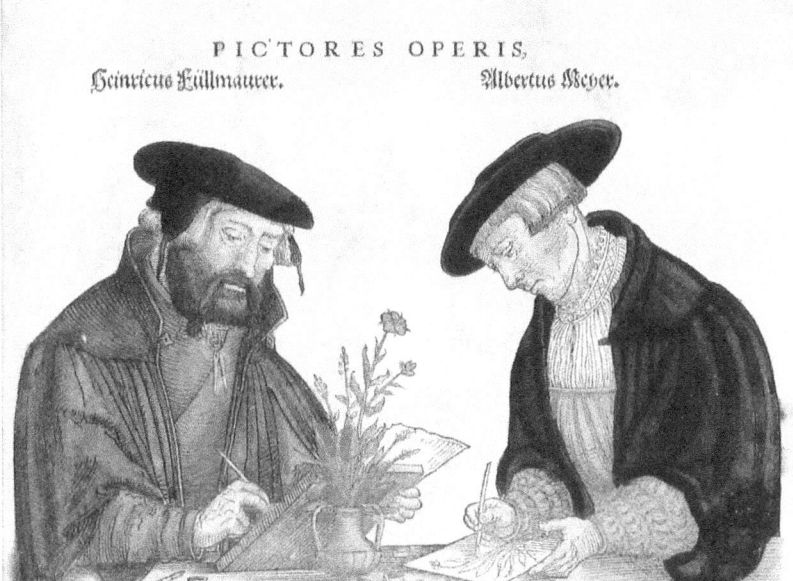

PICTORES OPERIS,
Heinricus Füllmaurer.   Albertus Meyer.

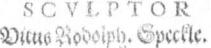

SCVLPTOR
Vitus Rodolph. Speckle.

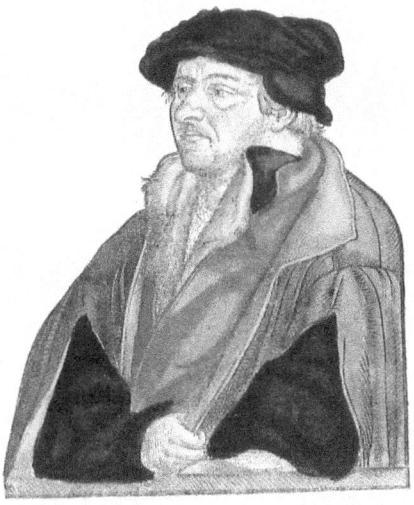

Figure 3.7   Albrecht Meyer, Heinrich Füllmaurer, and Veit Rudolph Speckle,
the painter, the copyist, and the engraver of the illustrations,
portrayed in Fuchs's *De historia stirpium* (Basel, 1542). London,
Wellcome Library

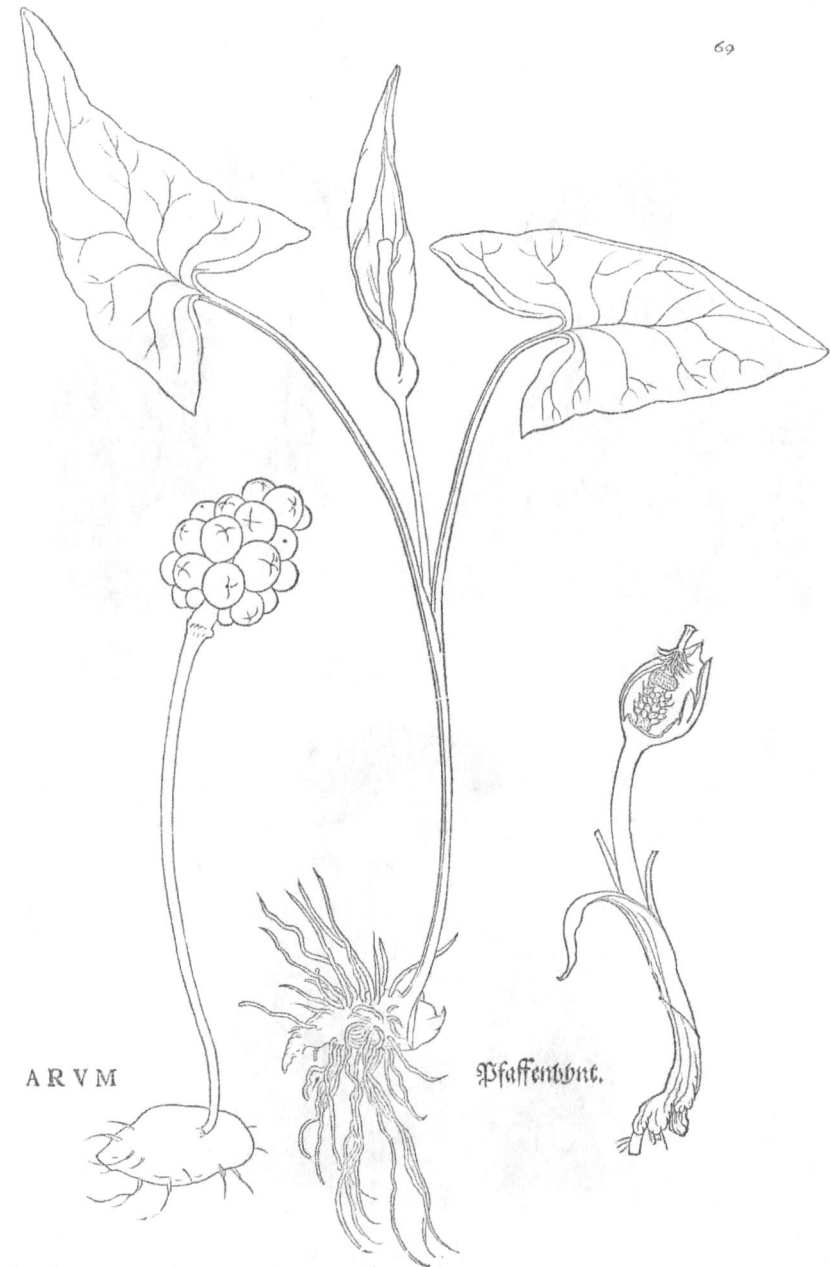

A R V M

Pfaffenwut.

Figure 3.8   'Dipsacus albus', woodcut from Leonhart Fuchs, *De historia stirpium* (Basel, 1542). London, Wellcome Library

This was precisely the difference between the botanical illustrations in the book of Brunfels and in that of Fuchs. The plants of Weiditz were portrayals of single plants, with all their 'accidental' features such as withered flowers, dried and damaged leaves or broken stems, while the plants of Fuchs were depicted to represent the species (Figure 3.8). To do so, under Fuchs surveillance, his artists could not confine themselves to imitating nature, they had to synthesize nature, representing only features that characterized a certain species, or even to elide the seasonal stages, as when a plant was depicted bearing both flowers and fruits at the same time.[77] To be of service to the study of plants, an illustration had to satisfy certain criteria that only the naturalist could establish. Fuchs was very careful to dictate the rules to which his artists had to conform; for example, he stated that the plants had to be painted without shading, and 'other unnecessary things through which the craftsmen sometimes try to achieve artistic glory', and underlined that he had not permitted 'the artists to follow their fancies so that the drawing should not accurately correspond to the truth'.[78]

If Benedetto Varchi could put on the same level the pictures of Vesalius, Fuchs and Bacchiacca, taking for granted that the mere ability to imitate nature could meet in the same way and at the same time the requirements of art and science, Fuchs points out the difference between a picture that has to satisfy an aesthetic criterion, and one that has a cognitive function. The phrase 'painted from life' or 'true to nature' acquires new meanings depending on the context.

The Debate on Images

The use of pictures to represent natural objects, however, was not approved of by all scholars. Some of them were not against it, but felt that illustrations could divert one's attention from the first-hand study of nature. Even the great anatomist Andreas Vesalius (1514–1564), who complemented his *Fabrica* with numerous and rightly famous illustrations, warns students of natural history and medicine that pictures cannot be a substitute for the direct examination of natural objects: 'These [herbs and parts of the body] must be studied not in drawings, but with a diligent work of dissection, and everything must be checked with one's own eyes'.[79]

The study of plants was pursued as part of natural philosophy, and plant representation implied a philosophical reflection on the definition of plants and

---

77   See for example, Giuseppe Olmi, 'Le raffigurazioni della natura nell'età moderna: "spirito e vita dei libri"', in M. Santoro and M.G. Tavoni (eds), *I dintorni del testo: approcci alle periferie del libro* (Rome, 2005), vol. 1, pp. 217–34. Zucchi, 'Brunfels e Fuchs'.

78   Fuchs, *De historia stirpium*, fol. 7v.

79   Andrea Vesalio, *De humani corporis fabrica. Libri septem* (Basel, 1543).

natural objects in general. The differing and contrasting positions taken up by classical authors on this subject (Dioscorides approved of it, Pliny and Galen did not), were at the basis of debates and controversies that had serious philosophical implications.[80] This passage from Fuchs's introduction to *De historia stirpium* reveals how lively the discussion must have been:

> Though the pictures have been prepared with great effort and sweat we do not know whether in the future they will be damned as useless and of no importance and whether someone will cite the most insipid authority of Galen to the effect that no one who wants to describe plants would try to make pictures of them. But why take up more time? Who in his right mind would condemn pictures which can communicate information much more clearly than the words of even the most eloquent men? Those things that are presented to the eyes and depicted on panels or paper become fixed more firmly in the mind than those that are described in mere words.[81]

Although the simple rhetorical question addressed by Fuchs to his readers seems to imply that the usefulness of pictures was self-evident, it is clear, from the passage that precedes it, that he was really concerned about his contemporaries' reactions. In fact Fuchs had been engaged in a polemic concerning the usefulness of illustrations since the publication of his *Errors of recent physicians* (1530).[82] This work, where Fuchs points out a series of wrong identifications of plants on the part of recent physicians, was criticized by the physician Sebastianus Montuus who published a series of very polemic 'annotations' in reply to Fuchs's work.[83] In his seventh annotation, 'Pictures of simple medicines are fallacious and the arguments derived from them are also fallacious', Montuus bases his very brief (less than thirty lines of a small book) and not perfectly clear condemnation of pictures on the grounds that the definition of a species must not be *ex genere et accidentibus* but *ex genere*

---

[80]   Reeds, 'Renaissance humanism and botany', pp. 530–31; Sachiko Kusukawa, 'Leonhart Fuchs on the importance of pictures', *Journal of the History of Ideas*, 58 (1997), pp. 403–27; Kusukawa, 'Illustrating Nature', p. 107; Jensen, 'Description, Division, Definition', pp. 185–206.

[81]   As quoted and translated in Pamela H. Smith and Paula Findlen, *Merchants and Marvels: Commerce, Science, and Art in Early Modern Europe* (New York and London, 2002), p. 8.

[82]   Leonhart Fuchs, *Errata recentiorum medicorum* (Haguenau, 1530); *Sessanta errori dei medici contemporanei con l'aggiunta delle confutazioni*, Italian translation and commentary by A. Morricone and V. Pedicino (Rome, 1963).

[83]   Sebastianus Montuus, *Annotatiunculae S Montui in errata recentiorum medicorum per L. Fuchsium* (Lyon, 1533).

et differentia essentiali.[84] Pictures are fallacious because they are based on accidents, that is to say on features that are susceptible of change with the seasons and other circumstances, as Pliny said. And this, he thinks, is the reason why Galen did not have simples depicted. In other words, pictures are useless, as they cannot define the essence of the plant. The controversy continued in another work of Fuchs's, *Three Books of Medical Paradoxes*, in which he gives a different interpretation of Galen and Pliny's view of pictures.[85] He also responds to the issues of the definition of a plant, distinguishing between different kinds of accidents, i.e. separable and inseparable accidents. Some of them, although not essential features (*differentiae*), are *accidentes* which are not separable from the natural object (for example heat and fire or hardness and stone). Definitions *ex genere et accidente inseparabili*, Fuchs states, are acceptable. Montuus replied and summarized the arguments and counter-arguments of the controversy in his *Two Books of Medical Arguments.*[86] Here he continues the discussion on pictures explaining his objections with greater clarity. The centre of his argument is that there is no correspondence between the external features of a plant and its inner essence, and therefore pictures are devoid of cognitive value.

This very schematic and very partial account of a long and complicated controversy on the theoretical legitimacy of pictures, shows that Montuus and Fuchs, although fierce enemies, agreed on a fundamental point. They both thought that the *differentia*, that is to say the true essence of the plant, was its medical power (*vis*). As Jensen points out, Montuus was interested *only* in the medical properties of plants, which obviously cannot be represented in a picture. Fuchs instead 'agreed that the *vires* of plants are their essential differences, but he also wished to pay attention to the physical shapes which make it possible to distinguish one type of plant from another'.[87] Fuchs believed in the usefulness of pictures, but was also seriously interested in finding a theoretical support for it. His attention to the philosophical side of the question and his knowledge of the opinions of the *antiqui scriptores* had a very direct influence on his book: they explain his efforts to produce plant pictures that would represent not an individual specimen, like those of Weiditz in Brunfels's book, but a species. To do so, the plant represented had to show all the features that characterized that particular species.[88]

---

[84] 'picturas simplicium medicamentorum esse fallaces, & inde ducta argumenta esse fallacia', Montuus, *Annotatiunculae*, folio V. See Kusukawa, 'Fuchs on the importance of pictures', pp. 418–19.

[85] Leonhart Fuchs, *Paradoxorum medicinae libri tres* (Paris, 1546).

[86] Sebastianus Montuus, *Dialexeon medicinalium Libri duo* (Lyon, 1537).

[87] Jensen, 'Description, Division, Definition', p. 189.

[88] Fuchs, after the publication of his *Historia Stirpium*, had another controversy with the Lutheran physician Janus Cornarius (1500–1558). Cornarius had written a commentary

Italian physicians and naturalists did not engage in vehement polemics on plant pictures, although their views were far from unanimous. They were aware of the different views of the authors of antiquity, and of the recent controversies, and they usually provided a justification for introducing or not introducing illustrations in their herbals.

Andrea Cesalpino who, as seen, thought that the medical properties of a plant were accidents, and had nothing to do with its true essence, was not against pictures in principle. In the dedication to Francesco I of his *De plantis* he seems to hold a somewhat ambiguous position as far as illustrations are concerned. Outlining the principles of his plant classification, he explained that he was attempting to determine the affinities of plant-groups and the differences between one group and the others. In this regard he maintained that pictures were of no use, as they could not make evident, as words could, affinities and differences of plant-groups at the same time. In spite of that, however, he regrets that the illustrations that had already been painted 'with such skill that they expressed all the most minute details' ('ea industria depictae ut minutissimas quasque differentias esprimant') could not be published, as the woodcuts had not been prepared.[89] His view, however, is better explained in a letter of 25 June 1579, in which he asks Francesco I's secretary Belisario Vinta to remind the grand duke of his oral promise ('fatta in voce') to have the woodcuts prepared for printing. In the letter Cesalpino also declares that his first intention was to publish his book without illustrations because 'such is the order and the description of each plant that there is no need of pictures, however they would bring much more beauty'.[90] This point is interesting, as it provides evidence that Cesalpino attributed a decorative more than a 'scientific' function to pictures. Information, in his opinion, is conveyed by words, and clarity and precision are assured by the exact order provided by the classification. The grand duke, anyway, did not keep his promise, and Cesalpino's book on plants came out without illustrations.

Pietro Andrea Mattioli, in the introduction to the 1550 edition of his *Commentaries on Dioscorides*, which did not contain any plant illustrations, explains why he does not think that they were necessary: 'with books alone no one can become a perfect 'semplicista', even if the pictures are executed and printed with the greatest possible art', because, as Galen and Dioscorides say, 'it really is necessary ... to see the plants from life with one's own eyes not only

---

to Dioscorides and had published it without pictures. He maintained that pictures were useless because no one who had not seen the plant in nature could get to know the plant from a picture. Pictures represent a plant in one stage of their life and in a certain place, and it is very unlikely that one could encounter it in the wild in the same form. See Kusukawa, 'Leonhart Fuchs and the importance of pictures', p. 426.

[89]   Cesalpino, *De plantis*, Dedication to Francesco I.

[90]   Quoted in Viviani, *Vita e opere di Andrea Cesalpino*, p. 87.

at one season of the year but in various and different [times] ...'. Pictures, he continues, are not of great use because they only show 'an image of one stage, and also because artful and painted things, never show perfectly their features, like natural, true, and living ones do'.[91] The idea that pictures can only grasp one moment of the plant's growth and life, which is so often referred to by the authors who are not in favour of pictures, is based on a famous and frequently quoted passage of Pliny about Greek botanical illustration:

> they [the painters] painted likenesses of the plants and then wrote under them their properties. But not only is a picture misleading when the colours are so many, particularly as the aim is to copy Nature, but besides this much imperfection arises from the manifold hazards in the accuracy of the copyists. In addition, it is not enough for each plant to be painted at one period only of its life, since it alters its appearance with the fourfold changes of the year.[92]

For this reason, in Mattioli's opinion, illustrations, as well as descriptions, are of no use to those who have not acquired previous knowledge of plants by other means. Like Cesalpino, however, although for different reasons, he is not against botanical illustration in principle, and very sensibly concludes: 'It seems to me nevertheless, that pictures impress on one's memory the simples that one already knows, and that they give no little pleasure to the eyes.'[93] In fact the following edition of his book (1554) appeared with a large number of small illustrations, and in the editions after 1562, new large illustrations were prepared by the painter Giorgio Liberale da Udine and the German sculptor Wolfgang Meyerpeck, as Mattioli himself informs us.[94] These pictures can be seen, for example, in the Latin edition issued in 1565. They are impressive pictures that fill the page leaving almost no white space, sometimes assuming a square shape to use all the possible surface of the woodblock. There is usually great attention to detail, and (unlike in Fuchs's pictures) there is a frequent use of shading (Figure 3.9).

---

[91] Mattioli, *Discorsi* 1550 (Venice, 1550), 'Discorso sopra il Prologo di Dioscoride', p. 7.

[92] Pliny the Elder, *Natural History*, translation by W.H.S. Jones (Loeb Classical Library), (Cambridge, MA, 1956), vol. 7, Book 25, iv. Quoted, for example, in Blunt, *History of Botanical Illustration*, p. 9; Gill Saunders, *Picturing Plants: An Analytical History of Botanical Illustration* (Berkeley and Los Angeles, CA, 1995), p. 17.

[93] Mattioli, *Discorsi* 1550, 'Discorso sopra il prologo di Dioscoride', p. 7.

[94] Mattioli, *Discorsi*, 1st edition in Latin (Venice, 1565), Preface: 'adiuvit nos quoque mirum in modum Giorgius Liberalis homo artis pingendi peritissimus, & post ipsum Volfangus Myerpeck misnensis ... nulli quidem labori, ac diligentiae pepercerunt'.

ARBVTO.

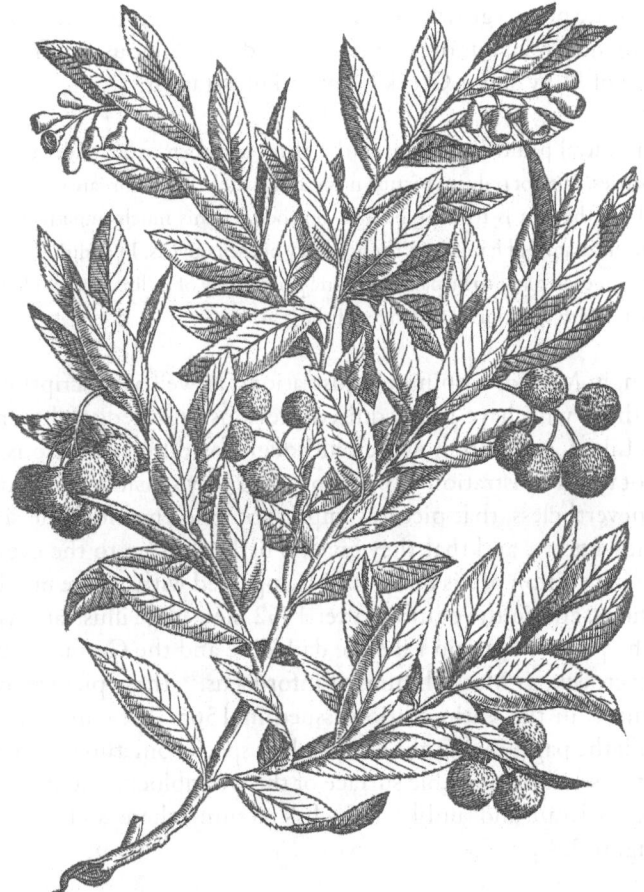

L O Arbuto in Tofcana, oue per ogni felua fi uede uerdeggiare il uerno, fi chiama Albatro. Et come che Diofcori- Arbuto, & fi·a
de lo raffembri al melo cotogno, penfò che piu alluda egli alla procerità, che alle frondi, & alla corteccia. Quan- effamin.
tunque io habbia non poco da fufpicare, che fia in quefto luogo corrotto il tefto di Diofcoride. Imperoche appreffo Sera-
pione, che ne toglie di parola in parola l'hiftoria da Diofcoride,non fi legge che fia l'Arbuto uniuerfalmente fimile al me
lo cotogno; ma che produce egli le frondi minori di quelle del melo cotogno. Ne manco fcriue egli, che habbi l'Arbuto
le frondi fottili, come fi legge ne i piu frequentati tefti di Diofcoride. Imperoche (come è chiaro à ciafcuno) le frondi
dell'arbuto fono piu groffe di quelle del lauro, & parimente dell'elice. fenza che fi ritroua un tefto antico fcritto à pen-
na, che legge λεπτόφιον, cioè di fottil corteccia, & non λεπτόφυλλον, cioè fi fottil fronde. Scriffe dell'Arbuto Theophra-
fto al X V I. capo del I I I. libro dell'hiftoria delle piante, cofi dicendo. L'Arbuto, il quale porta un frutto buono da
10 mangiare, non è troppo grande. ha la fcorza fottile, come il tamarigio, & le frondi mezane tra l'elice, e'l lauro. Fio-
rifce il mefe di Luglio. I fiori ftanno infieme à modo di racemo, attaccati con un fol picciuolo nella parte ultima loro.
                                                                         BB 2   E' ciafcun

Figure 3.9   Liberale da Udine, 'Arbuto'. Pietro Andrea Mattioli's *Discorsi*,
                1568, p. 192. Milan, Biblioteca Braidense

Ulisse Aldrovandi had no doubt about the usefulness of illustrations. So much so that he even blamed the ancients for not providing them, on the grounds that if they had painted all the things which they described, one would not find it so difficult to understand them.[95] A long series of comments on the importance of naturalistic illustrations and on his relationship with various painters, who worked under his strict surveillance, is to be found in his writings and in his vast correspondence.[96] Pictures of plants and animals played a leading role in his colossal attempt to record all the natural world, and were collected in his 'museum' along with natural objects.[97] Giuseppe Olmi reports that towards the end of the 1590s Aldrovandi had about 8,000 watercolour and gouache pictures, 2,000 of which had already been copied and engraved on woodblocks.[98] He was convinced that illustrations were indispensable tools for recording nature and they had to have a scientific and not a decorative function. Referring to his *Ornithologia*, he claimed that if the pictures aroused admiration for their beauty, they would completely miss the mark, and underlined that the skill of the painters and engravers would be useless without his constant control.[99]

Jacopo Ligozzi

Even if the leading role of the author-botanist was essential, the ability of the painter remained a sine qua non, and was very much admired and sought after. Aldrovandi himself had always longed for, and had occasionally succeeded, in having his plants painted by the Veronese painter Jacopo Ligozzi (1547–1627), who was invited to Florence by the Grand Duke Francesco in 1577, and was considered to be the most talented and refined painter of 'natural things'.[100] Jacopo Ligozzi served four grand dukes, and was involved in a vast series of

---

[95]   'Volesse Iddio che Aristotele, Thephrasto, Dioscoride, Plinio e tanti altri scrittori celebri havessero dipinto in queste historie questa varietà di piante e di animali, che' invero non penaressimo ad intendere molte cose.' Ulisse Aldrovandi, 'Discorso naturale', c. 557a, in Sandra Tugnoli Pattaro, *Metodo e sistema delle scienze nel pensiero di Ulisse Aldrovandi* (Bologna, 1981), pp. 173–232.

[96]   G. Olmi, *L'inventario del mondo*, pp. 21–157.

[97]   Ibid., p. 59.

[98]   Giuseppe Olmi, 'Il collezionismo scientifico', in Raffaella Simili (ed.), *Il teatro della natura di Ulisse Aldrovandi* (Bologna, 2001), pp. 28–9.

[99]   Ulisse Aldrovandi, *Ornithologiae, hoc est de avibus historiae libri XII* (Bologna, 1599). Quoted by Giuseppe Olmi, 'La raffigurazione della natura', p. 222.

[100]   Lucia Tongiorgi Tomasi (ed.), *I ritratti di piante di Jacopo Ligozzi* (Pisa, 1993); Mina Bacci and Anna Forlani (eds), *Mostra di disegni di Jacopo Ligozzi (1547–1626)*, Gabinetto disegni e stampe degli Uffizi (Florence, 1961).

works most of which are large encomiastic or devotional paintings that show very little of his exquisite skill in representing nature.[101] At the time he was in the service of Francesco I (1577–1587), however, he had his own workshop in the Casino di San Marco, and was asked to paint a large number of plants and animals, some of which have come down to us (Figure 3.10). Almost all of them are now kept in the Gabinetto dei Disegni e delle Stampe of the Uffizi where there are sixty-five pictures of animals and seventy-eight of plants; some others (about thirty, of which a small number are replicas), are among Aldrovandi's collection.[102] And it is Aldrovandi himself who provides us with information about the works of Ligozzi whom he defines as 'another Apelles'.[103] During his visit to the Casino di San Marco in June 1577, accompanied by the grand duke himself, he was shown 'all the pictures drawn from life by Signor Jacopo Ligozzi, which lack nothing but the breath of life itself'.[104] In 1586, after a second visit, he describes some miniatures of animals and plants by Ligozzi (he reports having seen eighty-four paintings of plants), and provides us with a list 'Catalogus plantarum quas nunc Magnus Dux habet depictas'.[105] Some of them are exotic plants, and there is one of the first portrayals of a pineapple, a replica of which is also among Aldrovandi's pictures.

Mina Bacci leaves no doubt as to Ligozzi's skill: 'By comparison with the pictures painted by the artists who were paid a salary by Aldrovandi (Lorenzo Benini from Florence, Cornelius Swint from Frankfurt, and also Jacopo's brother Francesco Ligozzi, Andrea Budano and Pastorino de' Pastorini) Ligozzi's paintings reveal at once a much higher quality that distinguishes them immediately even from the best of Aldrovandi's painters.'[106]

It has been pointed out that Ligozzi's masterly painting was based mostly on colour. The technique he used, as it is possible to see from his unfinished drawings, was to lay on a base of opaque gouache, a series of transparent layers of colours, using very fine brushes.[107] There were a few paintings by Ligozzi which were copied and carved on the woodblocks to be printed, such as the 'Bird of paradise and exotic finch on fig branch' that was prepared for Ulisse Aldrovandi's *Ornithologia* (1599).

---

[101] Large paintings by Ligozzi, for example, can be seen in the Salone dei Cinquecento in the Palazzo Vecchio.

[102] Tongiorgi Tomasi, *I ritratti di piante*, p. 24.

[103] Ulisse Aldrovandi, *Vita di Ulisse Aldrovandi cominciando dalla sua natività sin a l'età di 69 anni vivendo egli ancora*, 'Appendice al 1577', p. 142. Transcribed in R. Simili, *Il teatro della natura di Ulisse Aldrovandi*, pp. 131–43.

[104] Ibid.

[105] Tongiorgi Tomasi, *I ritratti di piante*, p. 22.

[106] Bacci and Forlani, *Mostra di disegni di Jacopo Ligozzi*, p. 21.

[107] Ibid., p. 19. Tongiorgi Tomasi, *I ritratti di piante*, p. 26.

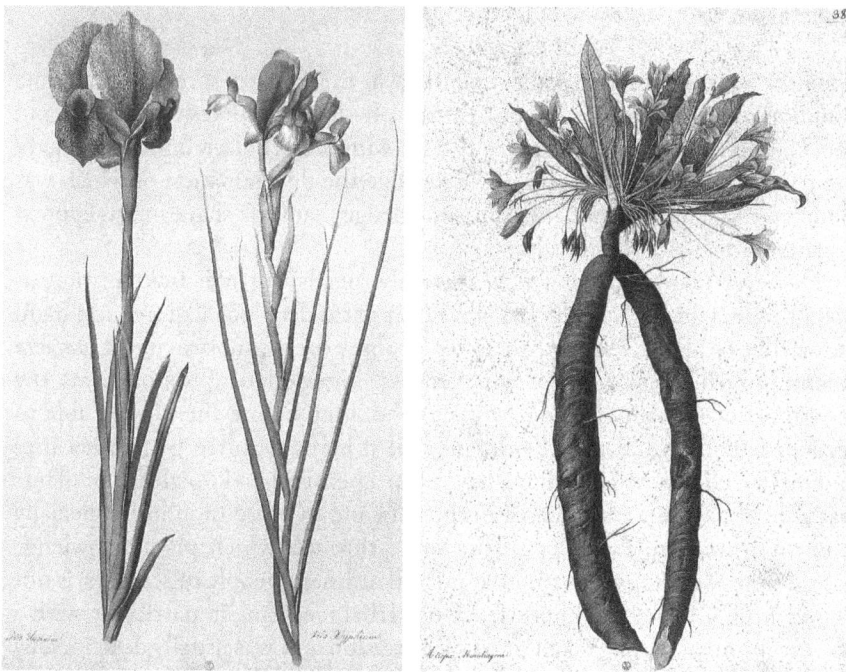

Figure 3.10   Plant illustrations by Iacopo Ligozzi: Mandrake; mourning
iris (Iris Susiana) and Spanish iris (Iris xyphium). Florence,
Gabinetto dei Disegni e delle Stampe degli Uffizi

Although the drawing and the *mise en page* maintain their elegance, the
rendering of the different consistencies of surfaces and the most minute details
obtained through subtle colouring, which are the distinctive mark of his
style, are clearly lost. Lucia Tongiorgi Tomasi hints at the possibility that the
illustrations referred to by Cesalpino in the dedication of *De plantis*, and in
the letter to Belisario Vinta mentioned above, might be pictures by Ligozzi.[108]
Although this is only a guess, as we do not have any further evidence, it is not
inconsistent with the above mentioned description of Cesalpino, and with his
view that they would lend great beauty to his book.

---

[108]   Ibid., p. 22.

Conclusion

The new ways of studying plants examined in this chapter spread and became common ground among scholars, learned physicians, university students and apothecaries. They were devised and used within a scholarly milieu and gave rise to a production of 'botanical' knowledge the dissemination of which was confined to a cultural elite. The plant knowledge that took shape in this context is mainly a form of learned culture.

However, one aspect which certainly needs further investigation is the process which initially led physician-naturalists to acquire first-hand knowledge of plants, enabling them to become expert connoisseurs of *materia medica*. At the beginning of this process, knowledge of simples was the monopoly of peasants and old women who, long before them, were able to recognize, collect and provide the medicinal herbs required by apothecaries and private clients.[109] There must have been a point when knowledge of plants was at least partially transmitted in the field and by word of mouth especially from herb women. Evidence of the route through which plant knowledge passed downwards to upwards, that is from ordinary people to scholars, is not easy to find. Old women's knowledge of herbal medicine in particular, with a few exceptions, was not taken into consideration and was usually described by learned physicians in a derogatory way.[110] One of the rare passages testifying to this transition is that from Euricius Cordus's *Botanologicon* quoted above. It is a significant passage, as it is one of the very rare cases (I did not find anything as explicit in Italian medical literature) in which a scholar admits to needing the advice of a wise woman to be able to select the right herbs.[111] Certainly women, who were used to gather herbs for their family, were also employed by apothecaries to collect medicinal plants for their shops. In the background of Gherardo Cibo's botanical illustrations women at work are sometimes depicted (Figure 3.11).

---

[109]   See above, Chapter 2, p. 100.

[110]   'For the doctor relies on the druggist and the druggist on a greedy and dirty old woman ... So it often happens that the patients' safety depends on the herbal knowledge of an ignorant and crafty woman'. This is a significant passage, from Thomas Johnson's *Descriptio itineris Plantarum* (1632). Quoted in Anna Pavord, *The Naming of Names: The Search for Order in the World of Plants* (London, 2005), pp. 5–6.

[111]   Another passage is by Anton Schneeberger, a Polish pupil of Konrad Gesner's: 'I was not ashamed to be the pupil of an old peasant woman'. *Catalogus Stirpium quarundarum latine et polonice conscriptus* (Krakau, 1557), quoted by Agnes Arber, 'Review: B. Hryniewiecki, *Anton Schneeberger (1530–1581), ein Schüler Konrad Gesners in Poland*', *New Phitologist*, 37(5) (1938), p. 480.

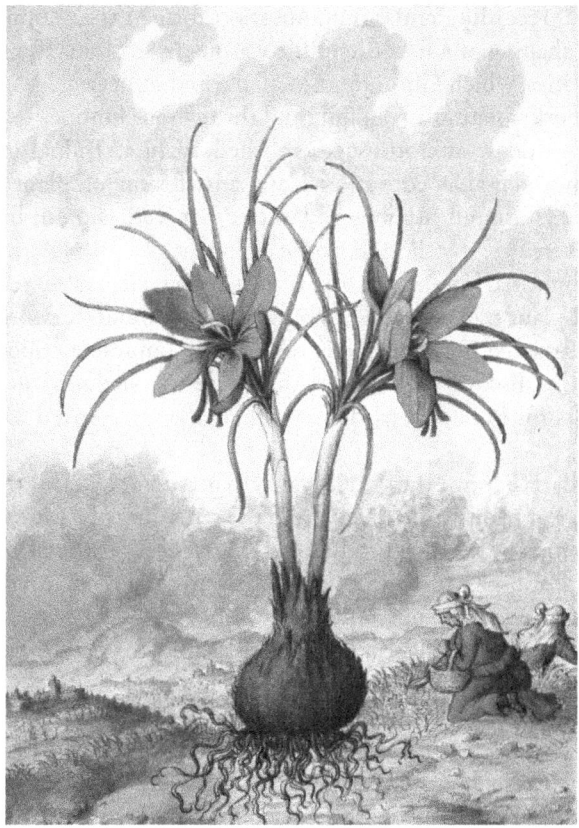

Figure 3.11   Gherardo Cibo, 'Zaffarano' (saffron). Women collecting flowers
can be seen in the background. British Library, MS Add. 22332

The various means and methods described above were all aimed at rendering observation of nature easier and more easily recordable, and constituted the common ground on which to organize the new findings. However, it is important to note that they also provided the ways by which naturalists began to communicate with each other. They permitted a relatively quick transmission of data supported by tangible evidence: seeds, dried specimens or plants painted from life. This way of disseminating plant knowledge became characteristic of botanists (humanists, physicians, pharmacists or amateurs) and bound together their emerging community. Unlike books they were flexible and separated data, and they did not have to make up a *summa* or to be all-inclusive. Although the mere accumulation of natural objects and data is per se insufficient to constitute a science, a fact of which Cesalpino was well aware, these specific ways and means of observation, recording and communication formed the common language on which the shaping of a new discipline was made possible. The series of new scientific activities, which Ghini most of all devised or perfected, spread among his pupils and other naturalists in Italy and throughout Europe.

Botanical gardens, after those established at Pisa, Padua and Florence, became an indispensable educational aid and forum of plant study, as is attested by the enormous number of gardens that were laid out by Italian and European universities: 'by the end of the eighteenth century, Europe possessed some sixteen hundred botanical gardens connecting scientific enterprises, plant acclimatation, plant transfers and experimentation around the world'.[112]

Field trips, started initially mostly to identify simples described in classical texts, led to the discovery of species that were not included in them. They supplied plants for botanical gardens and herbaria and proved to be essential didactic tools.

While herbaria became the standard way to preserve plants for the purpose of study, drawings of plants from life allowed the recording of nature in a different and more complex way. They produced a complete transformation of printed botanical texts, and provided, among other things, the most direct knowledge possible of vegetation from unstudied territories.

Botanists now shared the general belief that 'studying nature was a calling in its own right'[113] and pursued it through direct observation.

All the procedures and techniques described in this chapter could equally be applied to medicinal as well as to non-medicinal plants. For the first time plants could be studied as such, irrespective of their use. They are the tools by means of which botany took shape and became separated from medicine. This does not mean that plants were no longer the basis of pharmacology, but that plants were no longer studied *only* for their medicinal virtues.

---

[112] Londa Schiebinger and Claudia Swan, 'Introduction', *Colonial Botany* (Philadelphia, PA, 2005), p. 13.

[113] Findlen, 'Formation of a Scientific Community', pp. 370–71.

Chapter 4
Plants from the New World

The first descriptions of the luxuriant and unknown vegetation of the New World aroused great interest among naturalists throughout Europe. Enthusiasm, curiosity, eagerness to see and to possess, are all present in the vast correspondence between physicians, apothecaries, collectors and amateurs of the sixteenth century. Their letters contain frequent references and inquiries about the *plantae peregrinae* lately discovered in the New World. What is more, and peculiar to this field of inquiry, the correspondence was not confined to information, but included a constant exchange of specimens, seeds, leaves, dried plants and illustrations.

The question that first comes to mind is what kind of impact the discovery of a whole new world of unknown vegetation might have had on the understanding of plants of the time. The interest shown is per se significant, but it does not tell us whether, to what extent and for what reasons the new plants were accepted and introduced into Europe. Their reception in Tuscany is the subject of this chapter. It will examine which American plants were included in the Florentine Pharmacopoeia and in the medical texts and herbals of the time, in order to gauge their weight and importance from the pharmacological, the aesthetic, and from a more general point of view.

The works containing the first descriptions of American plants have been dealt with in recent extensive studies, mainly by Spanish historians. These studies, however, are mostly focused on the works of the Spanish writers of the time.[1] Not enough attention has yet been directed to the reaction to and acceptance of new exotic species in sixteenth-century Italy, not even with regard to some well-known works such as the *Discorsi* by Pietro Andrea Mattioli and *De plantis* by Andrea Cesalpino, each remarkable in their own right, although different in content and scope. In order to investigate some aspects of the acceptance of American plants in the sixteenth century, I will concentrate mainly, although not exclusively, on the above works, and the first Pharmacopoeia ever published

---

[1]   José Pardo Tomáš and Maria Luz López Terrada, *Las Primeras Noticias sobre plantas americanas en las relaciones de viajes y crónicas de Indias (1493–1553)* (Valencia, 1993); José María López Piñero and José Pardo Tomáš, *Nuevos materiales y noticias sobre la Historia de las plantas de Nueva España de Francisco Hernández* (Valencia, 1997). Huguet-Termes, 'New World Materia Medica in Spanish Renaissance Medicine', pp. 359–76.

in Europe, the *Nuovo ricettario fiorentino*, which appeared in various editions during the sixteenth century, between 1498 and 1597.[2]

During the first decades of the sixteenth century the fundamental texts on *materia medica* of the past had gone through a massive work of editing, translating and commenting. Dioscorides' *Materia medica*, in particular, came to be considered the fundamental book on medical botany, and was also prescribed as the textbook for the *lectura de simplicibus* at the University of Pisa.[3] Sixteenth-century physician-naturalists had to front and to appropriate a double renewal in the field of *materia medica* and *res herbaria*. As has been pointed out, both the re-discovery of the old world, and the discovery of the New World were regarded by the scholars of the time as an encounter with new realities and novel experiences.[4]

We have seen how the recovery and translation of the classical authors who wrote about *materia medica* not only brought new information, but also led to the re-appropriation of a whole set of notions and values. The study of medicinal plants was no longer confined to the theoretical discussion of the texts, but included first-hand observation, according to the recommendation of the ancient writers. The *lectores simplicium* of the University of Pisa commented on the plants listed in Dioscorides' book, but also showed them to their students in the botanical garden or in the wild. The encounter with the old world had been fertile and led to a rethinking of *materia medica* and a novel attitude towards plants. I will now focus on the encounter with the New World.

The New Plants

When Columbus, sailing westward, arrived in what we now know to be America, his first concern was to look for the most sought-after exotic plants in Europe in his time. Very significant is his despair in being unable to take advantage of the new plants he was encountering: 'I believe there are many plants and many trees which are worth a great deal in Spain as dyes, medicines or spices; but I do not recognize them, which causes me great grief'.[5]

---

2   See Chapter 5, pp. 156–62.

3   See Chapter 2, p. 57.

4   See for example, Fredi Chiappelli (ed.), 'Introduction', *First Images of America: the Impact of the New World on the Old* (Berkeley and Los Angeles, CA, and London, 1976), vol. 1.

5   Cristoforo Colombo, *Giornale di bordo (1492–93)* (Milan, 1968), p. 61. Quoted by Joseph Ewan, 'The Columbian Discoveries and the Growth of Botanical Ideas with Special Reference to the Sixteenth Century', in F. Chiappelli (ed.), *First Images of America, the Impact of the New World on the Old* (Berkeley and Los Angeles, CA, and London, 1976), vol. I, p. 807, and Antonello Gerbi, *Nature in the New World* (Pittsburgh, 2010), p. 16.

In his letter to Luis de Sant'Angel (1493), Columbus referred to pepper and aloe-wood, and wrote that he believed he had found cinnamon and rhubarb.[6] We know however, that none of them were the luxury spices the Europeans were used to, for the simple reason that they did not grow in the Americas. This fact tells us that the attitude towards a new natural world was not to observe and record unknown species, but rather to identify, among all this unfamiliar vegetation, the well-known and precious plant products, so much sought-after in Europe.

The accounts of voyagers and explorers of the time abound with descriptions of wonderful and luxuriant vegetation. The comparison is inevitably with the Garden of Eden, something totally uncontaminated, and lavishly beautiful where nature offers its fruits and man gets his food without the sweat of his brow.

Interest in the accounts of the New World is attested by the immediate spread of the first works about it, the so-called 'Columbian sources' (*fuentes colombinas*). The above mentioned *Carta de Colon a Luis de Santangel*, for example, published for the first time in Barcelona in 1493, appeared the very same year in eight Latin and three Italian versions.[7] As for American natural history in particular, the author who provided the greatest and most detailed information on plants and fruit in the first half of the century, was Gonzalo Fernandez de Oviedo (1478–1557), who was in constant correspondence with a circle of Italian intellectuals,[8] and whose works were published in Venice between 1529 and 1556.[9]

Apart from a general interest and curiosity for what was new and exotic, plants were considered under different points of view according to different interests. The ways natural science, medicine and trade approached unknown plants, although often interweaving, obviously did not coincide. While for the naturalist all new species were, at least in theory, interesting in themselves, from the medicinal and commercial point of view, they were interesting only in relation to certain characteristics. As far as medicinal plants are concerned, there

---

[6]   Cristoforo Colombo, *The Spanish Letter of Columbus to Luis de Sant'Angel* (London, 1891), p. 17.

[7]   López Piñero and Pardo Tomás, *La influencia española*, p. 24.

[8]   On the Italian relations of Oviedo see, for example, Stefano Grande, 'Le relazioni geografiche fra Pietro Bembo, Gerolamo Fracastoro, Giovanni Battista Ramusio e Giacomo Castaldi', *Memorie della Societa' Geografica Italiana*, 12 (1905), pp. 93–197. Gerbi, *Nature in the New World*, pp. 145–200.

[9]   Part of what Oviedo had written on guaiacum had already been published in the work of the Andaluse Francisco Delicado in Venice in 1529. His *Sumario de la natural y general historia de las Indias* was published in Italian for the first time in 1534; his major work *Primera parte de la historia natural y general de las Indias*, in 1556.

had to be a serious reason for any species, unknown to Europeans, to be taken into account and considered worth importing into Europe.

If one looks at the process through which a new exotic medicinal plant or substance was chosen, one realizes that the necessary condition was that it should be used as such by indigenous people in their place of origin. No new medicinal plants were discovered by European physicians among the new exotic species. This condition, however, was not sufficient; it also had to prove to be a remedy which was lacking in the European pharmacopoeia, and necessary to cure 'European diseases', a fact which would also guarantee a profit from a commercial point of view. The process had little to do with first-hand observation of or experimentation on new plants. It was first of all a matter of information and depended very much on the kind of contact explorers and merchants were able to establish with indigenous peoples. As José Pardo Tomáš and Maria Luz López Terrada have pointed out, when Spanish authors mention the indigenous use of some simple, they always associate it with a European one with an identical use. In early accounts there is hardly ever reference to indigenous medical practice or indigenous use of unknown medicinal plants in their own right. Some of the plants which were introduced into the European pharmacopoeia, as seen above, were plants similar to European known and sought-after species that these authors believed they had found in the New World.[10] The same attitude was pointed out by David Gentilcore referring to the late introduction into the diet of Italian people of some New World foodstuffs, which are now fundamental. He notes how chilli pepper and maize, for example, which were substitutes for existing foodstuffs (pepper and wheat), were accepted much earlier by Europeans than those considered completely new: 'the potato, like the tomato, would only come into its own when Europeans learned to treat it as something different and developed new culinary associations for it'.[11]

When information about a new plant reached the learned European physicians, before being accepted, it had to be adapted to the complex medical theory of the time. It was assigned, never without controversy, its qualities and relative degrees, according to the traditional Galenic theory. Physicians and apothecaries, especially in the second part of the sixteenth century, very often refer to the fact that they have personally employed and tested the remedies. The Latin word *experientia* or the Italian word *esperienza* appear over and over again.[12] When one finds mention of some of the New World's plants in the herbals and medical treatises of the time, moreover, one must keep in mind

[10]   Pardo Tomáš and López Terrada, *Primeras noticias*, pp. 198–9.

[11]   David Gentilcore, *Italy and the Potato: A History 1550–2000* (London, 2012).

[12]   Charles B. Schmitt, 'Esperienza ed esperimento: un confronto tra Zabarella e il giovane Galileo', in *Filosofia e scienza nel Rinascimento* (Milan, 2001), pp. 25–64.

that their introduction implied at least the admission, not always taken for granted in the sixteenth century, that a remedy not recommended by the ancient authors could be admitted in the pharmacopoeia.

Florence and Discoveries

Information about the plants of the New World reached Europe mainly through the works of Spanish authors. As José Pardo Tomáš has documented, however, 'Italy was undoubtedly the geographical area where [the diffusion of American natural history and *materia medica*] had the quickest and largest repercussions'.[13]

As far as Tuscany and Florence in particular are concerned, there is evidence of a constant interest in the news and products coming both from the West and East Indies. Florence could boast some prominent figures in the history of the discovery and exploration of the New World. The most famous among them are Paolo del Pozzo Toscanelli, Amerigo Vespucci and Giovanni da Verrazzano, who all played key roles in the first phase of that history. In successive decades, during the sixteenth century, groups of Florentine merchant-sailors founded colonies both in Seville and Lisbon. The Spanish crown had imposed a monopoly that established that all commercial traffic with the West Indies had to pass through Seville and could be conducted only by Spanish subjects. For this reason, some Florentine tradesmen had moved to Seville and settled there with their families. Although trade was their main interest, some of them, as for example Giuliano Fiaschi, Galeotto Cei, Niccolò del Benino, and Francesco Carletti were at the same time learned men and wrote accounts about the lands of the New World they visited that certainly were primary sources of information for Tuscan citizens. Galeotto Cei (1513–1579), for example, in his Viaggio e relazione delle Indie, provides a description of the life and costumes of Central American people, and a vivid account of plants and animals of those regions.[14] Francesco Carletti (1573–1636), who was the first to circumnavigate the globe, left Florence when he was 18 and returned at

---

[13] José Pardo Tomáš, 'Obras Espanolas sobre historia natural y materia medica americanas en la Italia del siglo XVI', *Asclepio*, 43(1) (1991), p. 51; note 1, p. 80: of the (roughly) ten works considered, eight were published in Italy for the first time out of Spain. Of the seventy-six foreign editions of these works in the sixteenth century, forty-two (more than 55 per cent) were Italian.

[14] Galeotto Cei, *Viaggio e relazione delle Indie*, ed. Francesco Surdich (Rome, 1992). See also Luisa D'Arienzo, 'I Toscani sulla via delle Indie all'epoca di Cristoforo Colombo', *Rivista Geografica Italiana*, 100 (1993), pp. 321–43. Among Tuscan merchants in the East Indies who left interesting accounts of their journeys, see the works of Giovanni da Empoli, Andrea Corsali, Filippo Sassetti, and Francesco Carletti.

the age of 42 as a poor man, having lost everything, even his travel notes. He was welcomed by Grand Duke Ferdinando and gave a public account of his 'immensa pellegrinazione' before him and his court.[15]

The grand dukes took a great interest in the various aspects of exploration and discovery. In Grand Duke Ferdinando's words to his ambassador in Spain, they were 'very curious (curiosissimi) of everything, but most of all of the Indies', and urged him to 'get to know in detail the things of New Spain and Peru'.[16] During Cosimo's rule Florence became a centre for geographical and cartographical research. The most extraordinary evidence that can be produced is the Sala delle Carte commissioned by the duke from the cosmographer Egnazio Danti for his apartments in Palazzo Vecchio. Danti and his successor Stefano Buonsignori, represented all the known world in more than fifty large maps, painted on the cupboard doors of the of the Guardaroba in the Palazzo Vecchio.[17]

Detlef Heikamp provides detailed information on the interest of Cosimo and his sons in new cultures. The outstanding collection of works of art from Mexico gathered by the grand dukes, is a significant proof of this interest.[18]

The large number of documents concerning new exotic plants is evidence of the attention the dukes devoted to them. Descriptions of the gardens of their villas often contain references to exotic and rare plants. In his report of 1561, Ambassador Vincenzo Fedeli tells us that Cosimo wanted to be informed about the new plants and wished to send a man of science 'to the Indies to bring back some simples from those regions, in order to prove if they are of the same virtue, or if there are other species which are of greater virtues than ours.'[19] The dedication of the 1597 edition of the *Ricettario fiorentino* praises the 'house of Medici' with regard to the study and introduction of foreign plants. 'Who - it asks - has sent the most expert men, despite the great expense, to every regions, including the most distant, to investigate and bring home the foreign plants? Who has set out such pretty and spacious gardens full of the rarest and unknown simples, for their conservation?'[20]

---

[15]   His written report was published only in 1701. Francesco Carletti, *Ragionamenti di Francesco Carletti Fiorentino sopra le cose da lui vedute nei suoi viaggi si dell'Indie occidentali, e orientali come d'altri paesi* (Florence, 1701).

[16]   'Essendo noi curiosissimi d'ogni cosa, ma particolarmente delle Indie ... cerchate di sapere a minuto le cose della Nuova Spagna e del Perù'. Quoted by Detlef Heikamp, *Mexico and the Medici* (Forence, 1972), p. 18.

[17]   For a description of the *Sala delle carte* see Galluzzi, 'Il mecenatismo mediceo e le scienze', pp. 196–7.

[18]   Heikamp, *Mexico and the Medici*.

[19]   'Relazione di Firenze di Messer Vincenzo Fedeli' p. 356.

[20]   *Ricettario fiorentino* 1597, p. 2r.

The Medici were interested in the new plants from different points of view. If the great commercial value of exotic species from the Indies had always attracted their attention, we have seen that Cosimo I, and his sons Francesco and Ferdinando, were personally interested in plants from the medical and ornamental point of view as well. Several American plants were seen and commented upon by naturalists who had visited the botanical gardens and the large gardens around their villas. Among the watercolours of the Veronese painter Jacopo Ligozzi, who was in charge of depicting the most significant animals and plants in their possession, we can still see the first European representations of pineapple, agave (American aloe), false jalap (Mirabilis jalapa), and Mexican convolvulus (Ipomea quamoclit). These drawings were shown by Francesco himself to Ulisse Aldrovandi, who mentioned them in his notes, and who obtained some copies by Ligozzi himself, from the grand duke.[21]

In sixteenth-century herbals, as we will see, the plants of the newly discovered lands were sometimes listed without a precise identification of their medicinal virtues, but on the basis of their novelty or beauty. The same can be said for the new species planted in the botanical gardens. Therefore, if we want to investigate the reception of American plants from a strictly medical point of view, we will have to examine texts which deal exclusively with plants used for therapeutic purposes.

American Plants in the *Nuovo ricettario fiorentino*

A good starting point is the various editions of the first pharmacopoeia, the *Nuovo ricettario fiorentino*, which was published for the first time in Florence in 1498.[22] I will deal at length with the Florentine pharmacopoeia in Chapter 5; here I will consider it only in order to investigate the attitude of Tuscan learned doctors and pharmacists towards the use of new exotic plants in therapy.

We find the first reference to American plants in the second edition, which was issued half a century after the first, in 1550. The first part of the 1550 *Ricettario*, included two new sections entitled 'Of foreign plants' and 'Of foreign plants that do not grow in our countries'.[23] Although they are very short generic sections, here for the first time an 'Indian balsam' is mentioned among balsam substitutes,[24] and guaiacum wood, the well-known remedy for

---

[21]   See Chapter 3, p. 143.

[22]   *Nuovo Receptario composto dal famosissimo chollegio degli eximii doctori della arte et medicina della inclita cipta di Firenze, Impresso Nella inclyta ciptà di Firenze per la compagnia del Dragho* (1948). The *Ricettario fiorentino* and its various editions are dealt with in Chapter 5, pp. 156–62.

[23]   *Ricettario* 1550, pp. 6–7.

[24]   Ibid., p. 190.

French disease, is added and described in the list of plants included in the first part of the book, and it is mentioned again, though in passing, in the section which dealt with oils. Curiously, however, there are not yet any recipes containing guaiacum in the 1550 edition.[25] This is surprising, as we know that remedies based on it had been known by physicians and apothecaries for a long time prior to that date.[26] Moreover, guaiacum was the only plant of the New World to be universally accredited (with the sole exception of Paracelsus), and had a place in all the books dealing with medicinal plants.

A brief diversion concerning the early reception and use of guaiacum will show how late it made its appearance in the Florentine Pharmacopoeia by comparison with other medical texts, and point out the extreme caution with which novelties were introduced in a text which had a prescriptive purpose.

A long series of authors had already written about the disease that had hit Europe and spread in epidemic form at the very beginning of the century.[27] The disease, which in Italy came to be commonly referred to as mal francese (morbus gallicus in the Latin texts), had been at the centre of interminable controversies, mainly concerning the question whether it was already a known illness, described by the ancient authors, or had to be considered a new one.[28] As to the treatment, all the authors referred to guaiacum, an American tree from whose wood a remedy, considered almost miraculous by some, was derived.[29]

---

[25] Ibid., pp. 27–8.

[26] The date of the introduction of guaiacum in Italy (1517) reported by Francisco Delicado is probably not far from truth, as he himself was allegedly cured of *mal francese* in the Hospital of San Giacomo in Rome in the 1520s. See Jon Arrizabalaga, John Henderson and Roger French, *The Great Pox: The French Disease in Renaissance Europe* (New Haven and London, 1997), p. 231. Antonio Musa Brasavola whose treatise on French disease is included in Luisini's collection, postpones it to 1525. We know that Fracastoro knew Hutten's book, and his famous medical treatise *De contagione* was published in 1546. Mattioli had written a booklet about the cure of the French disease *Morbi gallici novum ac utilissimum opusculum* as early as 1533, and included guaiacum and recipes for its preparation in the first edition of his *Discorsi* (1544). Alfonso Corradi reports that the Ospedale degli Incurabili in Florence had bought 990 pounds of *legno santo* in 1533, and 6,230 pounds in 1541. Alfonso Corradi, 'L'acqua del legno e le cure depurative nel Cinquecento', *Annali Universali di Medicina e Chirurgia*, 269 (1884), p. 53, note 3. See also Arrizabalaga, Henderson and French, *The Great Pox*, ch. 8.

[27] The most influential treatises were collected at the time by Luigi Luisini, *De Morbo Gallico omnia quae extant apud omnes medicos cujusque nationis ... in unum hoc corpus redacta* (Venice, 1566–67). The collection of Luisini included an impressive number of works (more than sixty), the most part of which written by Italian authors.

[28] See for example, Arrizabalaga, Henderson and French, *The Great Pox*, pp. 56–87.

[29] See Robert S. Munger, 'Guaiacum, the holy wood from the New World', *Journal of the History of Medicine and Allied Sciences*, 4 (1949), pp. 169–229. For the use of guaiacum in Italy, see Corradi, 'L'acqua del legno', pp. 49–82.

According to the Spanish priest Francisco Delicado, who as early as 1529 had published the booklet *El modo de adoperare el legno de India Occidentale*, guaiacum was first known in Spain in 1508, and introduced into Italy in 1517.[30] In that same year, according to Nicolaus Poll, physician to Emperor Maximilian, guaiacum wood had already cured almost 3,000 Spaniards suffering from French disease.[31]

In 1519 the prominent German humanist Ulrich van Hutten wrote a very influential treatise, De Guaiaci medicina et morbo gallico, in which he explained how he himself had been saved by this prodigious wood, and described in detail how to prepare and take the remedy. Hutten's book was translated into many languages and spread rapidly throughout Europe. After that, guaiacum acquired its fame of prodigious remedy, and the 'holy wood', as it was already referred to, was hailed as the perfect and decisive cure for the French disease.[32] The name syphilis, which is how French disease is now usually called, was coined by the Veronese humanist-physician Girolamo Fracastoro (1476–1553) who wrote the poem *Syphilis sive Morbus gallicus* (1530), where guaiacum was praised as 'hope of mankind' (*spes hominum*), and 'new glory of the world' (*nova gloria mundi*).[33]

The first edition of the *Ricettario fiorentino* which contains preparations of American plants is that of 1567, in which guaiacum wood, china root and sarsaparilla are included in the first part, where simples are described, and then appear in a series of decoctions in the third part. The description of guaiacum is more detailed than the brief one of the previous edition. It also contains a correction concerning its being a species of ebony: '... today it is clear that

---

[30]   Francisco Delicado, *El modo de adoperare el legno de India Occidentale, salutifero rimedio a ogni piaga & mal incurabile* (Venice, 1529).

[31]   Nicolaus Poll's report on French disease *De cura morbi gallici per lignum guaycanum* was published in 1535, but written in 1517. Munger, 'Guayacum, the holy wood', p. 197. Corradi, 'L'acqua del legno', p. 52.

[32]   Many authors (for example Antonio Musa Brasavola and Gabriele Falloppio) had distinguished between two species of guaiacum. One of them, usually referred to as guaiacum (Guajacum officinale) came from Santo Domingo, the other one, the true 'holy wood' (Guajacum sanctum), from S. John of Portorico. In Tuscany physicians usually refer to any remedies based on guaiacum simply as the 'cura del legno'.

[33]   Girolamo Fracastoro, *Syphilis sive morbus gallicus* (Verona, 1530). The third book of the poem by Fracastoro was devoted to guaiacum and was written after the publication of Ulrich von Hutten's book. The second book of the poem was written before, and it praises mercury, as a remedy for the French disease. See Munger, 'Guaiacum, the holy wood', p. 216, note 43. Fracastoro subsequently wrote other treatises about the French disease, where he deals with the medical explanation of the illness and its contagion, and the manner to prepare and administer guaiacum. See John Henderson, 'Fracastoro, il legno santo e la cura del "mal francese"', in A. Pastore and E. Peruzzi (eds), *Girolamo Fracastoro: fra medicina, filosofia e scienze della natura* (Florence, 2006), pp. 73–89.

it [guaiacum] is not ebony; but a tree of a species of its own, which grows in the West Indies.'[34] A short description of another exotic plant, the so-called 'cina', whose provenance is left uncertain, appears in the same section,[35] and finally, the description of the American sarsaparilla, which is said to be similar to the local Smilax aspera.[36] In the section dedicated to the recipes, guaiacum appears in three different decoctions: the first one of wood (without bark), the second of wood and bark (*scorza*), and the third of wood, bark, and Greek wine. A decoction of 'salsapariglia Magistrale' and a decoction of 'cina Magistrale' appear in the same section.[37] The decoction of holy wood ('Decotto di legno santo senza scorza magistrale') is a simple preparation. One pound of holy wood, freshly cut, must be put in infusion for 24 hours, and then boiled until it reduced by two thirds. The same wood, after filtering the first decoction, must be boiled again with another 12 pounds of water. This recipe, from which two decoctions of different strength are obtained, is the same as that described in the book of Hutten, and by all the authors who treated the subject. The other recipes, where bark and/or wine are added, are more recent and are variations of the original one. As far as sarsapariglia and china radix decoctions are concerned, the procedure is the same, while the quantities and proportions are adapted to the different substances.

In the 1567 edition there is also a short description of 'Western balsam' (balsamo occidentale), which is a substitute for the Eastern balm (balsamo orientale), whose 'wood, seed and liquor we lack.'[38] Both descriptions and recipes appear without variations in the following edition of 1573.

The edition of 1597, compiled by a group of two doctors and two apothecaries, was dedicated to Grand Duke Ferdinando.[39] Its dedication, as mentioned above, praises the grand dukes who, regardless of expense, had greatly contributed to the discovery, study and diffusion of foreign plants. Despite this, there is nothing significantly new in this edition of the *Ricettario*, with regard to preparations containing new exotic plants. The decoctions based on the three American plants (guaiacum, cina and sarsaparilla) were also included in the 1623 edition of the *Ricettario fiorentino*, which was identical to that of 1597. They do not appear again in the subsequent editions. It is worth noting that they were the only remedies against French disease,

---

[34]   *Ricettario* 1567, pp. 43–4.

[35]   Ibid., pp. 29–30.

[36]   As will be seen, some contemporary authors maintained that sarsaparilla and smilax were one and the same, and that the local plant was as good a remedy as the American one.

[37]   *Ricettario* 1567, pp. 125–7.

[38]   Ibid., pp. 18–19.

[39]   *Ricettario fiorentino di nuovo illustrato* (Florence, 1597).

since preparations containing mercury (the other traditional remedy for this disease) were not included in any edition of the *Ricettario fiorentino*.[40]

Luca Ghini on the French Disease

Before the first recipes based on guaiacum, china root, and sarsaparilla appeared in the Florentine pharmacopoeia, the use of the American simples against the French disease had already been described in various works by the professors of the medical faculty at Pisa. One of the rare writings of Luca Ghini that has come down to us, *Morbi gallici curandi ratio perbrevis*, is a small treatise on the French disease and its treatment written between 1548 and 1555, but published several years later in 1589.[41] Ghini knew the works that had been written before on this subject and refers to the most well-known authors such as Girolamo Fracastoro, Andreas Vesalius, Gian Battista da Monte, Giovanni Manardo and Guillaume Rondelet.[42] In the very brief preface to his treatise, Ghini tells us that he is not going to make any general comment on the disease. He does not tell us if he sided with those who considered it a new disease or with their opponents. The fact that he mentions only contemporary authors, however, suggests that he did not think that the French disease was known by the ancient medical writers. Ghini is almost exclusively interested in the treatment, and addresses immediately the heart of the matter. He describes the *intemperies* of French disease and then explains that it first affects the liver, then the brain, and eventually the heart. Different symptoms characterise each of these stages, and for each of them he proposes appropriate treatments.

Ghini refers to the small group of New World plants (china radix, sarsaparilla, guajaci lignum), usually adopted for the treatment of the French disease. As to the preparation and administration of the first one, china root (*china radix*), he simply advises conforming to Vesalius's prescriptions.[43] He then suggests that

---

[40] Corradi explains this fact by maintaining that mercury had fallen into disrepute for the abuse of the *empirici*, who had inconsiderately employed it, especially for the treatment of French disease; so much so that the use of mercury had been forbidden even in hospitals. Corradi, *Le prime farmacopee*, p. 52.

[41] Luca Ghini, 'Morbi Gallici curandi ratio perbrevis', in G. del Guerra e Pier Luigi Mondani (ed.), *I primi documenti quattrocenteschi sulla sifilide e le lezioni pisane di Luca Ghini* (Pisa, 1970); Sabbatani, *Morbi Gallici curandi ratio*.

[42] Several works on the French disease were written already before the end of the fifteenth century. See for example *The Earliest Printed Literature on Syphilis: Being Ten Tractates from the Years 1495–1498, in Complete Facsimile*. With an introduction and other accessory material by Karl Sudhoff; adapted by Charles Singer (Florence, 1925).

[43] Del Guerra and Mondani, *I primi documenti*, pp. 114–20.

china root can be replaced, as also Fracastoro believed, by *radix arundinis* and *calamo aromatico*, and proceeds to describe a series of recipes.

He next refers to sarsaparilla reporting that in Spain it was considered so powerful that all other medicaments had been forgotten. He is convinced that sarsaparilla is nothing other than Smilax aspera, which is easily to be found in Tuscany. He explains that he knows that for sure, because he had seen one of those plants sent to the duke and himself.[44]

The chapter on 'guajaci lignum' is much longer and more complex. In accordance with the Galenic medical theory, Ghini explains that guaiacum can be prepared in many different ways to suit different temperaments, stages of the disease, and circumstances. Different preparations result in different qualities, cold, hot and temperate.

Ghini does not comment on the fact that these are plants from the New World, unknown to Dioscorides and Galen. He is certainly not against them in principle, but he does not seem to find them indispensable. As far as sarsaparilla is concerned, he even denies it is a new plant, maintaining that in Italy you can easily find the same plant under another name, thus making fun of Spanish doctors. As to china root, he thinks that it can be easily substituted by local simples. He does not suggest a substitute for guaiacum but, contrary to most of his contemporaries, he does not claim that it works wonders. The criteria by which the various recipes are to be prepared and administered are the traditional ones.[45] He adds that he was the first one in Bologna to add various drugs to the guaiacum decoction (*decocto ligni*) in order to treat other symptoms, such as coughing, breathing difficulties, fever etc.

Although Luca Ghini did not leave explicit comments on exotic plants, it is quite clear that he did not object to their medical use. That he does not mention them in his *Lectures*, that have come to us in the form of manuscripts included in Aldrovandi's collection,[46] is easily accounted for by the fact that the teaching of medical botany, as the statutes of the University of Pisa prescribed, had to be based on Dioscorides' *Materia medica*.[47] With regard to information about their medical use, he refers to other contemporary Europeans authors, and does not seem to have tried to get first-hand information on their use in their places of origin.

He was certainly very interested in new exotic plants, as is shown by the fact that he collected a number of them in Pisa's botanical garden. Ghini, in his entry

---

[44]   'Ex ramulo illius plantae ad nostrum ducem et ad me missae', ibid., p. 116.

[45]   In this period the treatment, which sometimes was considered by the patients even worse than the disease itself, had become more tolerable. See for example Corradi, 'L'acqua del legno'.

[46]   See Chapter 2, pp. 87–90.

[47]   'Deputati ad lecturam de simplicibus legant Dioscoridem', Gli Statuti di Cosimo I', *Storia dell'Universita' di Pisa*, p. 616.

on sarsaparilla, informs us that he was able to observe *ex vivo* a twig of that plant and compare it with Smilax aspera, reaching the conclusion that they were one and the same. It is interesting to note that in his *Discorsi*, Mattioli expresses the same opinion, and backs it up with Ghini's, adding some interesting information. The passage is worth quoting:

> because he [Luca Ghini] affirmed that he had seen a plant of sarsaparilla brought from Spain to the most illustrious Cosimo Duke of Florence; which in all respects was not at all different from Smilax aspera ... as shortly after he was able to experience for himself. In fact, having had the Smilax aspera uprooted, and having given the decoction to some patients who were suffering from the French disease, they were all cured by this remedy.[48]

Therefore Ghini did not confine himself (contrary to what Mattioli confessed to have done, as will be seen) to looking at a twig of this new plant and comparing it with a known one, and asserting that they were one and the same. He proceeded to prove his assumption (at least this is what he meant to do) testing its curative power on some patients. Mattioli, on the other hand, justifies his adherence to Ghini's belief 'because he [Ghini] (as I can sincerely bear witness) at his time not only was a most singular herbalist, but also candid, sincere, true, and faithful in any other respect.'[49] Again from Mattioli, we know of another American drug that Ghini knew and probably used. It was Indian balsam that was adopted by the Florentine pharmacopoeia as a substitute for the Oriental balsam. Mattioli, referring to this plant in his *Discorsi*, reports that he had first heard of it through Luca Ghini.[50]

Other sources provide evidence that Ghini was very active in obtaining as many exotic plants as he could, and planting them in Pisa's botanical garden. Some American herbs that are included in Aldrovandi's herbarium or among his illustrations were obtained by him directly at (during his visits in 1549 and 1553) or sent from the *orto pisano*. To mention a few of them: *Planta maxima* or *Pianta del sole* (sunflower), *Canna Indica*, *Herba turca* or *Frumentum turcicum* (maize), various types of pumpkin, *Opuntia* or *Ficus indica/peruviana* (prickly pear) (Figure 4.1).[51] It is clear from the variety of plants, that the criteria on the basis of which Ghini collected them were not only those of medicinal usefulness. Food plants, ornamental plants, etc., were all looked for and planted.

48 Mattioli, *I discorsi di Pietro Andrea Mattioli* (Venice, 1568), p. 201.
49 Ibid.
50 Ibid.
51 Ubrizsy Savoia, 'La biodiversità Americana nell'opera di Aldrovandi', pp. 84–5; Ubrizsy Savoia, 'Le piante pisane nei manoscritti di Aldrovandi', pp. 363–80.

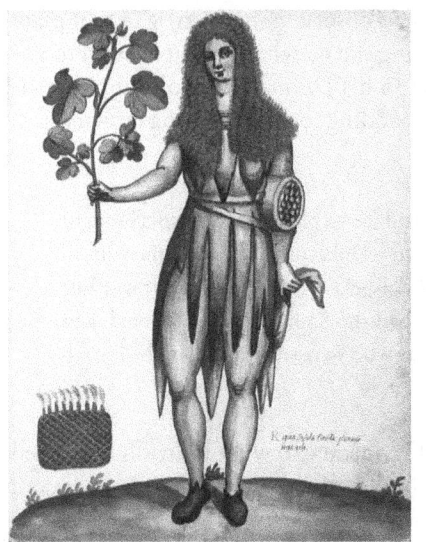
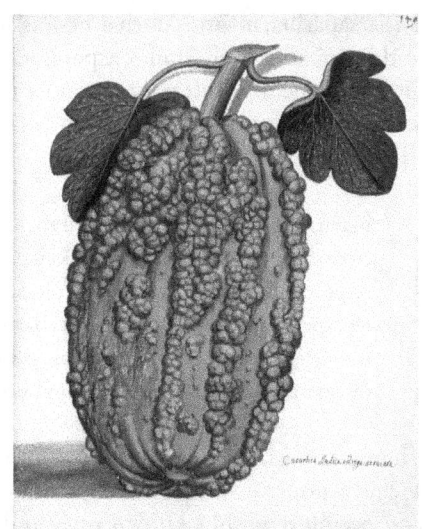
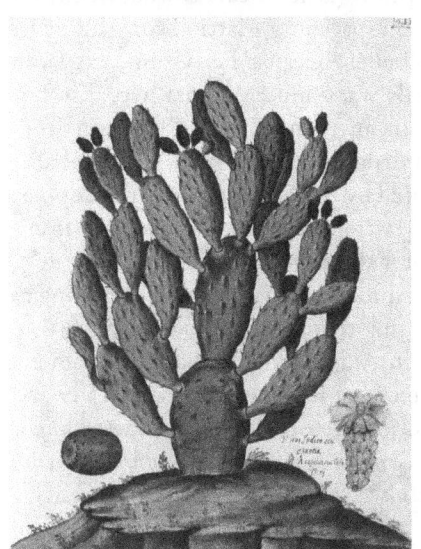
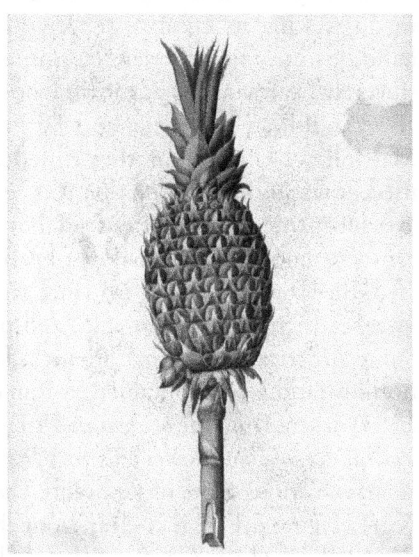

Figure 4.1   Some illustrations of American plants among Aldrovandi's.
1: Regina Insula Florida holding the leaves of Indian pumpkin;
2: Cucurbita indica oblonga verucata (Indian pumpkin) 3: Ficus
indica seu opuntia (Indian fig); 4: pineapple (painted by Iacopo
Ligozzi). Biblioteca dell'Università di Bologna

One can be certain that Ghini had tried to transplant in Pisa more plants than the ones about which we know. The letters of the time are full of accounts of plants which arrived at their destination in very poor condition or of plants that could not survive in a different soil or climate. Moreover, identification was often very difficult and description imprecise. Among Aldrovandi's manuscripts kept in Bologna, for example, there is a list of some plants Ghini sent to Mattioli along with the so-called *Placiti*. The list included some exotic plants, probably of the genus *palma*, coming from Brazil and the Island of Saint John, the identification of which remains somewhat vague.[52] They do not seem to appear in the list of plants of the botanical garden, therefore presumably if they had been planted, they had not survived.

Gabriele Falloppio's *Tractatus de morbo gallico*

Gabriele Falloppio (1523–1562), professor of anatomy at Pisa from 1548, is the author of another treatise on the French disease (*Tractatus de morbo gallico*, 1563).[53] His approach is more philosophical than Ghini's, but he is also very precise and attentive to details. He, unlike Ghini, discusses at length, with subtle arguments, whether the disease had to be considered new or extant, and finally reaches the conclusion that it is new.

He devotes a long section of his work to guaiacum. He distinguishes between two different species; one is guaiacum and the other holy wood. He seems to be very interested in the plants themselves. For their description he refers to the authors who had personally seen them, and he also reports that he had some fruits of guaiacum from a monk, and a twig of holy wood with yellow flowers from a merchant. He reports Oviedo's opinion that, although both species are a good cure for the French disease, holy wood is more efficacious (habet maiores vires) for other diseases. Falloppio proceeds to attribute to guaiacum its qualities according to the usual Galenic theory. As it is bitter to the taste, it is necessarily hot (omnia amara necessario calida sunt). Since it dries up ulcers and pustules, it is dry. As to the degree, it is hot in the third degree, but fades in the second (in secundo finiente), and is dry in the same degree.[54] Then he adds an interesting detail; he believes that guaiacum cures the French disease not because 'it dries or heats, but because such is in the nature of that wood.' In other words, guaiacum has an intrinsic property which cures this illness. It is, according to Falloppio, what we would

---

[52] De Toni, 'I Placiti', p. 14.

[53] The book, based on his lectures, was published posthumous. I will refer to Gabriele Falloppio, *De morbo gallico liber absolutissimus* (Venice, 1574).

[54] Falloppio, *De morbo gallico*, ch. 41 'De qualitatibus, & viribus ligni Indici', pp. 85–6.

now call a 'specific' for French disease. Only God, he declares, knows this essence (*substantia*), and men cannot have knowledge of it.[55]

Next Falloppio describes the treatment proper. Which wood is the best, how it must be prepared, how it must be administered, and what kind of regimen the patient suffering from the French disease must follow. There is no doubt, he says, that the most efficacious is holy wood; however, guaiacum, which is more easily found, can substitute it.[56] As holy wood and guaiacum do not grow in our woods, although several parts of the plant might be used, we will use the trunk and the cortex. The wood must be broken into tiny pieces and the best way is to use a rasp, as the *speziali* from Venice do, and obtain very fine filings to make a decoction.[57] The decoction can be simple or composed, according to the patient and the stage of the disease. Each phase of the process is discussed at length, the way to obtain the rasping, the maceration, the ratio between wood and water, the temperature of water, the kind of vessels that must be used, the boiling methods, etc. To summarize, a simple decoction, according to Falloppio's prescriptions, must be prepared soaking the wood filings in warm water (the ratio depends on various circumstances) for twenty-four hours. Then it must be boiled, possibly in glazed jars. Usually a simple decoction requires a double boiling and a meticulous filtering. When a patient is particularly debilitated, a broth of chicken, veal or kid can be used instead of water.[58] A series of recipes of composed decoctions are then described. These always contain cortex, besides wood, sometimes combined with other simples such as blessed thistle, wall germander, betony, rosemary, stecado and fennel. He reports that in Tuscany the most common recipe is to bring to the boil 18 pounds of water with 1 pound of guaiacum rasping and half the quantity of bark, and let it reduce to one third. This decoction will subsequently be boiled again with 3 pounds of strong white wine. Falloppio then refers to Mattioli and Musa Brasavola, who suggested adding purges in the decoction. He also describes a preparation for small children and suckling infants. He ends by saying that it is better to use simple decoctions, which are most efficacious for the French disease.

The section in which Falloppio treats of china root is a short one. He only says that it is not known if it comes from the East or the West Indies, and that Emperor Charles V made it famous. He provides a recipe for a decoction, but he says that he uses it for curing the ailments of the viscera, ulcers, and inflammations, but he does not employ it for the French disease.[59]

---

[55]   Ibid., p. 86. Although guaiacum is considered a specific, the treatment described by Falloppio seems all centred on heat and sweat, through which the bad humours are to be expelled.

[56]   Ibid., p. 89.

[57]   Ibid., p. 92.

[58]   Ibid., p. 95.

[59]   Ibid., pp. 109–12.

As far as sarsaparilla is concerned, he (like Ghini and Mattioli) says he had seen a whole specimen which was brought by a Spanish man to the Duke of Florence. Therefore he can affirm that it is one and the same with Smilax aspera, which is confirmed by *experientia*. In fact, he had found this plant on mount San Giuliano near Pisa, had had it reproduced, and subsequently, he had always used it with great success for the cure of the French disease.[60]

According to the texts on the French disease that we have examined, it is clear that guaiacum, china, and salsapariglia were considered a useful acquisition from the New World. But they were useful as remedies of a disease that also came, according to most physicians, from that part of the world. These remedies were certainly not enough to compensate the great sufferings that this disease (which did not seem to hit the American natives with the same terrible symptoms) had caused the old world. Given the spread of the disease and its gravity, it is comprehensible that the importation of these plants, and most of all guaiacum, was considered of great importance from the medical point of view, and that it came to be at the centre of paramount economic interests. From the reading of the *Ricettario fiorentino*, which deals with the whole range of existing pharmacological products, one can see that these, with the only exception of 'Indian balsam', were the only American plants considered.

New Plants in Mattioli's *Discorsi*

Our investigation into the reception of American plants will now turn to herbals, which, although traditionally written for medical purposes, seem to be the genre more apt to take in new unknown plants.

We will first consider the Italian translation of and commentary on Dioscorides' *Materia Medica* of the Sienese physician Pietro Andrea Mattioli, the so-called *Discorsi*, which was undoubtedly the most read book on plants of the century. As said above, Mattioli's work appeared in many different editions. As far as New World plants are concerned, some new ones appeared over the years, some entries were expanded or modified, and illustrations introduced and added. In the first edition of 1544, for example, the only plant he deals with at length is guaiacum, but in the edition of 1568 (which contained 'large pictures') many other new exotic plants are dealt with. Between this edition and that of 1573, which is considered to be the last one published under the supervision of the author, there are no major differences, as far as American species are concerned. Therefore I will mainly refer to the 1568 edition.

---

[60] Ibid., pp. 112–18.

Since Mattioli's *Discorsi* was meant as a commentary on Dioscorides, the addition of plants from the New World does not appear to be consistent with the general scheme of the book. He mentioned and described a certain number of American plants and inserted them into his comment on a plant that, in his opinion, bore a certain resemblance to the new one. Mattioli translates the entry 'Ebony' in Dioscorides and then, in his commentary, he includes a description of guaiacum.[61] To introduce it, he says that it is thought that the wood called Guaiaco, Guaiacane or Legno Santo, used for the treating of the French disease, might be some sort of ebony. He then adds that he could neither reject nor support this opinion, because he did not find any ancient writers who say which leaves, flowers, or fruits ebony produces. He proceeds by quoting Giovanni Manardo and explaining that there are three kinds of guaiacum, a fact that he can confirm, having used all of them. In his opinion, they do not come from different trees, but from trees at a different stage of growth. His description is based on what he has heard from people 'coming from the regions where it grows', and it is likely that he had seen nothing but pieces of wood and bark kept in apothecary shops (Figure 4.2). Also the provenance of guaiacum is very uncertain, as he maintains that it comes from the 'newly found Indies', but also from Calicut, and from Taprobana Island and, as somebody says, even from Ethiopia.' He then expresses an opinion which is very frequently reiterated, that 'being a truth universally acknowledged that the medicaments and aromas which grow in the Oriental regions are better than all the others, it is to be believed that the one [guaiacum] that is brought to Spain from the West, is much less effective than the one that grows in the East or in the South.'[62] He attributes to guaiacum hot and dry faculties, and adds that it contains a resin (*ragia*) that opposes the contagion and the putrefaction of the French disease. He then explains how guaiacum should be used and maintains that he was the first to use a decoction of guaiacum in wine to treat the French disease.

He relates that when guaiacum was first discovered, and for many years since, the remedy was administered with great fear, as it was believed that if the patient did not follow some very strict rules, he would be in danger of death. These rules involved seclusion for at least forty days in a room in the dark, with a diet of a little bread and raisins. Wine and meat were considered mortal poisons. He warns against those 'empirici' who are ignorant of the rules of medicine and who, regardless of whether the complexion or the disease is warm or cold, or whether it is winter or summer, and whether the person they are treating is a man or a woman, young or old, they administer guaiacum wine in a glass of hot water every morning, curing one merely by chance, and killing ten.

---

[61]   Mattioli, *Discorsi* 1568, p. 199.

[62]   Ibid., p. 200.

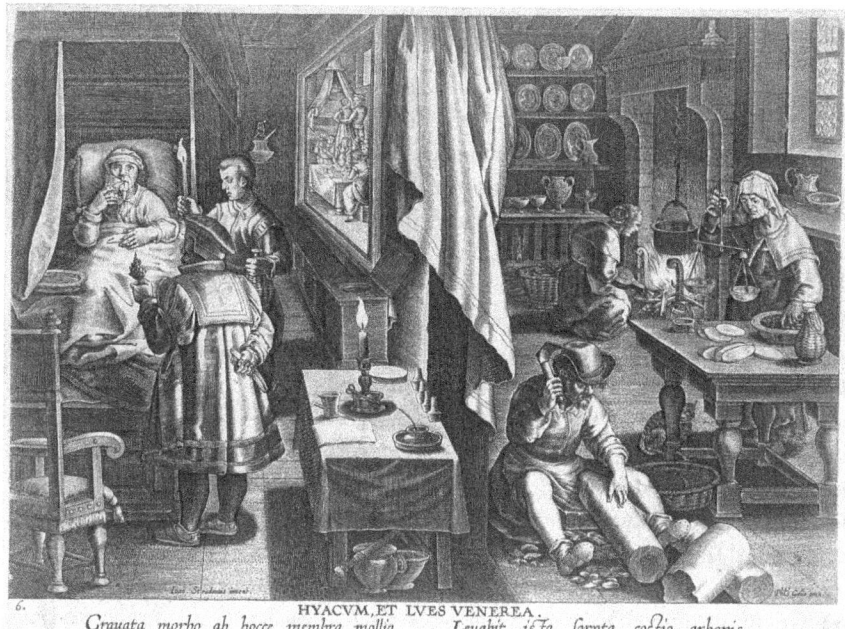

Figure 4.2   Print from Giovanni Stradano's *Nova reperta* (1587–89), a
patient suffering from 'mal francese' and the preparation of
'acqua del legno'. London, Wellcome Library

He then provides a recipe, as well as indications of how and when the remedy
is to be administered. To make the true wine of guaiacum you have to take 4
pounds of wood very subtly rasped, and 2 pounds of its bark. You then add
blessed thistle, maidenhair, scolopendra, cordial flowers, cinnamon, anise and
Madeira sugar. You put all these substances in a barrel and then pour 150 pounds
of hot white wine on it. This is a simple recipe for a guaiacum wine, that is to be
taken at meals. In the morning and in the evening the patient must be given a
weaker decoction of guaiacum made of water and various other substances with
the addition of purgative substances such as senna and rhubarb.[63] During the
treatment, the patient can eat roast chicken or partridge, raisins and bread.

Neglecting the fact that he is commenting on ebony, Mattioli then proceeds
to deal with other exotic remedies against the French disease. The first one he
considers is the root of cina or china, brought to Europe by the Portuguese and
the Spanish from the 'southern regions', much praised by the Emperor Charles V.[64]

---

[63]   Ibid., pp. 200–201.
[64]   Ibid., p. 201.

He describes the root (but not the plant) and refers to the fact that Vesalius despised it and was against its use on grounds he did not know. However, and this is his conclusion, the root of china would not have been held in such great esteem by the emperor had it not been of great utility.

Then, still in the same entry, he considers sarsaparilla. I have already reported how Mattioli relies on Ghini's opinion and experience to jump to the conclusion that sarsaparilla is one and the same as Smilax aspera, a plant growing in many parts of Italy and also in the *orto pisano*. Mattioli points out that there are many who are not of the same opinion and think that the two plants are different in many respects. It is interesting to note that he explains this diversity by referring to Theofrastus's belief that the same plant found in a different climate, soil, etc., can vary in 'many ways, such as taste, smell and shape'. He also uses, as further evidence, the etymology of the Spanish word, which is the same of that of the Tuscan one. He then adds that it is a good remedy not only for the French disease but also for a series of other 'cold' diseases. The recipe consists of a simple decoction of roots in water. It is to be administered very hot, so that the patient, well covered, may sweat for about two hours. The treatment must be repeated twice a day for forty days, although sometimes thirty days might be sufficient. The patient, moreover, must be purged every ten days. The diet is similar to that prescribed for guaiacum: bread, raisins, and if necessary, chicken.[65]

We have seen that Mattioli does not confine himself to comment on Dioscoredean *materia medica*. His research is based on the simples Dioscorides has included in his work, but his ambition is to exceed the master. His comments are always longer (and sometimes enormously longer) than the original entries by Dioscorides and the plants unknown to him are always included. Mattioli therefore refers to several plants from the New World, usually for their supposed medical qualities, but sometimes just for the novelty they represented. The 1568 edition includes a letter from the Paduan physician Iacomo Antonio Cortusio with a large illustration and an accurate description of *Pianta massima* (sunflower), the seeds of which he had received from the Flemish botanist Carolus Clusius (Charles de l'Escluse, 1526–1609). Cortusio's letter also contains an explanation of how the flower turns its corolla according to the different positions of the sun in the sky, and how indigenous people (from Peru) proceeded to sow the plants.

Another plant Mattioli takes into consideration is chilli pepper (Capsicum annuum), which appears under the entry on pepper,[66] for the obvious similarity of strength between the two plants. He reports that Indian pepper (*pepe d'India*) had become quite common in Italy (*hormai fatto per tutto volgare*), probably because of its interest as a food plant rather than for its medicinal qualities.

---

65   Ibid.
66   Ibid., p. 608.

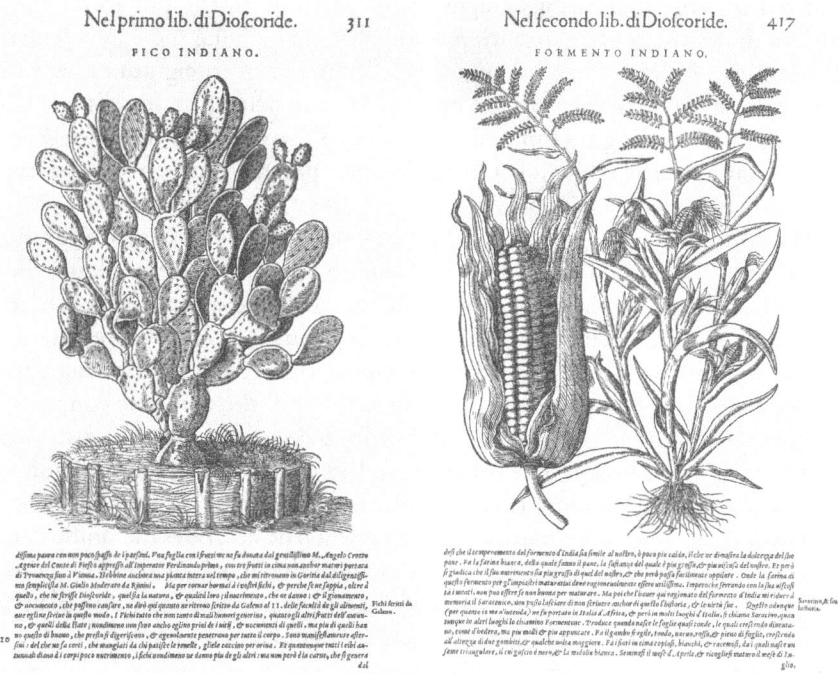

Figure 4.3   Two American plants in Mattioli's *Discorsi*, 1568. Fico indiano (Indian fig); formento indiano (maize). Milan, Biblioteca Braidense

It never became a substitute for pepper, which was one of the most common ingredients in medicinal recipes.[67]

Other new plants included in Mattioli's *Discorsi* are maize (*formento indiano*),[68] prickly pears (*fico indiano*),[69] a type of pumpkin (*zucche indiane*),[70] tomato (*pomi d'oro*).[71] In the edition of 1568, almost all of these plants are

---

[67]   Pepper (Pepe lungho, pepe nero, pepe biancho) was mentioned not less than in 87 recipes in the first edition of the *Ricettario fiorentino*. Huguet-Termes, 'Approximacion Historico-farmacologica', p. 96.

[68]   Mattioli, *Discorsi* 1568, p. 416, illustration p. 417. (Here Mattioli points out that this plant comes from the West Indies and must be called Indian corn and not Turkish corn, as Fuchs calls it. It is peculiar that in Italian maize is still called Turkish corn (*granoturco*).

[69]   Mattioli, *Discorsi* 1568, p. 310, illustration p. 311.

[70]   Mattioli, *Discorsi* 1568, p. 541.

[71]   Tomatoes (*pomi d'oro*) are mentioned in the entry on mandrake and are considered a species of eggplant. They are just mentioned, as in the previous editions, but no picture is provided. Mattioli informs us that they can be eaten, usually with salt, pepper and oil, and that they are sometimes red like blood, and at other times the colour of gold. Mattioli,

depicted in large illustrations (Figure 4.3). Mattioli, in the preface of this edition, draws the reader's attention to the fact that among these new larger illustrations of plants there are 'not a small number of foreign ones, which neither by me nor by any others have been ever printed or published ...'. Particularly interesting are some editions where the woodcut prints have been hand-coloured, such as the one Gherardo Cibo painted for Francesco Maria della Rovere, Duke of Urbino.[72]

Mattioli is always fully conscious that his book is to be considered a comment on Dioscorides, thus he keeps his attention centred on the therapeutic aspect of plants, even when he describes new plants which have little to do with medicinal properties. Although in his preface he maintains that he would have liked to visit foreign lands, as Galen did, regretting that the 'weak complexion of the body, the marital bond, the domestic concerns, and the medical profession' did not allow him to undertake a long journey, he did not seem to be bound, like other naturalists, by the spell of an unknown plant world. He very seldom speaks of plants as 'beautiful', or remarkable in their own right, as for example does Cortusio when he describes the sunflower, or, as will be seen, Cesalpino when he describes the flower of the American aloe. However he is willing to include in his *Discorsi* as many American plants as possible. When he deals with French marigold, for example, which is considered to be the first ornamental American species to be grown in Europe, he knows that it had not been attributed any medical virtue. In his book, two species of French marigold are illustrated in large pictures, under the names of *Cariophillus indicus maior* and *minor*, and in his comment Mattioli explains that he does not know anything certain about the qualities of this plant, but that being bitter of taste, 'it is not to be doubted that it has hot and dry faculties'.[73]

Much more interesting from the medical point of view at the time is Indian balsam (*balsamo indiano*).[74] The precious balsam described by Dioscorides and the other ancient authors, which originated in Egypt and the Middle East, had become extremely rare and it could no longer be obtained through the usual trade routes. Here Mattioli refers to a new balsam which was a

---

Discorsi 1568, p. 1136. David Gentilcore, *Pomodoro! A History of the Tomato in Italy* (New York and Chichester, 2010), pp. 1–2.

[72] This edition, kept in Rome (Bibl. Alessandrina, rari 278) has been partly reproduced in Arnold Nesselrath (ed.), *Discorsi sulle piante e sugli animali. Il Dioscoride colorito e miniato da Gherardo Cibo per Francesco Maria II della Rovere Duca d'Urbino* (Rome, 1991). Another one is kept in the Wellcome Library. The Latin edition of 1583, kept in the British Library, is also hand-coloured.

[73] I found mention and illustrations of the French marigold in the Latin version of Mattioli, *Discorsi* 1583.

[74] Mattioli, *Discorsi* 1568, p. 67.

'most odorous liquor' coming from the West Indies. He adds that he first heard about 'this precious liquor' from Luca Ghini.[75] This certainly was a very interesting substance for the physicians and apothecaries of the time, as balsam was considered one of the most precious and rare ingredients in European pharmacopoeia, and also a very sought-after component of theriac. In a letter sent from Pisa on 7 January 1573 by Cosimo I to his son Francesco, there is reference to the controversy that took place among Florentine apothecaries on the use of a newly found balsam coming from the Indies in the recipe for theriac. It also reports that Baccio Baldini, as a representative of the Arte degli Speziali, had authorized the speziale al Moro to use the new Indian balsam instead of the traditional balm.[76] Although a *balsamo occidentale* (coming from the West Indies) was already described in the *Ricettario fiorentino* of 1567 and indicated as a substitute of Oriental balsam, it is apparent that this was not approved of by all apothecaries, especially when theriac was at stake.[77]

From this brief survey of Mattioli's description of the new exotic medicinal plants that he included in his *Discorsi*, a few observations can be made. First of all, the inaccurate indication of their provenance should be noted. Guaiacum, in Mattioli's opinion, can be found both in the West and East Indies.[78] On the grounds of this statement, and on the assumption that Eastern remedies are best, he even reaches the conclusion that an improbable 'oriental guaiacum', must be more effective than the Western one.[79] In his accounts, Mattioli often points out controversial issues, such as the uncertainty about the identification of the plant, as in the case of sarsaparilla, the discussion about the effectiveness of the remedy, as in the case of china root, the conflicting opinions about the way of preparing and administering the decoction, as in the case of guaiacum. Since there was no authority of ancient masters to refer to, Mattioli had to rely on information that was evidently very imprecise, on the often conflicting opinions of the 'moderns', and, when possible, on his own experience, that did not always coincide with that of others. The overall impression is one of vagueness and imprecision, all the more if one remembers that the edition of the *Discorsi* from which I have taken these examples is the one of 1568, fifty years after the first appearance of guaiacum in Europe.

---

[75] Ibid.

[76] ASF, vol. 241, f. 84 (Medici Archive Project).

[77] *Ricettario fiorentino*, 1567, pp. 18–19.

[78] Falloppio, in his treatise, points out Mattioli's mistake. See Falloppio, *De morbo gallico*, p. 83.

[79] No picture of guaiacum is provided.

Nicolas Monardes's *Historia medicinal*

In the latter part of the sixteenth century, information about new plants became wider and more precise. This was due principally to the *Historia medicinal* by the Spanish learned doctor Nicolas Monardes (1493–1588).[80] This work, written between 1565 and 1574, had a great influence on the medical works of the time, and made a substantial difference.[81] We can appreciate this difference, for example, between the first edition of Mattioli's *Discorsi* (1544), and the edition of 1568, when the first part of Monardes's work had been published. Cesalpino's information about New World plants relies almost exclusively on Monardes's work.

Monardes lived all his life in Seville, where he became a prominent physician, and where at the same time he engaged in the African slave-trade with America.[82] He never visited the New World, but established a botanical garden in Seville where he sowed, planted and grew the plants that arrived at that port with other American goods. His book was translated into Latin, shortly after its appearance, by the prominent botanist Carolus Clusius.[83] Clusius's version was not a literal translation, but rather a rearrangement of the whole book in a more conventional herbal. He did not report all the anecdotes and comments that characterised Monardes's book. Annibale Briganti's Italian translation, which appeared in 1576, was not based on the original, but on the Latin version of Clusius.[84]

This is not the place to go into the details of Monardes's work; nevertheless, I think that at least one example of how he proceeded to account for an unknown American drug can provide some insight into how information passed from the new to the old world. Although it is very likely that Italian scholars would have read the book in Clusius's or Briganti's versions, it is worthwhile referring to Monardes's original, where many more anecdotes and details are reported. Reading Monardes's book one can actually see how he was able to gather information about plants without moving from Seville and, what is more

---

[80]   Nicolas Monardes, *Primera y segunda y tercera partes de la historia medicinal de las cosas que se traen de nuestras India Occidentales que sirven en medicina* [1565–74]. (Facsimile edn, Seville:, 1988; English translation, John Frampton, *Joyfull Newes Out of the Newe Founde Worlde*, London, 1596).

[81]   José Pardo Tomáš and Maria Luz López Terrada, in *La influencia Española*, divide the works that deal with *materia medica* 'before' and 'after' Monardes.

[82]   Charles Ralph Boxer, *Two Pioneers of tropical medicine: Garcia d'Orta and Nicolas Monardes* (London, 1963).

[83]   *De simplicibus medicamentis ex Occidentali India delatis, quorum in medicina usus est*. Auctore D. Nicolao Monardis Hispalensi medico; Interprete Carolo Clusio Atrebate (Antwerp, 1574).

[84]   Nicolas Monardes, *Delle cose che vengono portate dall'Indie occidentali pertinenti all'uso della medicina* (Venice, 1575).

important, one can find significant examples of how information about the medicinal use of American plants reached Europe. In his account of the plant called 'michoacan', Monardes tells how he discovered it while curing a sick friar coming from New Spain, who refused to be purged with any other medicine but the root of michoacan. After having witnessed its indubitable beneficial action, Monardes experimented with it on many other patients.[85] Michoacan, he found, was different from other medicines of the kind, as its purgative effect stopped as soon as the patient resumed taking food or liquids. Monardes also tells us about the difficulties he encountered in gathering information on the plant's appearance.[86] He asked merchants coming from the region the plant took its name from, but the descriptions of the plant that he got, and that he punctiliously recorded, were very vague, and the most interesting detail he was able to get hold of was that the plant was 'very green'. In the second part of the book, however, in a subsequent entry on 'the flower michoacan', he seems to have gathered all the necessary information to furnish a complete description, and it appears evident that he had actually managed to see the plant. This is one of the rare cases in which one can follow the process through which information was obtained, verified, and published.

American Plants in Cesalpino's *De plantis*

In the dedication of his work *De plantis libri XVI* (1583), Cesalpino mentions Nicolas Monardes ('most learned Castilian doctor'), who provided information on New World plants.[87] The new plants he deals with are in fact, apart from some exceptions, based mostly on information drawn from Monardes.[88]

Cesalpino's work on plants had little in common with Mattioli's *Discorsi*. First of all it was not a commentary on an ancient author, but a completely new herbal. Cesalpino, moreover, did not intend to confine himself to a description of plants and their faculties, but, as has been seen, approached *historia plantarum* from the point of view of systematics, which had been long neglected.[89] The occasion that attracted his attention and convinced him of the need of a new classification of plants was provided, as he himself declares, by the enormous number of new species discovered in the New World, which were unknown to Pliny, Dioscorides and Galen, and that had continued to increase. That 'disorderly

---

[85] Monardes, *Historia medicinal*, pp. 30r–30v.

[86] Ibid., p. 31r.

[87] Cesalpino, *De plantis*, 'Dedication', pp. III–IV.

[88] López Piñero and López Terrada, *La influencia española*, p. 113.

[89] See Chapter 2, pp. 101–103.

multitude appals the mind', he maintained, and therefore a reorganization of whole *materia medica* was called for.[90]

The most extensive and detailed entry is, as usual, the one on guaiacum, which apparently is based on previous sources.[91] He mentions that guaiacum originates in the Island of Santo Domingo, from where Columbus brought it together with some indigenous men and women, and with a kind of 'lues' which was called 'Buua' by the natives, and was later called French disease. So the disease and the remedy came from the same place. He distinguishes guaiacum from 'holy wood' that comes from the Isle of Saint John and is more efficacious in the cure of the French disease. He adds that the root of that plant cures not only the French disease, but also other diseases due to an excess of cold humours that other remedies could not cure. He finally describes at length the recipe and method of its administration.[92]

The preparation of the remedy described by Cesalpino is very simple and consists of a decoction of guaiacum bark in water. He maintains that guaiacum is best used alone, because any mixture seems to diminish its heating power. The patient, after being purged has to stay in bed, protected from cold and air. He has to take ten ounces of very hot guaiacum decoction a first time in the morning, and be immediately covered with heavy blankets. This will induce sweat for at least two hours. Then, after drying the sweat, he will wear a warm *linteum* and other cloths. After four hours he can eat some sultanas, almonds, and a small quantity of *biscoctum* bread, and drink water sufficient to quench his thirst. Then at about *hora octava* (2 p.m.), he will take again ten ounces of hot guaiacum decoction and repeat more or less the same sequence. A moderate quantity of the same food and water can be ingested for dinner. This treatment will last for fifteen days. Weak patients might add some chicken to their diet, on the ninth day. On the sixteenth day the patient must be purged with 10 drachmae of cassia pulp. Then the cure of *acqua del legno* begins again and must be continued for twenty days. Half a chicken can be added to the diet, but the patient must not leave the bed. After that, he can gradually restart his usual life, but with some precautions, among which abstinence from Venus and wine.[93]

Another very long entry is the one on sarsaparilla. Here Cesalpino refers to the Spanish as having learnt the use of this plant from the natives of New Spain, who used it to treat many different diseases. He explains that 'sarzaparilla' is the Spanish word for a West-Indian root used for many different diseases. Although he finds some resemblance between sarsaparilla and Smilax aspera,

---

90   Cesalpino, *De plantis*, 'Dedication', p. III.
91   Ibid., pp. 105–107.
92   Ibid.
93   Ibid., p. 211.

he does not maintain, as Ghini and Mattioli had done, that they are one and the same. He adds that there is another species, coming from Honduras, which is very different. As far as its qualities are concerned, Cesalpino says that it is a remedy for the French disease and other ailments and that it cures them through sweat (*sanat sudorem provocando*). A very long explanation of the way it used to be administered by the natives, very similar to that of guaiacum, follows. Sarsaparilla being warmer and guaiacum drier by temperament, they are sometimes more efficacious when mixed together.[94]

There is also a short entry on maize. He says that it is named *maiz* after the Indian name, and that the seed has been recently brought to Italy. There is no reference to the fact that it was erroneously called Turkish corn as Mattioli points out. It is described accurately, and no medical use is specified.[95] Cesalpino also mentions the 'Mala insana' (this is what he calls the tomato) which is of two species, both *peregrinae*, one is of the colour of gold (and they call it 'malum aureum'), and the other one is red. It is grown, Cesalpino points out, more for his peculiar aspect than for its use (ad spectaculum potius, quam usum).[96]

Another American plant Cesalpino describes is the sunflower (*helenium indicum*, or *flos solis*). Sunflowers were grown in the botanical garden at Pisa, therefore we know for certain that Cesalpino had seen them. Although he does not mention this fact, he says that the plant could now be seen in our part of the world, and his description is particularly accurate. As to its medicinal faculties, he says, they have not yet been found.[97]

Two plants that he says he has personally seen are American aloe (*aloe indica*) and tobacco (*tornabona*). They were both grown in the Tuscan garden of Bishop Alfonso Tornabuoni, to whom Cesalpino had given one of his herbaria of dried plants. The description of the gigantic flower of the American aloe conveys the sense of marvel that this wonderful vision (*spectaculum pulcherrimum*) must have occasioned the first time it was seen.[98]

Tobacco's entry is under the name of *Tornabona*. Cesalpino informs us that the plant takes its name from the fact that some seeds had been given by Nicolò Tornabuoni, Tuscan ambassador to France, to his uncle Bishop Alfonso Tornabuoni who planted them in his garden. This is one of the first times that the plant appears in an Italian herbal. We know that the cultivation of tobacco, which was of some importance to Tuscan agriculture, was begun in that period

---

[94] Ibid., pp. 219–21.
[95] Ibid., p. 181.
[96] Ibid., p. 211.
[97] Ibid., pp. 499–500.
[98] Ibid., p. 418.

by the Grand Duke Cosimo.[99] Cesalpino states its temperament, deciding that it is dry in the third degree and hot in the first degree. It has many different healing powers, and different uses. Its main use, we are told, is against malignant ulcers, including in the lungs, but it also cures tumours and cancers. As Monardes had mentioned, if a small ball of tobacco (*globules ex ea*) is kept in the mouth, it increases the strength in the body. Cesalpino finally adds that it is said that 'its fumes inebriate' and are a remedy against fatigue.[100] It is interesting to note that Cesalpino, consistently with what he had stated in the Preface of *De plantis*, indicates the medical qualities of plants only when he describes the new species, unknown to the ancient authors.[101]

Another plant Cesalpino refers to is Indian balsam (*balsami arbor*). He reports that a new genus of balsam was recently imported from the West Indies. It was extracted from a tree in an island of New Spain and the natives called it *Xilon*. The Indians used it in fumigations for head-aches or made decoctions with its oil. There is no reference to the use of American balsam as a substitute of Oriental balm, by that time unobtainable.[102]

Cesalpino deals with 'michoacan' (*meciacan*), the purgative drug that was described by Monardes, only in a very short account contained in his *Appendix* to *De plantis*.[103] He reports that Monardes's description coincides with that of *Tamarus vulgaris* which was called 'wild vine' by Dioscorides. He does not refer to the supposed unusual properties of this purge.

Cesalpino's *De plantis* had other features that rendered it very different from Mattioli's *Discorsi*. It was written in Latin, and therefore was meant only for learned physicians and naturalists, and, as far as we know, it had only one edition (1583). It was not given much attention and was not often mentioned by his contemporaries. An aspect that made Mattioli's *Discorsi* so attractive, especially in the editions after 1568, was its beautiful illustrations, which in the case of unknown plants, were obviously of paramount importance. *De plantis*, on the contrary, despite the fact that a set of drawings had been ordered and prepared, came out without illustrations.[104] Therefore Cesalpino did not have any significant influence in regard to the diffusion of new exotic plants. It is also interesting to note that notwithstanding his mentioning so often the vast number of plants that had been discovered, and the fact that he was clearly interested in plants in their own right, he included in his book a very limited number of American species.

---

[99] Antonio Targioni Tozzetti, *Cenni storici sulla introduzione di varie piante nell'agricoltura e orticoltura toscana* (Florence, 1853), pp. 118–27.

[100] Ibid., pp. 344–5.

[101] Cesalpino, *De plantis*, p. VI. See also Chapter 2, p. 101.

[102] Cesalpino, *De plantis*, pp. 60–62.

[103] Andrea Cesalpino, *Appendix*, in Boccone, *Museo di Piante rare*, p. 19.

[104] Cesalpino, *De plantis*, 'Dedication', p. VII. See also Chapter 3, pp. 139–40.

Conclusion

The fact often pointed out by historians who have dealt with the subject, that only very few American medicinal plants were introduced into the pharmacopoeia of the time, was certainly confirmed by the survey of the works I have examined.[105]

One of the reasons put forward to explain this point was the difficulty connected with the fact that a new plant was never accepted as such, but had to be adapted to the complex medical theory of the time.[106] From what I could see, however, this aspect did not seem to constitute a particular problem. The attribution of qualities (hot-cold-dry-moist), based mainly on taste, and the attribution of the relative degrees, in a range between one and four, had always been a matter of controversy, even when known plants were concerned. Also the uncertainty of provenance, the conflicting opinions on identification, the different evaluations of the curative power, the discussions on the ways to compose a recipe and to administer it to a patient, cannot be considered peculiar to New World plants. The above mentioned pharmaceutical reform that was based on the search for and identification of the plants Dioscorides had described, was characterized by the same sort of controversies. The literature of the time provides evidence that all these issues were controversial, and a constant object of debate between physicians. Pointing out the supposed mistakes made by other authors was a constant concern of the scholars of the time.

An aspect that might have had some influence, and is worth taking into consideration, is the fact that the Italian physicians never seemed to take any interest in the medical notions embedded in different cultures. All information about American drugs and the way they were used was gathered and recorded by Europeans and then filtered by learned doctors through Galenic theory. The only exception of a herbal written at the time by a native about the plants of New Spain, is an illustrated book written by the Aztec healer Martino de la Cruz in the Nahuatl language and translated into Latin by Juan Badiano with the title *Libellus de medicinalibus indorum herbis* (1552). This herbal, however, intended as a gift for Charles V, remained unknown until the last century, when it was rediscovered.[107] Teresa Huguet-Termes, in her article about New World *materia medica*, suggests that this herbal might have been seen in manuscript form

---

[105] Guenter B. Risse, 'Transcending Cultural Barriers: The European Reception of Medicinal Plants from the Americas', *Botanical Drugs of the Americas in the Old and New Worlds* (Stuttgart, 1984), pp. 31–42; J. Worth Estes, 'The European reception of the first drugs from the New World', *Pharmacy in History*, 37(1) (1995), pp. 3–23.

[106] Risse, 'Transcending Cultural Barriers', pp. 31–2. Palmer, 'Medical botany in northern Italy'.

[107] The codex is reported and translated by Emily Walcott Emmart, *The Badianus Manuscript (Codex Barberini, Latin 241, Vatican Library): An Aztec Herbal of 1522* (Baltimore, 1992).

by some learned doctors, and thus might have influenced learned medicine.[108] However, no reference either to this manuscript or to the indigenous medical system as a whole is to be found in the works I have examined.

A reason why so few plants attracted the attention of learned medicine was probably inherent in the medical theory at the basis of therapeutics. The major part of remedies it employed were remedies with properties that helped to get rid of what, within the humoral theory, was called the 'peccant humour', that is the humour in excess, which caused an unbalance. Purging, urinating, vomiting, sweating, etc., were the effects that remedies were expected to have. Plants with these properties were already present in the European pharmacopoeia. Therefore, to be considered useful, they had to have some additional property that rendered them different and worthy of note. Michoacan, among purgative drugs, for example, was one of these cases, although, only Castore Durante seems to have emphasized its exceptional qualities.[109] Guaiacum, as Falloppio affirms, besides being hot and dry, had a specific intrinsic power that cured the French disease.

In fact, as pointed out above, Europeans were not in search of new medicinal plants, which is per se a good reason that they did not find them. Rather, they were looking for an easier way to get hold of some precious Oriental drugs, used in food recipes, and sometimes also in medicinal recipes. That is how, for example, chilli pepper was discovered, although it never took the place of pepper as a medicinal substance. Balsam was the most significant example of a very precious drug that was lacking in the European pharmacopoeia, and thus eagerly sought after, until something that could be substituted for it was found, and called Indian balsam. Apart from balsam (which was inserted in the section of 'substitutes'), the only American medicinal plants that entered the official Pharmacopoeia of Tuscany were the three used as a remedy for the French disease. Even if not all the learned doctors agreed that French disease was a new disease, this opinion seemed to have been shared by all the Italian authors of the period under discussion who have dealt with the question. The fact that the disease and its remedy (guaiacum) were brought at the same time from the West Indies, as the first Spanish authors had affirmed, is repeated many times in the Italian herbals of the period, as in the case of Cesalpino and Falloppio. If one asks oneself why only the simples for curing the French disease were introduced into the *Ricettario fiorentino*, a very simple but not unreasonable answer would be

---

[108] She refers also to the so-called Florentine Codex, a collection of writings on Aztec life and costumes, which was held by the Medici. She points out that Aldrovandi, who had heard of it by Mercuriale, had tried to see it. Huguet-Termes, 'New World materia medica', p. 367.

[109] Castore Durante, 'Compendiosa narratio de usu & praxi radicis Mechoacan', in Giles Everard (ed.), *De herba panacea, quam alii tabacum, alii petum aut nicotianam vocant, brevis commentariolus* (Antwerp, 1587), pp. 57–73.

that only a new disease, brought from America, would justify the introduction of new American remedies.

From what I could observe, Italian learned physicians were not against foreign remedies in principle, nor did they reject them on the grounds of the commonly held opinion that God had provided each country with local remedies for its own diseases. Neither can it be maintained that learned medicine, based on classical sources, would not accept remedies because they had not been approved of by the ancient masters. It seems rather that physicians and apothecaries did not find substantial reasons to add other New World remedies to the extant pharmacopoeia.

In Mattioli's and Cesalpino's works a certain number of American plants appear, but only some of them are considered as medicinal plants. For some of them, the authors confess that they do not know of any medicinal properties. Other medicinal plants which are taken into account do not seem to be considered essential. Even as far as the three remedies against *morbus gallicus* are concerned, only guaiacum seems to be appreciated by all the authors I have considered. On china root the opinions were conflicting, and sarsaparilla was usually considered useless, as it could be easily substituted by the local Smilax aspera.

The fact that interest in New World's nature was closely connected with interest in its economic value and commercial exploitation sometimes led to privilege the point of view of merchants and entrepreneurs, which might not always coincide with that of learned physicians. The case of the great success of guaiacum could probably be linked with its commercial history and the economic power of the Fuggers who held the monopoly on its trade. However, it cannot be denied that it was backed up by the approval of almost all European prominent physicians.[110] From a strictly medical point of view, therefore,

---

[110] For the monopoly of guaiacum in the hands of the Fuggers, see Munger, 'Guaiacum, the holy Wood', pp. 209–10. The famous Swiss physician Paracelsus, who was fiercely against the use of guaiacum, accused the physicians of conniving with the Fuggers: 'The spiritual and worldly traders have brought you doctors a wood, and you have taken your medical theory and practice from them'. Quoted ibid., p. 210. See also Claudia Stein, 'The meaning of signs: Diagnosing the French Pox in early modern Augsburg', *Bulletin of the History of Medicine*, 80(4) (2006), pp. 617–47. Particularly interesting is the case of Indian balsam, which was discovered in Santo Domingo by the Spanish entrepreneur Villasante through his Taino wife. The Spanish crown granted him a monopoly for its commercialization, but was challenged by the Spanish doctor Barreda living in the island, who called into question Villasante's credibility and his right to export a drug which was not approved of by Spanish learned physicians. As a consequence, the Spanish crown ordered a series of experiments to ascertain the virtues of Indian balsam. Antonio Barrera, 'Local Herbs, Global Medicines: Commerce, Knowledge, and Commodities in Spanish America', in Paula Findlen and Pamela Smith (eds), *Merchants and Marvels: Commerce, Science, and Art in Early Modern Europe* (New York, 2002), pp. 163–81.

we can but conclude that the plants which were accepted into the European pharmacopoeia were very few, and that their introduction did not have any significant impact on the medical theory and practice of the time.

However, if we now re-insert the question into the more general one, with which we started, of whether the discovery of such a great number of unknown species had some influence on the general understanding of plants, our investigation has perhaps taken us a step forward.

If no change was produced by the few single species that were introduced into the pharmacopoeia, and that were incorporated in the traditional scheme of the Galenic theory, the discovery of the existence of a completely new flora, unknown to the ancient authors, certainly had an impact on the understanding of plants of the time. As long as the vegetable kingdom coincided with the few hundreds of plants known and described by the *antiqui* on the basis of their usefulness to man, God's design was unquestionable, and was before everybody's eyes; plants were a gift of God intended to provide mankind with the remedies it needed. After the discovery of America it became clear that the plants created by God were by far more numerous than those mentioned by the ancient authors. The vegetable kingdom was not known as it was thought to be, and its limits were constantly extending. Cesalpino found a rational way to control that disorderly multitude of plants, which, in his words, 'appals the mind', and channelled it through a new systematization. From a more general perspective, however, the vastness of the unknown species 'appalled the mind' because the certainty that plants existed only for men's use was no longer supported by evidence. Men simply did not know anything yet about the greater part of American flora. In the meantime, however, the new plants could well be included in the herbals of the time. The fact that new species, even if not considered significant from the point of view of their utility, began to appear in the works of prominent physicians of the time is a sign of change in the attitude towards plants. The study of plants did not coincide any more with the study of medicinal plants, and herbals began to distinguish themselves from the more specific pharmacological works.

Chapter 5

The *Nuovo ricettario fiorentino* and the Understanding of Therapy

Right at the end of the fifteenth century something new occurred on the Tuscan medical scene. An official pharmacopoeia, the first to appear in Europe, was published in Florence, under the title *Nuovo ricettario fiorentino*.[1]

Although a pharmacopoeia should, by definition, represent the state of the art of pharmacy and therapy in the place where it is in force, it is difficult to gauge to what extent a prescriptive text reflects reality. Therefore, an examination of the *Ricettario fiorentino* and its various editions over the sixteenth century will be the starting point for our survey of the current views on the therapeutic use of plants, which is the subject of this chapter. In order to evaluate to what extent the *Ricettario* reflected the understanding of therapy of the time, we will then broaden our context and examine a series of other texts.

Leaving out the multifarious world of empirics, quacks, and wise women, which would not provide an easy comparison with an official pharmacopoeia, I will concentrate instead on the works of learned doctors and the circle of intellectuals connected with the university and the court.[2]

The grand dukes themselves and the members of the Medici family are leading characters on the Tuscan medical scene. The activities that the Medici undertook in their workshops and *fonderie*, which often included the preparation of remedies, are recorded in a number of documents and manuscripts that are valuable sources for inquiry.

The books circulating among physicians and in the intellectual circles of the Medici court, which are listed in inventories, such as that of the botanical garden in Pisa, closely connected with the university, and that of the Casino di San Marco, site of Francesco I and his son Antonio's *fonderie*, provide information

---

[1]   *Nuovo Receptario composto dal famosissimo chollegio degli eximii doctori della arte et medicina della inclita cipta di Firenze, Impresso Nella inclyta ciptà di Firenze per la compagnia del Dragho* (1948). This edition bears the date 21 January 1498 according to the Florentine calendar which established the beginning of the year on 25 March. That is why often the date of the first *Ricettario* is recorded as 1499.

[2]   For the remedies sold by charlatans, see David Gentilcore, *Medical Charlatanism in Early Modern Italy* (Oxford, 2006), ch. 6. Gentilcore's analysis shows that the remedies sold by charlatans, which had to be approved and licensed by public authorities, tended to resemble those prescribed by physicians and prepared by apothecaries.

about current cultural interests and the penetration of medical notions and ideas from other milieu and countries.

The First Edition of the *Nuovo ricettario fiorentino*

In the *Prohemio* of the first edition (1498) the purpose of the *Nuovo ricettario fiorentino* is clearly expounded. The request for a new book of recipes, addressed to the *Collegio dei Medici*, came from the *Arte degli speziali*, who were aware of the risks of having to follow different prescriptions, often contradicting one another.[3] The novelty, and a very significant one, was in the idea that it was 'necessary to compile a new book of recipes', which would include in one text all the prescriptions of the ancient *auctores* and would become the authority to which all apothecaries and physicians conformed. Corradi, in his essay which is perhaps still the most complete and accurate account of the first Italian pharmacopoeias, points out that it is not that previously there had been no *receptari* or *antidotari* to which to refer. The problem was rather that there were too many, written by individual authors from different periods and countries, in editions originating from manuscripts that were likely to contain all sorts of errors.[4] This was the first time that a public authority placed itself above all the ancient authors to decide what was best for the common good.

The content of the book is strictly pharmaceutical. All the information contained in it is practical, from the guidelines of what an apothecary shop should be like, of when and how the simples are to be collected and kept, to the various kinds of preparations and recipes. Even the usual information on the 'qualities' (hot, cold, dry and humid, and in which degree) of the various simples is omitted.[5] The first *Ricettario* is made for apothecaries, but written by physicians. It is clear that the intention of the authors was to make sure that the demarcation line between the two professions was maintained. Therapeutic decisions were the prerogative of doctors; apothecaries had to confine themselves to putting into practice the doctors' prescriptions. This is very clear from the scheme of the work and is confirmed by a passage which is placed at the conclusion of the second part of the book. Allowing that some of the recipes may be changed by

---

3   On *Collegio dei Medici*, see Lucia Sandri, 'Il Collegio medico fiorentino e la riforma di Cosimo I: origini e funzioni (secc. XIV–XVI)', *Umanesimo e università in Toscana* (1300–1600), in S.U. Baldassarri et al. (eds), *Umanesimo e università in Toscana* (Florence, 2012), pp. 183–213.

4   Corradi, *Le prime farmacopee*, pp. 3–4.

5   Charles de L'Ecluse, in his translation of the 1550 edition of the *Ricettario*, adds the 'qualities' of each plant. Carolus Clusius, *Antidotarium, sive de componendorum miscendorumque medicamentorum ratione libri tres ex Graecorum, Arabum & recentiorum medicorum scriptis collecti. Nunc vero primum ex Italico sermone Latini facti* (Antwerp, 1561).

physicians according to the needs of the patient, the *Collegio dei Medici* is careful to ensure that 'no ignorant and presumptuous apothecary could presume to be able to proceed by himself, without the expertise of a physician, thus causing infinite scandal; and therefore in this collection of recipes of ours we have not given any indication of what they are for, because we hope that he who has to use it knows it, and he who does not know it will learn it and then will use it appropriately'.[6] In fact, in the *Ricettario* there is no mention of the diseases the recipes are to cure, and this is announced here as a precaution to avoid an improper use of them. The reference to the 'ignorant and presumptuous apothecaries', however, is not repeated in the subsequent editions, which seem to be the result of a greater collaboration between physicians and apothecaries (the authors of the 1597 edition were two physicians and two apothecaries). However, a long appendix, containing the Statutes and Provisions which governed the relations between doctors and apothecaries, was added to these editions.

The *Ricettario* is divided into three books. The first contains the rules concerning an apothecary's shop, which had to be in a suitable place, far from wind, dust, sun, humidity and smoke. The *speziale* had to keep in his shop some books, which were more or less the ones mentioned in the *Prohemio*, with some others. There follows an explanation of when the *speziale* had to collect the herbs, flowers, seeds, roots and bark to be kept in the shop. The instructions are furnished month by month, beginning from March, according to the Florentine calendar, and seem to be based more on the seasonal growth of plants, than on astrological assumptions. How to preserve the vegetable material is then specified. The first book continues with a section on the falsification of some of the substances used in pharmacy, 'not in order that the apothecaries could falsify them, but so that they could recognize those that have been falsified'. There is then a list of the simples that had to be kept in the shop, divided into seeds, fruits, flowers, leaves, woods, bark, roots, juices, gums, bones, entrails and flesh of animals, fats, galls, excrements, precious stones, salts, metals and earths. Finally all the 'electuaries' according to the ancient authors, and the indication of how long they can be kept are noted.

The second book is a pharmacopoeia in the proper sense of the word, divided into eighteen different classes of remedies and their compositions, such as electuaries, syrups, pills, oils, ointments, powders, cataplasms, collyria, etc.

The third book is a miscellany of rules and information about various compositions and the way of preparing them, and ends with a section on weights and measures.

Although the *Nuovo ricettario fiorentino* arose from a new necessity, it does not represent anything particularly new from the point of view of its medical content. Almost all the prescriptions, rules, and recipes are based on the authors

---

6   *Ricettario* 1498, second section, XVIII.

from antiquity, which are quoted in the *Prohemio*. The *Collegio dei Medici* underlines that they did not intend to leave anything out, or add anything to the ancient masters, and everything included in the new book had to be based on them: 'it is necessary to compose a new book of prescriptions neither leaving out nor adding, but rather following the instructions of Mesue, Niccholao, Avicenna, Galeno, Lalmansore, and all the authors who have written ...'.[7]

The Evolution of the *Ricettario*

If we cannot find anything significantly new in the content of the first *Ricettario*, its evolution through the different editions which were published during the sixteenth century, reveals some important changes. Comparing the 1498 edition to that of 1550, we can see that there was a substantial change of direction. The prevalence of Arab medicine gave way to that of Greek and Latin medicine. A series of new medicaments were added, and others excluded. For example, all the preparations based on excrement (*sterchi*) were rejected. This constituted quite a novelty, since all herbals of the time, Mattioli's famous *Discorsi* included, still listed a number of *sterchi* in their recipes. A very significant change was also that the *preparazioni magistrali*, that is to say the preparations of recent or contemporary masters, became much more numerous. In this edition there is a series of recipes by modern, especially Tuscan, physicians, such as Dino del Garbo and Gentile da Foligno.[8] The fact that relatively 'new' remedies were now being taken into account, shows that the ancient authors were no longer the only authority. In the 1550 edition of the *Ricettario*, an American plant, guaiacum, is mentioned for the first time, although there are no recipes for its use.[9] As is explained in the introduction to this edition, a new book of recipes was necessary because 'time had shown new sorts of medicines' and for that reason the Collegio dei Medici was given the task of reviewing the old *Ricettario* adding all that 'had come to light either through the passage of time or for other reasons'.[10]

The 1567 edition contains a further development in the same direction.[11] More '*magistrali*' recipes are included, among which there are preparations by

---

[7]   'essere necessario componere uno nuovo riceptario non passando ne aggiungendo: immo seguendo l ordine di Mesue, Niccholao, Avicenna, Galeno, Lalmansore e tutti gli auctori li quali hanno scripto ...'. *Ricettario* 1498, 'Prohemio'.

[8]   Corradi, comparing the 1498 edition with the 1567 edition, points out that the *preparazioni magistrali* were 69 in 1498 and 123 in 1567 and that 58 new preparations were added. Corradi, *Le prime farmacopee*, p. 50.

[9]   *Ricettario* 1550, pp. 27–8. See above, Chapter 4, p. 129–30.

[10]   *Ricettario* 1550, 'Dedication'.

[11]   The edition of 1567 is not drawn up by the Collegio di Medici, but by 12 'reformers' appointed by Cosimo I.

sixteenth-century physicians, such as Montano (Giambattista Monti), Giovanni da Vico, Berengario da Carpi and Gabriele Falloppio.[12] Three American plants appear, with the recipes for their use.[13] In this edition, moreover, a small change was introduced that seems to lead in a new direction.

Paolo Galluzzi draws attention to the fact that in this edition there is 'a more massive presence of "mineral" drugs and medicaments'.[14] Although the adjective 'massive' does not seem appropriate, a slight shift towards chemistry actually took place. In this edition there is a very brief section on distillation, complemented by one engraving. In the section on the preparation of simple medical substances 'How to distil water by humid furnace' and 'how to distil water by dry furnace' can be found.[15] The emphasis is on the practical side. The description of how to make a furnace for distillation and how to use it is very accurate, and the illustration, complete with a legend, is very detailed. A new entry on 'distilled waters' is also introduced and a small number of recipes containing chemical substances is added. In the classes of medicaments [*distinzioni*] the class of 'composite waters' is for the first time included, which lists eight 'waters', the major part of which are distillates containing chemicals. Another new class, entitled '*Capitelli ovvero Rottorii*' includes four recipes, all of them based on non-organic substances. In the section of 'powders', four new *magistrali* recipes based on chemical substances are listed.[16]

Corradi, unlike Galluzzi, underlines the scarcity of the chemical content of this edition.[17] He points out that one of the few chemical preparations introduced, the water recorded in the class 'Composed waters' as 'Falloppio's alum water' ('*Acqua d'allume del Falloppio*') containing alum and corrosive sublimate, very useful against Gallic ulcers, had been sold for years in the apothecaries' shops while Falloppio was still alive, and he had died five years previously.[18] Corradi also stresses the fact that most recipes containing minerals and metals were only for external use, and that some of them had to be considered as part of the traditional Galenic therapy, as concoctions such as '*lettovario di gemme*', '*diacorallo*', etc. made up of precious stones and coral could certainly not be considered among new chemical recipes. In fact, looking at the simples that appear in the first part of the *Ricettario* of 1567, which are defined as 'those simple medicaments which are most important for the compositions' only about

---

[12]   Corradi records that in the edition of 1498 the *preparazioni magistrali* were 69 and had become 123 in the 1567 edition. Corradi, *Le prime farmacopee*, p. 50.

[13]   See above, Chapter 4, p. 132.

[14]   Galluzzi, *Firenze e la Toscana*, p. 197.

[15]   *Ricettario* 1567, pp. 97–100.

[16]   Ibid., pp. 180–82.

[17]   Corradi, *Le prime farmacopee*, pp. 50–51.

[18]   Ibid. The recipe is in G. Falloppio, *De morbo Gallico, Opera Omnia* (Venice, 1606), vol. 2, p. 195.

10 out of 137 are minerals or metals.[19] Mercury, one of the ingredients often considered fundamental for the cure of French disease, does not appear in this edition or in any other edition of the *Ricettario Fiorentino*.[20] Mercury had always been considered a dangerous substance. Dioscorides puts it in the section about poisons (the sixth book of his *Materia medica*) and Mattioli in his comment on it describes the terrible effects caused by mercury when ingested. He indirectly admits, however, that it was used when he says that 'it always produces a terrible stink on the breath, as we manifestly see in those who use it for the French disease'.[21] Quicksilver appears in some recipes of the *Ricettario*, but only in the form of a precipitate (calcinated mercury) to render it harmless. Cesalpino in his book on 'metals' introduces the idea that its being poisonous is controversial, as recent scholars say that it is not a harmful genus, but it can be, depending on the quantity used.[22] He then describes a preparation with calcinated quicksilver for external use on putrid ulcers caused by the French disease.[23]

Ottaviano Targioni Tozzetti refers to this edition of the *Ricettario* (1567) saying that the 'reformers' had introduced many new preparations, with many drugs and herbs that were not known. Then a certain Filippo da Firenze, a minor friar native of Bagno a Ripoli, he explains, 'thought to oblige the apothecaries and the physicians' providing them with a compendium and an explanation of the simples and drugs used in medicine, including those recently added by the reformers.[24]

The work by Friar Filippo, however, although referring explicitly to the 'reformers' in the title and elsewhere in the text, has little to do with the *Ricettario Fiorentino*.[25] The book is divided into five parts. The first four parts are devoted to medicinal plants (also including 'many plants necessary for human food'), according to a rather disordered criterion. The fifth part is dedicated to

---

[19]   The list is reported by Corradi, *Le prime farmacopee*, p. 35.

[20]   Arrizabalaga, Henderson and French, *The Great Pox*. Luca Ghini, for example, in his *Morbi Gallici curandi ratio perbrevis*, recommended a treatment with mercury, in the most difficult cases of French disease.

[21]   Mattioli, *Discorsi* 1573 edition, p. 935.

[22]   This could be read as a reference to Paracelsus who had declared that a substance could be useful or poisonous depending on the quantity used. This idea is clearly expounded in a booklet by Paracelsus where he confutes the accusations made against him by his detractors. Paracelso, *Contro i falsi medici. Sette autodifese*, ed. Massimo Luigi Bianchi (Bari, 1995).

[23]   Andrea Cesalpino, *De metallicis libri tres* (Rome, 1596), p. 194.

[24]   Ottaviano Targioni Tozzetti, 'Di alcune opere relative alle scienze composte in volgare o in esso tradotte sotto il regno di Cosimo I Granduca di Toscana. Lezione tenuta il 9 agosto 1825', *Atti dell'Imperiale e Reale Accademia della Crusca*, p. 6.

[25]   Filippo da Firenze, *Compendio della faculta de' semplici di tutte quelle cose, che sono piu in uso nell'arte della medicina, con le ordinationi nuovamente fatte da riformatori, poste a' proprii capitoli di detti semplici* (Florence, 1572).

non-organic substances. As far as the sections dedicated to plants are concerned, there is nothing worthy of note except for a particular attention paid, mainly in the first part, to plants usually found in Tuscany. There is some effort at accuracy in the descriptions, the 'temperaments' of plants (hot-cold-dry-moist) and therapeutical indications are sometimes recorded, but Fra Filippo's work does not help apothecaries and physicians any more than the other herbals of the time. Fra Filippo does not seem particularly keen on describing 'not known' plants either, since in his book there is no mention of the three American plants included in the *Ricettario fiorentino* of 1567, not even guaiacum.

The section on mineral substances is very brief (pp. 174–89 of a volume in octavo), and refers mainly to Dioscorides and Mattioli, not adding anything new or especially useful.

Another edition of the *Ricettario*, almost identical to the one of 1567, was published in 1573. The only difference from the previous edition worth noting is that it contains a longer section on distillation, with three engravings instead of one.

The subsequent edition was drawn up by two doctors and two apothecaries appointed by Grand Duke Ferdinando I and appeared in 1597 with a long dedication in which the grand dukes are praised for their knowledge of *materia medica* and their activities connected with medicine. The new edition brought about very marginal changes. As far as the simples listed in the first section are concerned, only a few details were added. No remedies of the previous edition were omitted and sixteen new remedies were included. Of these five are '*magistrali*' and one is a distilled water, but none of them contains mineral ingredients or are worthy of note in any other respect. A new edition of the *Ricettario fiorentino* was issued in 1623, which was, however, identical to that of 1597.

Long after the first edition of the Florentine pharmacopoeia, in the second half of the century, various official pharmacopoeias were compiled and published in other Italian towns. The first one was the *Antidotarium Bononiense*, which appeared in Bologna in 1574 with an introduction by the prominent physician and naturalist Ulisse Aldrovandi.[26] Giovanni Fantuzzi, the biographer of Aldrovandi, recounts the various mishaps and the contrasts between him and the *Collegio dei Medici* that preceded its publication.[27] Aldrovandi is the recognized author, despite the fact that it appeared as the work of the '*Collegio* of physicians and philosophers of the town of Bologna'.

The pharmacopoeia of Bologna has different formal characteristics, compared to the 1574 edition of the Florentine *Ricettario*. The fact that it was the work of a

---

[26]   *Antidotarii Bononiensis sive de usitata ratione componendorum, miscendorumque medicamentorum epitome* (Bologna, 1574).

[27]   Giovanni Fantuzzi, *Memorie della vita di Ulisse Aldrovandi* (Bologna, 1744), pp. 30–36.

single author, and this was the very learned Aldrovandi, is evident, as it is written in Latin, and after each recipe, its therapeutical use is noted. On first sight, as far as the content is concerned, few points are worth noting. The major part of the remedies is from ancient Arab and Greek authors, although there are some which are by recent physicians. The classes of medicaments are more or less the same as those of the *Ricettario fiorentino*, and they are largely based on plants. There does not seem to be a wider use of chemical substances. No special emphasis on distillation is given (there is no specific section), although there are some remedies based on it, especially in the class of oils where there is a distilled 'oleum ex Ligno Guaiaco' which 'ad tumoures gallicos, & gallica ulcera optimum est'.[28]

The survey of the different editions of the *Ricettario fiorentino* in the period between its first publication (1498) and that of 1623 shows a development that brought about some changes. The most significant was that of a certain (but by no means definitive) detachment from Arab medicine and a wider use of remedies devised by recent or contemporary physicians. It cannot be maintained, however, that there was a significant shift in the primary matter on which therapy was based. We know that in the first *Ricettario* about 500 simples were included; of these 375 were vegetable, 68 animal, and 57 mineral substances.[29] This proportion does not seem to have changed significantly. Nor can it be argued that the recipes were significantly altered in their composition or in the way they were prepared and assembled. The only novelty was the use of distillation, which, however, was moderate.

The Penetration of Paracelsus's Ideas into Tuscany

Tracing the development of Florentine pharmacology through the comparison of the various editions of the *Ricettario*, however, only tells part of the story. A prescriptive book is likely to offer only a partial view, leaving out significant aspects which are necessary to complete the picture. Thus we need to look beyond the *Ricettario* and try to take an overall look at the understanding of therapy of the time.

If we look beyond the Florentine pharmacopoeia, Corradi is clearly right in his statement about the scarcity of chemicals in the editions of the second half of the sixteenth and early seventeenth centuries. In fact, this is surprising for more than one reason. First of all, remedies based on minerals, though less numerous than those based on plants, had always existed. They formed a section of Dioscorides's treatise, and were taken up and commented on at length by Mattioli in his *Discorsi*. The teaching of *materia medica* in the

---

28   *Antidotarii Bononiensis*, p. 372.
29   Huguet-Termes, *Approximacion historico-farmacologica*, p. 99.

Universities, although primarily focused on plants, usually included lectures on 'metals'. As far as the *Studio pisano* is concerned, we know from a passage of Benedetto Varchi's *Questione dell'Alchimia*, that Luca Ghini gave a series of lectures on minerals.[30] All sixteenth-century treatises on medicaments had at least one section on minerals, and Andrea Cesalpino, devoted an entire book to them (*De metallicis libri tres*, 1596). Aldrovandi wrote a *Museum Metallicum* which was published posthumously, but that certainly proves his interest in the subject. The famous treatise by the German scholar Georgius Agricola *De re metallica* was translated 'into Tuscan language' in 1563, and the Sienese Vannoccio Biringuccio often refers to it in his book *Pyrotechnia*, which contains a large section on metallurgy.[31]

That so little attention was given to non-organic substances in the *Nuovo ricettario fiorentino* is even more surprising if one considers that throughout Europe, during the second half of the century, therapy based on minerals or 'iatrochemistry' was widely adopted, especially after the spreading of the ideas of the Swiss philosopher, alchemist and physician Paracelsus. Although Paracelsus's ideas and their penetration into Tuscany may appear to be irrelevant to the subject under discussion, I believe they cannot be left out as they are a true novelty on the European medical scene of the time, both from the theoretical and the practical points of view. The emphasis Paracelsus placed on minerals represents a completely new approach to the use of remedies, and the principles according to which he used them called into question the whole Galenic theory. Even when he used medicinal plants, as we will see below, his criteria are completely different from those with which we are familiar. If and how Paracelsus's ideas reached the Medici court, and in what way the circle of physicians responded to them is a necessary part of an investigation into the understanding of the therapy of the time in Tuscany. Moreover, it is important to note how some therapeutic practices and views which are often associated with Paracelsus, such as distillation and the 'doctrine of signatures' had a development of their own and were used and expounded by Italian authors without contradicting the humoral theory.

Paracelsus's medical theories are embedded in a vast, intricate and not always consistent or comprehensible philosophical-religious system. To understand this system as a whole, as the historian and physician Walter Pagel has pointed out, nothing is more misleading than trying to separate the non-scientific from the scientific aspects within his complex vision, pointing out a series of elements that can be seen as steps forward along an imaginary path that leads from ignorance to science.[32] The complexity of his philosophy,

---

[30]   Varchi, *Questione* sull'Alchemia, p. 34.

[31]   Vannoccio Biringuccio, *De la Pyrotechnia (1540)* (Milan, 1977).

[32]   Walter Pagel, *Paracelsus, an Introduction to Philosophical Medicine in the Era of the Renaissance* (Basel and New York, 1958), pp. 50–53.

often obscure to his own contemporaries, however, produced different levels of comprehension and reception. As Debus and Thorndike underline (and Galluzzi after them), Paracelsus's followers adhered sometimes to the whole of his vision, others to parts of it. Some rejected his cosmological-philosophical ideas but supported his medical innovations, or just some of his chemical preparations. Others tried to combine his medical views with the Galenic tradition. Paracelsus's medical ideas, strongly against Galenic principles, were in particular the object of endless controversies and arguments in many European countries, with the possible exception of Italy. The penetration of Paracelsus's ideas into Italy has been long overlooked and has been studied only recently. Neither A.G. Debus in his work The *Chemical Philosophy*, nor Thorndike in the chapter of his *History of Magic* devoted to this subject, nor Walter Pagel in his various studies on Paracelsus mentioned Italy.[33] It has also been pointed out that Paracelsus's thought is founded for a great part on themes and theories already present in earlier magic, mystic, hermetic and alchemical traditions. The hinge of his vision, the idea of a mutual correspondence between macrocosm and microcosm stood also at the centre of Neo-Platonism and its formulation by Marsilio Ficino and was therefore familiar to the circle of Florentine intellectuals.

Since the 1980s, the issue of the diffusion and understanding of Paracelsus's work in Italy has been given some attention and a number of studies on this subject have appeared.[34] Giancarlo Zanier's long and exhaustive essay outlines the penetration and diffusion of Paracelsus's ideas throughout Italy. Particular emphasis is placed on the prominent physicians Leonardo Fioravanti (1518–1588) from Bologna and Tommaso Zefiriele Bovio (1521–1609) from Verona who were familiar with Paracelsian works, but who were interested, in his opinion, almost exclusively in its practical side.[35] He underlines the fact that the work of Paracelsus, in the period under discussion, was accepted as the work of a chemical physician, and author of new *remedia*, not necessarily contrasting

---

[33]   Allen G. Debus, The *Chemical Philosophy: Paracelsian Science and Medicine in the Sixteenth and Seventeenth Centuries* (Mineola, NY, 2002); Thorndike, *A History of Magic*, vol. 5, pp. 617–51; Pagel, *Paracelsus*.

[34]   Giancarlo Zanier, 'La medicina paracelsiana in Italia: aspetti di un'accoglienza particolare', *Rivista di storia della filosofia*, 4 (1985), 627–53; Paolo Galluzzi, 'Motivi paracelsiani nella Toscana di Cosimo II e di Don Antonio dei Medici: Alchimia, medicina 'chimica' e riforma del sapere', in *Scienze, credenze occulte, livelli di cultura* (Florence, 1982); Perifano, *L'Alchimie*; Antonio Clericuzio, 'Chemical Medicine and Paracelsianism in Italy, 1550–1650', in M. Pelling and S. Mandelbrote (eds), *The Practice of Reform in Health, Medicine, and Science, 1500–2000: Essays for Charles Webster* (Aldershot, 2005).

[35]   For Leonardo Fioravanti see William Eamon, *The Professor of Secrets* (Washington, DC, 2010).

with the Galenic doctrine, and that this was consistent with the alchemical Italian tradition, which was essentially a laboratory activity.[36]

Paolo Galluzzi's article, which deals with the spread of Paracelsus's ideas into Tuscany, is particularly interesting in this context. Galluzzi refers to a series of documents which show how the grand dukes and their circle were interested in chemistry and in its medical applications. He draws attention to the figure of Don Antonio, son of Francesco de' Medici and Bianca Cappello, who inherited the Casino di San Marco and its *fonderia*, where he devoted himself to all sorts of alchemical, chemical and medical experiments. A vast number of recipes and 'secrets' deriving from Don Antonio's intense activity are preserved in the Biblioteca Nazionale di Firenze in two manuscripts.

The first is a manuscript in four volumes containing thousands of recipes and 'secrets'.[37] Although there are sections that deal with different subjects, as for instance a manual of alchemy and a treatise on breeding horses, the greater part of them is made up of long collections of medical recipes. They are likely to have been the transcription of pre-existent *ricettari* and do not seem to record any of the laboratory activities performed in the *fonderia*. Paracelsus, even if mentioned in the title, is very seldom referred to, and although a much more accurate examination is required, the remedies described appear to be traditional remedies.

The second manuscript is a small parchment codex of only 26 leaves.[38] The first part of the manuscript (cc. 1–18), which does not have any introduction, contains thirty-five Galenic and chemical recipes sometimes with reference to their authors. The name of Paracelsus is never mentioned, and some comments in the text of the recipes, such as references to their qualities of hot-cold-dry-moist, provide evidence that they belong to the Galenic tradition.[39] The compiler is very careful to stress that all the recipes included have been experimented on, and with regard to 'oil for poison' (*olio da veleno*) he reports a case where the people treated with this oil were cured and 'the others died'.[40] The second part of the codex (cc. 18–26) contains explanations of how and in what dosage the remedies are to be employed.

Galluzzi points out that in these collections no direct Paracelsian influence can be found, and that 'never, not even implicitly was there awareness that it

---

[36]   Zanier, 'La medicina paracelsiana', pp. 631–5.

[37]   BNCF, XVI, 63. *Apparato della Fonderia dell'Illustrissimo et Eccellentissimo Sig. D. Antonio Medici. Nel quale si contiene tutta l'arte spagirica di Teofrasto Paracelso et sue medicine e altri segreti bellissimi.*

[38]   BNCF, Magliab. XV, 140. *Segreti sperimentati dall'Ill.mo et Ecc.mo Sigr. Principe D. Antonio de' Medici nella sua Fonderia del Casino San Marco.*

[39]   c. 21r: 'La qualità di questo olio non sappiamo noi ben discernere se è di proprietà calda o fredda in suo operare'; or c. 22v: 'Si può usare così nelle malattie fredde come nelle calde'.

[40]   c. 21v.

implied a radical break with Galenic medicine'.[41] This assertion, however, is contradicted by a very interesting book of 140 pages printed at the Casino di San Marco in 1604.[42] Galluzzi was probably not aware of this publication, which is now kept in the British Library, and the content of which must have been carefully considered by Don Antonio, as he decided to have it printed. The book, which is entirely devoted to chemical medical recipes, is divided into three parts. The first one entitled 'Of philosophical minerals and metals' deals with mercury, sulphur, salt, nitre, antimony, tin, copper, steel and lead. The second book treats the 'Oils of metals', and the third is about 'Salts of the principal herbs and of some minerals'. Each part contains a substantial number of recipes with the indication of their therapeutical use. All the authors of the preparations, when noted, are contemporary authors such as Gesner, Della Porta, Cardano, Bovio, Andernaco, etc. Some recipes are by Paracelsus. Even if the name of Paracelsus is mentioned only every now and then, the text is full of Paracelsian statements and not only as far as the content is concerned but also in tone and language – for example, when, in the section on mercury, it attacks physicians, philosophers and all other practitioners.[43] Or when a definition of mercury is given that refers to mercury as one of the three primary elements (the Paracelsian *tria prima*) on which both the macrocosm and microcosm are based: 'Mercury is nothing but corporeal spirit made in the entrails of earth, which attracts all the faculties, either animal, vegetable or mineral ... mercury receives all the properties of natural things.'[44] This definition of mercury is per se a proof of adherence to Paracelsus's theories, although there is no direct reference to an anti-Galenic position. In the third book, however, in a section about salt, there is a very explicit statement on the side of Paracelsus, overtly against one of the foundations on which the Galenic theory was based: '... and salt can be solved by salt only ... And so you will know that it is not true that contrary cures contrary, but that like cures like'.[45]

This statement provides evidence that Don Antonio and his circle did not only take into account Paracelsian recipes and 'secrets'. They were also perfectly aware that these recipes and secrets were founded on a theory that was in manifest contradiction with the Galenic principle that a disease is cured by its contrary.

Alfredo Perifano in his book *L'Alchimie à la Cour de Côme Ier de Médicis* draws attention to another important document, which is worth mentioning.

---

[41]   Galluzzi, 'Motivi paracelsiani', p. 36.

[42]   *La fonderia dell'Ill.mo et ecc.mo Sig. Don Antonio Medici Principe di Capistrano – Nella quale si contiene tutta l'arte spagirica di Teofrasto Paracelso, & sue medicine. Et altri segreti bellissimi*. Stampato nel Palazzo del Casino di S. E: Illustrissima (Florence, 1604).

[43]   Ibid., pp. 2–3.

[44]   Ibid., p. 4.

[45]   Ibid., p. 140.

It is the dedicatory letter that the Swiss Paracelsian alchemist and physician Adam von Bodenstein wrote to Cosimo I for his Latin translation of Paracelsus's *De tartaro*.[46] This letter is particularly significant for two reasons. First, because it was written as early as 1563, in a period when we do not have much evidence that Paracelsus's ideas were circulating in Italy. Second, because the letter was an accurate attempt to summarize Paracelsus's theories. Bodenstein states that he had realized that the medical books written up to that moment lacked remedies essential for medicine and that physicians declared some diseases incurable because they did not have the capability or the medicines to cure them; that he was able to solve this problem only after practising the *arte chymica* according to the books of the great physician Paracelsus, who had made such progress in medicine that 'no mortal in all philosophy had known and taught secrets so hidden and difficult'. He then says that he will briefly expound the points on which Paracelsus is in disagreement with the other physicians of the day, and recommends that the grand duke and the other readers should examine these points with the aid of great philosophers who knew how to compose bodies in imitation of nature and de-compose them again, according to the spagyric art, into their primary elements.[47] He proceeds then to illustrate them: the elements on which all things are based, the so-called *tria prima*, sulphur, mercury and salt; the four pillars on which medicine leans: philosophy, astronomy, alchemy and virtue; the theory of macrocosm and microcosm. He then goes on to explain in a rather confused manner how the substances drawn from minerals and metals are the best remedies, and how he himself, following Paracelsus's instructions, had produced a remedy based on gold that could cure in a short time even the gravest form of the French disease. Finally, he traces a brief outline of *De tartaro*.

It is very likely that Cosimo read this dedicatory letter, as he was personally interested in medical matters. Anyway, some of his secretaries would certainly have read it, and, given the peculiarity of its content, would have informed the grand duke. No comment on it has come down to us. In this case, as in others, there is no evidence that Paracelsus's ideas produced any sort of reaction. Contrary to what had occurred in other countries, his views were passed over in silence, without provoking any major controversy.

---

[46] The letter is transcribed in Latin and translated into French by Perifano, *L'Alchimie*, pp. 150–70. See also Alfredo Perifano, 'Considerations autour de la question du Paracelsisme en Italie au XVIe siècle: les dédicaces d'Adam de Bodenstein au Doge de Venise et a Côme Ier de Médicis', *Bibliothèque d'humanisme et Renaissance*, 62 (2000), pp. 49–61.

[47] The term 'spagyric', coined by Paracelsus, refers to the division of bodies into their primary elements, but is very often used in the medical literature of the time to define Paracelsian chemical remedies.

The books kept at the Casino di San Marco, of which an inventory has come down to us, provide further evidence of the fact that Don Antonio was familiar with Paracelsus's theories, and had also followed with great interest the debate that these theories had given rise to in Europe.[48] Paolo Galluzzi examines thoroughly the inventory of Don Antonio's books on this subject, pointing to a series of works by Paracelsus himself and many other books by Paracelsians and anti-Paracelsians.[49]

Another inventory of books which confirms that Paracelsus's work and ideas had spread through Tuscany is that of the books belonging to the botanical garden of Pisa, an institution directly linked with the university.[50] The whole collection of Paracelsian and chemical works, amounting to about eighty books, was acquired in Venice in 1614, at Cosimo II's request.[51]

Plants and Chemistry: Distillation

A practice that is traditionally regarded as characteristic of Paracelsus's medicine is that of distillation. Medicine based on chemistry is usually associated with metals and minerals. Plants are viewed as the traditional part of Galenic/herbal medicine, while iatrochemistry is often considered to be the 'new medicine' based on non-organic elements. However, and this point has not been paid much attention, in the second half of the sixteenth century, the chemical process of distillation was largely applied to plants and had a development which had little to do with adherence to Paracelsian views. Although existing since the beginning of the thirteenth century, it was often regarded as a novel method to obtain more effective medicaments, and new and more sophisticated alembics and apparatus were devised and produced (Figure 5.1).[52]

---

[48]   ASF, Guardaroba 399.

[49]   Galluzzi, 'Motivi paracelsiani' pp. 37–47; Paolo Galluzzi, 'La rinascita della scienza', *La corte, il mare, i mercanti. La rinascita della scienza. Editoria e societa'. Astrologia, magia e alchimia* (Florence, 1980), scheda n. 7.35, p. 202.

[50]   ASP, Università, 531, 5. The inventory of the botanical garden in Pisa is published in C. Sbrana and L. Tongiorgi Tomasi, 'Una biblioteca scientifica a Pisa durante il granducato mediceo: I libri del giardino dei semplici', in *Livorno e Pisa, due città e un territorio* (Pisa, 1980), pp. 556–68. See also Paolo Galluzzi, 'La rinascita della scienza'.

[51]   Galluzzi, 'Motivi paracelsiani', pp. 56–7.

[52]   As we will see below (p. 173) Mattioli regarded distillation as new; Giovanni Stradano included distillation in the series of his *Nova reperta*.

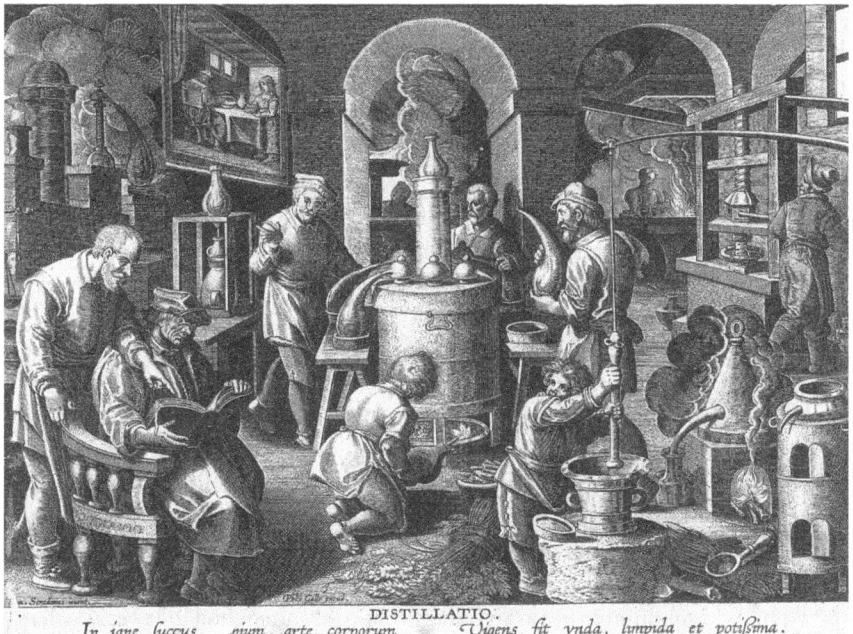

DISTILLATIO.
In igne succus .nium, arte, corporum   Vigens fit vnda, limpida et potißima.

Figure 5.1   Print from Giovanni Stradano's *Nova reperta* (1587–89),
'Distillatio'. London, Wellcome Library

Allen G. Debus provides a survey of chemically prepared medicines from the thirteenth to the sixteenth centuries.[53] He points out that 'interest in alchemy as a source for new medicine' was already present in the works of Roger Bacon (1214–1294), Arnaldo da Villanova (1235–1311), and John of Rupescissa (mid fourteenth century). Alchemy was already strictly associated with medicine by these authors, and the alchemical process most used was that of distillation. Distillation was considered essential to extract the pure virtues ('quintessences') from the gross matter of natural substances and particularly plants, and was largely adopted within the traditional Galenic scheme.[54] This tradition was continued and greatly expanded in the sixteenth century.

The first to devote a book to the distillation of plants was the German physician Hieronymus Brunschwig. His *De arte distillandi*, published in

---

[53]   Debus, *The Chemical Philosophy*, pp. 19–25. See also Robert Multhauf, 'The significance of distillation in Renaissance medical chemistry', *Bulletin of the History of Medicine*, 30 (1956), pp. 329–46; Bruce T. Moran, *Distilling Knowledge: Alchemy, Chemistry and the Scientific Revolution* (Cambridge, MA, 2005).

[54]   Debus, *Chemical Philosophy*, p. 21.

1512, became very popular and had a great influence on the dissemination of this pharmaceutical technique. Conrad Gesner devoted to distillation a long section of his *Thesaurus Euonimy Philiatry, de remediis secretis* (1552–1569) which also included metallic preparations. As Debus points out the process of distillation was applied mainly to medicinal plants: 'This sixteenth century interest in chemicals of medicinal value was to become more closely identified with the herbal tradition; in fact, both Brunschwig's and Gesner's texts can be characterized as chemically modified herbals.'[55]

A completely different use of distillation, applied to plants, was that of waters used to quench iron and render it harder.

In her *The triumph of Vulcan*, Suzanne Butters draws attention to a great number of herbal recipes obtained through distillation which were used as a 'temper' for hardening armour or steel tools. Many of these recipes were included in medical *Compendia* or 'Books of Secrets', and prepared by apothecaries (two recipes were recorded by the Florentine apothecary Stefano Rosselli), and some were experimented on in the ducal workshops. Suzanne Butters provides evidence that both Francesco and his son Antonio produced tempers in their *fonderie* at the Casino di San Marco. One of these herbal tempers was attributed to Cosimo I by Vasari who maintains it was so potent that tools quenched in it became hard enough to work a stone as hard as porphyry. The sculptor Francesco del Tadda was able to execute his porphyry statues, among which was the famous 'Justice' in the Florentine Piazza santa Trinita, using this recipe to harden his tools.[56]

That distillation applied to pharmacy had become a recognized practice and was widely used appears evident from the space devoted to it in the Italian medical literature of the time. As far as the Medici court in particular is concerned, there is evidence that it was one of the procedures largely employed in Cosimo I and his son Francesco I's *fonderie* in the preparation of medicaments. Two reports of Venetian ambassadors quoted above, for example, one concerning Cosimo, and the other Francesco, refer explicitly to their use of distillation:

> [Cosimo] has these simples processed with distilled waters and oils in order to
> experiment with them on different diseases and wounds ... and the place where
> so many admirable things are done is called the *fonderia* of the Duke of Florence,
> where work is continuously carried out with an infinite variety of fires, forges,
> furnaces and alembics ...[57]

55   Ibid., p. 23.
56   Butters, *The Triumph of Vulcan*, pp. 218–39 and 260–67; ch. 9 'A new Florentine recipe for hardening steel tools to work porphyry' (pp. 149–54) discusses the inventor of the recipe. While some authors (Vasari, Bocchi and R. Galluzzi) attribute it to Cosimo I, Benvenuto Cellini and Agostino del Riccio attribute it to Tadda himself.
57   'Relazione di Firenze di Messer Vincenzo Fedeli', pp. 356–7.

[Francesco] takes great delight in working with alembics producing many waters and oils suitable to treat many diseases, and he has a remedy for almost each of them.[58]

A small manuscript of sixteen *carte*, which bears the date 1556, preserved at the Biblioteca Nazionale di Firenze, provides more specific evidence, as it contains the record of some of the medical activities that took place in Duke Cosimo's *fonderia*.[59] The main part of the text deals with the distillation of herbs: 'The true way of making waters and then oils, and how substance of flowers, herbs, roots, seeds, gums and woods is drawn, and the way to preserve it'.[60] It is interesting to note that distillation is here described as 'the true way of curing' and that physicians are accused of hindering it because it would shorten the cure, which would be unprofitable. Doctors use medicaments that cannot cure, it is said, as they let all the useful substances evaporate, giving their patients only the dregs (*fecce*).[61] By distillation only what is good is extracted from plants and used as medicament, and the useless residue is discarded. A practical description of how to extract 'waters' from simples is then provided, recommending the use of a *bain-marie*, and glass vessels, and explaining how to extract oil from these 'waters'. A section is devoted to the preparation of oils, which can be made in various ways, provided they are not made in the way used by the *speziali* of the time, which is 'absolutely detestable, as they do nothing but put the herbs in an infusion or boil them in common oil'.[62] Though the focus is almost exclusively on medicinal plants, there is no prejudice against minerals. Further on it is specified that there will not be a section on minerals and metals in general because the subject is too vast 'as we want to write only about experiments and things that have been proved ....'[63]

It is very likely that the manuscript that has come down to us is only part of a more extensive one, at least in the intention of the compilers. It records only five recipes. The one entitled 'how to make oil for poison', containing thirty-six ingredients, is the famous '*olio di scorpioni*', also called 'oil of the Grand Duke', a very popular remedy mentioned by many doctors of the time and present in many collections of recipes.[64] It was made up of scorpions, gathered when the

---

58   'Relazione del clarissimo messer Andrea Gussoni', p. 226.

59   BNCF, Palatinus 1139, *[Li]bro nel quale si scriveranno esperimenti e cose certe per mano del duca di Fiorenza o vero in sua presentia, ne' ci sara' su cosa che non sia certissima per utile comune* (1556).

60   Ibid., c. 10r.

61   Perifano, *L'alchimie*, p. 51.

62   BNCF, Palatinus 1139, c. 12v.

63   Ibid., c. 13v.

64   The recipe of this oil, mentioned by Giovanni Targioni Tozzetti in his *Selve* (cc. 185–6), is the same reported in the small manuscript of recipes of the Casino di S. Marco.

Sun was in Leo, and fed on fresh basil for fifteen days. The scorpions had to be put (still alive) in very old olive oil. Another thirty-five ingredients were then added. The other recipes include an '*Elisir vitae probatissimo*' prepared by distillation and containing seventy-four ingredients, '*olio da spasmo*' '*matre balsamo*' and '*olio da tutte le gomme seche*'. All these recipes, except for the latter, are also present in the small manuscript (Magliab. XV, 140) where the 'secrets' experimented on by Antonio de Medici at the Casino di S. Marco are listed.

That distillation was a common medical procedure and that Cosimo was personally seen as an expert and producer of remedies is proved by a curious letter of 1559 written by Secretary and Diplomat Lorenzo Pagni to Cosimo I himself, where he tells him of his eye problems and describes in detail his urinary troubles. He specifically requests from the grand duke two remedies (one a distilled 'water' of asparagus, the other not specified) and even asks him directions on how to use them:

> ... often the urine stops, and in great pain I cannot urinate, and in the space of
> half an hour I urinate ten or XII drops with the most intense desire to urinate,
> and this happens to me six or eight times a day. Because Concino himself told me
> that his Excellency [Cosimo] had some water distilled from asparagus which he
> maintains is a perfect thing for the urine, and that he also has I know not what
> good water for the eyes, I beg you that he be kind enough to give me some of both
> and advise me how I have to use them ...[65]

A similar letter which at the same time provides evidence of how chemical recipes were considered effective, how distillation was held in high esteem, and how the members of the grand-ducal family were considered medical advisers, is that written by Caterina De' Ricci, a Dominican Florentine nun who was to become a saint, to Giovanna d'Austria, grand duchess of Tuscany (wife of Francesco I):

> I beg you to send me some distilled steel, the kind that is taken for oppilation;
> a niece of mine, a nun in this monastery, needs to take it, and doctors say that
> ordinary steel is dangerous, and that the distilled one is much surer ...

There are other recipes of oil of scorpions, among which one by Mesue. In this manuscript there is mention of an oil of scorpions by Mattioli, but – it is said – 'this recipe is reported, because it has been experimented'. Corradi comments on an oil of scorpions introduced into the *Ricettario fiorentino* only in 1670 (*Le prime farmacopee*, p. 72). This is the oil of grand duke Francesco I, described in the Relation of Ambassador Gussoni in 1576. Francesco Redi reports that this remedy was so popular that every year in Florence 400 pounds of living scorpions were used to prepare it. Francesco Redi, 'Esperienze intorno alla generazione degli insetti', *Opere* (Milan, 1810), vol. 3, p. 64 (quoted in Corradi).

[65]   ASF, MdP, vol. 479, f. 62 (Medici Archive Project).

And she also wants to know 'how it must be administered, the quantity, the time, which rules must be followed ...'[66]

It should be noted that steel (*acciaro*) does not appear in the *Ricettario fiorentino*.

Evidence that distillation had been already known about and used for a long time, but during the sixteenth century was in a sense rediscovered and its use greatly increased, is furnished by the inventories of pharmacies. We know, for example, that already in the 1370s 'two lead bells for distilling' were in use at the *spezieria* of the Florentine hospital of S. Maria Nuova, and that by the sixteenth century they numbered twenty-two.[67]

In this period new methods of distilling were devised, and a series of new apparatuses for distillation came into use, as can be seen in the illustrations of six different 'furnaces' included by Mattioli in the 1568 edition of his *Discorsi*, where an 'Appendix' on this subject was included.[68] Mattioli does not mention the medieval or contemporary authors who had discussed this subject. In the brief introduction to his 'Appendix' he says that he does not know of any ancient physician who wrote about distillation (they used infusions or decoctions instead), and thus it must be a recent invention. The process is said to have been discovered by alchemists, he adds, but there are also those who maintain that it was found accidentally by a physician while boiling some vegetables. Only the practical side of distillation is taken into account. Mattioli traces a short history of stills and techniques, warning against the use of lead and recommending *bain-maries*. No particular recipes are recorded. He does not seem to attribute much therapeutical value to the 'waters' obtained by distillation. In contrast with Brunschwig and other contemporary physicians, who attributed a much more effective power to distilled plants, he thinks that distillation maintains the taste and the perfume of herbs and flowers, but not their curative virtues as much as decoctions or infusions. Distillation is therefore useful to render medicines more pleasant, if less effective. In Mattioli's opinion, stilled waters are particularly suitable for the '*gentilissime madonne*' who will use them for perfumes and creams. He ends his introduction with a recipe for a beauty cream made out of lemon water. The most notable part of this section is the six very detailed large illustrations of six different furnaces, each with an accurate description.

Much more exhaustive are the writings of the Neapolitan Giambattista Della Porta on this subject. His book *De distillationibus* was first published in

---

[66]   *Le lettere spirituali e familiari di S. Caterina De' Ricci Fiorentina Religiosa domenicana in S. Vincenzo di Prato* (Prato, 1861), pp. 103–104.

[67]   John Henderson, *The Renaissance Hospital: Healing the Body and Healing the Soul* (New Haven, CT, and London, 2006), pp. 294–6.

[68]   Mattioli, 'Appendix', *Discorsi* 1568.

1608, but he had already dedicated the tenth book of the expanded edition of his *Magia naturalis* (1589) to distillation.[69] We know that Della Porta's books were known to the Medici circle, as they appear both in the inventory of the library of the Casino di San Marco in Florence and in that of the botanical garden in Pisa.

In the preface to *De distillationibus*, Della Porta mentions, among others, the grand dukes Cosimo, Francesco and Ferdinando who 'had brought to its apex an art still coarse and imperfect, sparing no diligence, study, labour or expense'.[70] In the same preface, Della Porta mentions the authors who had dealt with the subject before him, including Brunschwig, Gesner and Mattioli. What Mattioli had said about the fact that distilled waters were much more pleasant to ingest is repeated by Della Porta, but with much more convincing arguments. He says that his patients had sometimes to swallow a great quantity of matter that they could not retain and that made them vomit. This problem is avoided by taking a small amount of distillate, so that they are restored to health with a 'light stomach and a sweet mouth'.[71]

I will focus on the section on distillation of *Magia naturalis* (1589) rather than on the book entitled *De distillationibus* (1608) as its date of publication is within the period I am considering, and there are not any fundamental changes between the two works.[72]

Della Porta begins his treatise with a brief proem where he defines distillation as 'an invention of later times, a wonderful thing, to be praised beyond the power of man'.[73] Della Porta examines thoroughly the process of distillation and its medical applications mainly in relation to plants, although a few chapters of the book are devoted to non-organic substances. The book is essentially practical. Distillation for medical purposes was seen as an application of alchemy to pharmacology, and a practical laboratory activity, not easy to perform, but with no theoretical anti-Galenic implications. The only chapter where Della Porta mentions Paracelsus is that 'Of the Extraction of Essences' in which he includes a definition of 'Quintessence': 'The Paracelsians define a Quintessence to be the Form, or Spirit, or Vertue, or Life separated from the gross and elementary impurities of the Body ...'[74]

---

[69] Giambattista Della Porta *Magiae naturalis libri viginti* (Frankfurt, 1591); Giambattista Della Porta, *De distillationibus Libri IX* (Strasbourg, 1609).

[70] Della Porta, *De distillationibus*, 'Proemium', page III.

[71] Ibid.

[72] All quotations are from the anonymous translation into English of *Natural Magick by John Baptista Porta* (London, 1658).

[73] Ibid., 'Proeme', p. 254. In the first chapter, however Della Porta observes: 'yet there is another Kind of Art to be read in Dioscorides, then what we use', and describes how Dioscorides extracted an oil from pitch using a very simple method of distillation. *Natural Magick*, p. 254.

[74] Ibid., p. 267.

Always referring to quintessences, Della Porta adds: 'for being separated from the grossness of their Bodies, they become spiritual, and put forth their Power more effectually and strongly when they are freed from them.'[75]

In Paracelsus and his followers the separation of the pure from the impure by means of fire, i.e. distillation, was usually associated with the notion, in contrast with the Galenic theory, that like cures like. The remedy for an organ affected by a disease had to be sought in the essence of something that had a correspondence with the diseased organ, that is to say not contrary, but similar to it. This idea does not appear in Della Porta's writings on distillation. The theoretical side of it, the attempt to separate what is pure from the gross matter, is not seen by Della Porta as contradicting current medical ideas, and could be perfectly adapted to humoral theory.

What is interesting here, however, is that Della Porta uses distillation to support one of the more controversial points of the humoral theory, that of identifying, for each medicinal herb, its *facultates* or qualities. As is well known, the qualities attributed to a simple were 'hot', 'cold', 'moist' and 'dry', and usually assigned in pairs, so that a plant could be hot and dry, hot and moist, cold and dry or cold and moist. Each quality, moreover, was assigned a grade, from one to four, so that a plant could be, for example, hot in the second, and dry in the first degree. The qualities of hot, cold, dry and moist also characterized the four humours that constituted the body (blood, phlegm, yellow bile or choler, and black bile or melancholy) and represented the link with the universe at large as they also characterized the Aristotelian four elements that constituted the physical world (earth, water, air and fire).[76]

Traditionally, the quality of a plant and its degree were decided by tasting it. Bitterness, for instance, was indicative of a hot quality, and the degree was decided according to its intensity. The attribution of the qualities to simples, being based on a hardly definable sense like taste, had always been controversial. Many medical texts discussed the question, explaining and adding new considerations and precepts. Authors of herbals usually referred to what the writers from antiquity had said, relying on their own taste when the qualities of a new exotic plant had to be determined. Della Porta was clearly unconvinced by this method, and was in search of new parameters. He was certain that they could be found through the chemical process of distillation, as he declares in the 'Proeme' of the book 'Of distillation' of his *Magia Naturalis*: 'We can by Chymical Instruments, search out the Virtues of Plants, and better then the ancients could do by tasting them.'[77]

---

[75]   Ibid.

[76]   Wear, *Knowledge and Practice*, pp. 37–9.

[77]   Della Porta, *Natural Magick*, 'Proeme' of the Tenth book, 'Of distillation', p. 254.

In the twenty-first and last chapter, 'How to find out the Virtues of Plants', he returns to this argument, explaining:

> There are no surer Searchers out of the Virtues of the Plants, then our Hands and Eyes. The Taste is more fallible: for, if in Distillation, the hottest parts evaporate first, we may conclude, that it consisteth of hot and thin parts: and so of the rest. You may easily know by the Separation of the elements, whether a plant has more of Fire, or Water, or Earth, by weighing the Plant first: then afterward, when the Water and Oil are extracted, weighing the Foeces, and by their proportion you may judge the degrees of each Element in the Composition of it, and from thence of their Qualities. But the narrow limits of this book will not give me leave to expatiate further on this Subject ...[78]

Here Della Porta maintains that hands and eyes are much more reliable than taste. And for hands he does not mean touch, but the manual art of chemistry. Although the process used to identify the virtues of plants is not very clear, it is evident that Della Porta proposes a 'scientific' method in place of the traditional one. It is interesting to note that he refers to the eyes as the other 'sure searchers out of the virtues of plants', since, as will be seen, he will propose the so-called 'doctrine of signatures' as another effective, though completely different method to determine the qualities of plants.

Plants and Therapy in Paracelsus's *Herbarius*

Although Paracelsian medicine was mainly associated with mineral substances and the use of distillation, Paracelsus by no means excluded the use of plants in therapy. What is interesting in this context is to see how medicinal plants could be used on the basis of principles different from those of the traditional humoral theory. The only work by Paracelsus on this subject that has come down to us is his *Herbarius*.[79] The title should not mislead us. It is a very small treatise describing the virtues and uses of just six medicinal substances, only three of which are actually plants. In fact, only hellebore, persicaria, and angelic thistle are taken into account. The *Herbarius*, moreover, is probably nothing more than a collection of notes and fragments put together and published (Strasburg 1570) in a rather casual order.[80] Despite its brevity and lack of system, however,

---

[78]   Ibid., p. 279.

[79]   *The Herbarius of Theophrastus* [Paracelsus], *Concerning the Powers of the Herbs, Roots, Seeds, Etc. of the Native Land and Realm of Germany* has been translated by Moran in 'The *Herbarius* of Paracelsus', pp. 99–127.

[80]   Ibid., p. 99.

the content is more than sufficient to furnish a perfect picture of what the use of plants in therapy could mean in a Paracelsian vision.

It is worthwhile to look briefly at the 'Prologue', which accounts for the title and contains some attacks on the medical theory of the time, so typical of Paracelsus, and in this case especially centred on what he calls the 'Italian doctrine'.[81] He deprecates the fact that German medicines, although much better than any other medicines, are despised by physicians who seem to prefer those coming from other European countries, or even from far-off lands. This, he argues:

> is the fault of Italy, the mother of ignorance and inexperience. For the Italians saw to it that the Germans thought nothing of their own plants, but rather took everything from Italy itself or from beyond the sea. This they realized was to their own advantage and thus they pursued it, not out of brotherly love to be sure, which in them has wholly or almost entirely grown cold.[82]

Each land, Paracelsus continues, 'gives birth to its own special kind of sickness, its own medicine and its own physician. For this reason the Italian seduction must be rooted out, like a tree that bears no fruit.' He laughs at those German doctors 'who want to practise medicine in Italian and know nothing in German. They want to prepare medicines from across the seas while there are better medicines to be found in front of their noses in their own gardens.'[83] Paracelsus continues by saying that in his book, a herbarium, he will report what he has learnt 'about plants, roots, seeds and leaves'; that other German writers have described herbs and plants in books, but 'their work is like the coat of a beggar, patched together from all sorts of things' ... and goes on to attack them violently: 'All these raving sorts, these seducers, false informers, and teachers of medicine should not concern me. They are really of use to no one except to the printers of books who get rich and very fat in their kitchen ...'.[84]

These are but a few expressions of Paracelsus's animosity towards those whom he scornfully calls 'the doctors of humours'. Paracelsus then declares that he has resolved to supply plant recipes that can really offer relief to those who are suffering. To do so he will write how '*simplicia* are not sufficient in their qualities alone, but [also] in their *arcana*. On that account, there follows a double procedure: on the one hand, having to do with qualities, on the other, with *arcana*.'[85]

---

[81]　*The Herbarius*, 'Prologue', p. 104.
[82]　Ibid.
[83]　Ibid.
[84]　Ibid., p. 105.
[85]　Ibid.

He then introduces a system of therapy based on a constant interweaving of forces and influences between astral spirits and terrestrial elements. Paracelsus is very keen to point out that these forces and influences operate according to the laws of nature, and that they have nothing to do with magic. A good physician is one who acquires the capacity to recognize them, which is attainable only through experience. Nothing can be learned from the Greek, Arabic or Hebrew texts: one has to be able to read the Book of Nature.

But let us look briefly at how Paracelsus actually deals with a specific plant and its therapeutical uses. Among the three plants treated in the *Herbarius*, 'persicaria' is perhaps the best example, as, despite some inconsistencies and repetitions, the section on this plant seems to be the most orderly and systematic.[86]

'Persicaria', Paracelsus informs us, 'is a plant useful for treating the open wounds of men and beasts.' He then proceeds to explain how it must be employed:

> one takes the plant and draws it through a fresh stream. Thereafter, one lays it on that [injury] which one wishes to heal, and this for as long as it would take to eat half an egg. Then one buries the plant in a moist place so that it will decay. In this way, the injury is made healthy.

There are people, he adds, who make a cross over the wound or pray. These things, however, are unnecessary, as 'they do not belong to the cure, for there is [in the plant] an action which works naturally, not superstitiously and magically. Therefore, 'such phantasies should be abandoned and one should proceed according to the order of nature ...'. 'Here is nature that operates, not magic', he underlines, 'persicaria operates on the flesh in the same way as the magnet affects the compass needle. But understand that there must first be a unity that is a concordance between the flesh of the injury and this plant.' But why, one wonders, after having applied it on the wound, the plant should be buried? For this also, Paracelsus explains, 'there is a natural reason'. It is because persicaria 'is supposed to heal injuries. That is its obliged *labor* at which it works until it is entirely decomposed. Then its *labor* is completed and the injury healed. For that reason, if the plant takes longer to decay, the longer it takes to heal.'[87] This, then, is what a 'concordance between the flesh of the injury and persicaria' means.

---

86   Ibid., 'Concerning persicaria', pp. 110–13.
87   Ibid., p. 112.

The Doctrine of Signatures

If the Paracelsian therapeutic use of plants expounded above does not seem to have had many followers among Italian physicians, another theory founded on the medical transposition of the idea of a correspondence between macrocosm and microcosm had a large following in the second half of the sixteenth century. It was the so-called doctrine of signatures based on the assumption that the outer features of things, if read by a man of knowledge and experience, are signs of their inner nature.[88] Even if this doctrine is often associated with Paracelsus, who was one of its supporters, its systematic exposition and application to plants is not to be found in any of Paracelsus's works.

That the traits of a face revealed the inner qualities and vices of men was an ancient notion, as Giambattista Della Porta notes in his *Phisiognomonia*, the famous book he devoted to this subject.[89] In the case of plants, however, the correspondence between the external aspect and the inner qualities was a recent discovery and had an evident medical connotation. While the inner qualities of men had a series of implications, usually being 'good' or 'bad' from a moral and social point of view, the inner qualities of plants were strictly connected with therapy. The examples used to illustrate this theory are countless, since many different aspects of a plant, such as the shape of its roots, leaves or flowers, its colour, or even its smell can be the signs that reveal its qualities. Leaves which are similar to the claws of a scorpion are a remedy against a scorpion's bite, a root vaguely resembling a heart will be good for heart diseases, a yellow flower cures an excess of yellow bile, and so on. Paracelsus was an advocate of this theory, although he did not write at length on this subject. In his *De natura rerum*, there is an entire book ('De signatura rerum naturalium'), where he expounds extensively the theory of signatures, although he does not refer to plants in particular. Like all kinds of knowledge, the science of signatures is a consequence of original sin, since Adam, in the Garden of Eden, was not signed (*unbezeichnet*) until he had 'fallen into nature', which does not leave anything not signed).[90] All natural objects are signed; chiromancy and physiognomy are the sciences through which one can learn to read the signs that the stars have impressed on the faces of men, or on the lines of their hands, and that reveal the secret of the 'inner man'.[91]

We find some examples of the doctrine of signatures applied to plants in other works of Paracelsus, mainly in his medical works. Often quoted among these

---

[88]   On the doctrine of signatures see: Michel Foucault, *Le mots et les choses* (Paris, 1966), ch. 2; Massimo Luigi Bianchi, *Signatura rerum: Segni, magia e conoscenza da Paracelso a Leibnitz* (Rome, 1987); Giorgio Agamben, *Signatura rerum: Sul Metodo* (Torino, 2008).

[89]   Giambattista Della Porta, *Physiognomonia* (Vico Equense, 1586).

[90]   Agamben, *Signatura rerum*, p. 35.

[91]   Ibid., p. 3.

examples are *satyrion* which has the shape of men's *pudenda* and can therefore restore lost virility, eufrasia which has a mark in the shape of an eye and can cure eye diseases, and thistle that being thorny and sharp can cure sharp pains.[92] All natural things are 'signed', but as far as plants are concerned, the interpretation of signs becomes one and the same with medical knowledge, and the science of therapy. The physician aware of the connection between the stars and the natural things must have the capacity to interpret the signs and, as we have seen in the example of persicaria, recognize the correspondence between the plant and the body, and operate according to 'nature'.

The first to expound the doctrine of signs applied to plants in a systematic way, in order to be able to recognize their therapeutical virtues was, once again, Giambattista Della Porta. Della Porta had already written his *Physiognomonia*, which explained how the outer features of men's faces and bodies revealed their inner nature. In *Phytognomonica* (1588), he starts from the same assumptions, transposing them to plants. In the 'proemium' and in the first section of the book, where he outlines how the idea for writing this book took shape, and deals with the subject from a theoretical point of view, he never mentions Paracelsus, and does not use the term 'signatura'.[93] He mentions, instead, many ancient sources, from Pliny, Marcello Empirico, Theofrastus, and Dioscorides to the hermetic and astrological treatises, and refers to the science of signs as a personal discovery.[94] He states beforehand that one of the noblest tasks of philosophy is to investigate the hidden things of nature and that, as Herophilus has maintained, only some of the powers of plants can be numbered, the major part being unknown;[95] the power of God is in fact immeasurable. And he furnishes examples of the miraculous virtues of some herbs discovered by ancient authors. Why then, he argues, should we not continue to investigate and search for other unknown plant virtues? Even animals recognize and use plant virtues according to their needs. Often, Della Porta continues, he has noticed that when a plant is fine, its scent sweet and its colour lovely, so that 'it seems to reflect a divine splendour and, like a magnet it urges the eyes of spectators to contemplate the magnificence of nature, it will also have powers which are beneficial to men and of great utility to doctors'.[96] On the contrary, when a plant is repellent to the eye, it will usually have bad inner qualities.

He has also noticed, he says, that usually two plants similar in aspect had similar virtues, and plants which are very different from one another, usually

---

[92]   Bianchi, *Signatura*, p. 64.

[93]   Della Porta, *Phytognomonica octo libris contenta. In quibus nova, facillimaque affertur methodus, qua plantarum, animalium, metallorum, rerumquedenique omnium ex prima extimae faciei inspectione quivis abditas vires assequatur* (Naples, 1588).

[94]   Bianchi, *Signatura*, pp. 90–92.

[95]   Della Porta, *Phytognomonica*, 'Proemium', p. I.

[96]   Ibid., p. V.

provide different remedies. On these grounds, and considering the fact that the outer features of men corresponded to their inner qualities, Della Porta had come to wonder if the same assumption could be applied to plants. He then undertook research (*nihil inexploratum relinquendo*), comparing what he found with what was written on the medical treatises, to see if new qualities of plants could be discovered; and he achieved great results. He underlines the fact that everything included in this book has been accurately examined. He is not going to repeat the plant qualities of hot, cold, dry and moist as they were described in the books of other philosophers and physicians, but only what he had found personally.[97] Once again, as in his writings about distillation, Della Porta seems to refer to the Galenic qualities of hot, cold, moist and dry, traditionally attributed to medicinal plants, as something that must be reconsidered.

This book, Della Porta says at the end of the Proemium, is a very arduous and difficult undertaking, never attempted before.[98] It is clear that Della Porta refers to the whole thing as a personal discovery. Actually, although Paracelsus had mentioned, in passing, that the outer qualities of plants corresponded to their inner therapeutical virtues, this is the first time that the 'science of signatures' applied to plants was expounded in a systematic pharmacological work.

In the first book of *Phytognomonica* Della Porta tells how the ancient writers proceeded to find the qualities of plants on the basis of taste.[99] In the following chapter he points out the contradictions and inaccuracies into which those physicians who confine themselves to relying on what the ancient writers have said, run. Della Porta constantly refers to his *Physiognomica* pointing out similarities and differences between the investigation of the moral character of men through their outer aspect, and that of the *vires* of plants through their external *signa*. The outer signs will be interpreted by means of similitude, which is a 'depicted discourse' (*pictus sermo*) or a 'speaking picture' (*pictura loquens*). Similitude is how nature expresses itself, representing on plants the parts of the body or the diseases corresponding to their qualities.[100]

The last chapter (22) of the first book ('Quid sit phytognomonica') summarizes in a very clear way the terms of the subject. Della Porta first gives us a definition of the theory of signs applied to plants: 'Phitognomonia is a method for investigating the forces of plants through the signs, mobile or fixed, that appear on a part of them or in their life.'[101] Then he explains each part of it. He speaks of '*vires*' (forces) because both good qualities (*virtutes*) and bad qualities (*vitia*) are considered. He says '*partis*' and '*vitae*' because there is not

---

[97] Ibid., p. VII.

[98] Ibid., p. VIII.

[99] Ibid., Book 1, ch. 3, p. 6.

[100] Bianchi, *Signatura*, p. 92.

[101] 'Est autem Phytognomonica virium plantarum vestigandi methodus, ex partis & vitae, quae insunt signis fixis, & mobilibus.'

only a similarity between the parts of the plant and that of the human body and its diseases, but also the life of the plant, i.e. the way of germinating, bearing fruit, its longevity, etc. has to be taken into account. He says that some signs are 'mobile' and some others 'fixed', because some of the signs, such as seeds, roots and flowers are always the same, while others such as smell, colour, taste and shape depend on climate, soil, temperature and cultivation.

Another book, dealing with plants from the same point of view, but wider in scope as it includes Galenic and chemical recipes, remedies based on distillation, astrological considerations and much more, is Leonhart Thurneysser's *Historia sive descriptio plantarum*.[102] Thurneysser was a Swiss Paracelsian alchemist-physician who travelled all over Europe seeking patronage of various sovereigns of the time. Grand Duke Ferdinando welcomed him at his court where Thurneysser, in his presence, transmuted an iron nail into a golden. This episode had an international resonance.[103]

The *Historia sive descriptio plantarum* was certainly known and appreciated by the Medici. The edition of 1578 was published with the privilege of Francesco I, and the book appears in the inventory of the books of Don Antonio at the Casino di San Marco. That it was held in great esteem by the Medici is proven by the fact that they ordered a translation into Italian, and also a *Compendio* written by the Florentine chaplain Jacopo Carpi, which are preserved at the Biblioteca Nazionale of Florence in manuscript form.[104]

When one opens Thurneysser's herbal, one is at once impressed by the very complex and sophisticated layout of the book. The page is divided into two columns with a number of boxes written in smaller characters illustrating the various aspects being considered, while the margins are crammed with alchemical symbols. Each plant is accurately drawn within an ornamental frame, and there are other small illustrations in the various boxes. Some diagrams are added, to indicate the best astrological period under which the plant should be gathered. The German part of the edition extant in the British

---

[102] Leonhart Thurneysser, *Historia sive descriptio plantarum omnium, tam domesticarum, quam exoticarum* (Berlin, 1578). Both the copy kept at the British Library and that kept in the BNCF are published with the privilege of Francesco I of Tuscany.

[103] *Firenze e la Toscana*, p. 202. The golden nail was preserved in the 'stipo di Ferdinando' in the niche of the Tribuna degli Uffizi. Unfortunately it has not come down to us. John Evelyn saw the nail when in Florence in 1644 and commented on it in his *Diary*: 'An yron nayle, one halfe whereof being converted into gold by one Thornheuser, a German chymist. looked up as a great rarity, but it plainly appeared to have been soldered together'. John Evelyn, *Diary and Correspondence*, ed. William Bray (London, 1906), p. 81. Quoted in Partington, *A History of Chemistry*, vol. 2, p. 153.

[104] BNCF, Magliab. XIV, 8 and Magliab. XIV, 9.

Library, moreover, is coloured by hand.[105] One soon realizes, however, that the complexity of the form of the book is consistent with the complexity of its content, and represents an effort of clarity. To give an idea of the scope of the book it is worth quoting the 'subtitle' that Iacopo Carpi writes on the frontispiece of his manuscript:

> Work divided according to each member of the human body, by Lionardo Tornesseiro from Basel, Ordinary Physician of the Elector of Brandenburg.

> On the names, genera, and occult sympathy or correspondence with the human body, by means of signatures, and with heavenly bodies (constellations), of roots, woods, herbs, flowers, fruits and seeds, quality, temperament, birth, form, nature, virtue and efficacy; with the addition of the very ingenious division of the parts of the noble essence and of the purest prime matter of the subtle spirits, so that through their signatures and with the help of God it is easy to establish a rule for the cure of any disease or illness affecting each member of the human body, both internal and external ...[106]

Thurneysser's pharmaceutical treatise on plants is based, as he himself declares, on Paracelsus's ideas, and also on ancient and recent authors, and his own experience. Alchemy, astrology, doctrine of signatures, distillation and Galenic preparations are all present. The book, which the author intended to be followed by nine other books, deals only with plants of the family *umbelliferae*. It is interesting to note that as there are no parts of these plants that bear a resemblance to an organ of the human body, the whole plant is considered as a *signatura* of the whole human body:

> erect and tall is the species that has a single stem the top of which is ornate with a white umbrella of flowers; and it must be understood that the white head of flowers represents the disposition of the parts of the male human brain, the capital or mouth from where the flowers and stamen come out represents the disposition of the liver; the major leaves represent the lungs; the minor the spleen; the root the stomach ...[107]

The passage goes on to describe very accurately the 'correspondences' with all the other interior parts, and then the outer parts of the human body.

---

[105] The *Historia sive descriptione plantarum* kept in the British library (Berlin 1587) contains both the German and the Latin versions.

[106] Magliab. XIV, 8, frontispiece.

[107] Ibid., c. 1v.

Another pharmacological book in which the doctrine of signatures is expounded is the *Basilica Chymica* (1609) by Oswald Croll. It had a remarkable success, and it is curious that it does not appear in the inventory of the Casino di San Marco. We know, however that it was known to Tuscan physicians and very probably also to the Medici circle as it is listed in the inventory of books belonging to the botanical garden of Pisa. The book is divided into three parts: a long theoretical preface, a chemical pharmacopoeia and a treatise on signatures.

The 'Preface to the readers' where Croll refers to Paracelsus and Della Porta as his predecessors, is a vivid and eloquent *summa* of the theory in which the doctrine of signatures finds its place.[108] It opens with an attack on the herbalists of his time who 'are ignorant of the internal form, knowing only the matter, substance, and corporeity of herbs', and who:

> are at length wholly occupied about the exterior bitter rind: hence it is that many
> nomenclatures of herbs are found, which magnificently describe the receptacles,
> habitations, and external vestments of plants ... But the foot-steps of the invisible
> God in the creatures, the shadow and image of the creator impressed in the
> creatures, or that internal force, and occult virtue of operation ... is by the prudent
> physician only inquired into ...

And this is because 'in all external things the exterior case is only the receptacle of innate and inherent virtues, infused by God, as the soul into the human body'. '... herbs magically by their signatures bespeak the physician's thorough introspection, and to him by similitude manifest their interiors, concealed in the occult silence of nature'. In the case of herbs, the interpretation of the outer signs is strictly connected with their medical virtues and therefore, as in Paracelsus, the physician is called on to perform a crucial role. 'All herbs, flowers, trees, and other things which proceed out of the Earth, are books, and magick signs, communicated to us by the immense mercy of God, which signs are our medicine.' The physician therefore had to acquire the ability to read these 'books', which are the vessels of true medicine.

The 'Preface' goes on to describe in Paracelsian terms the link between astral and earthly dimensions, explaining that 'every herb is a terrene star growing towards heaven; and every individual star is a celestial herb in spiritual form. The seed is an example of how hidden things can all be comprised in a single unit: 'In the seed the whole tree is latent, viz. root, trunk, boughs, leaves and fruit.' Hence 'the seed is a tree complicate, the tree is a seed unfolded ... Unity is

---

[108] Oswald Croll, *Basilica Chymica*, 'Tractatus novus de signaturis rerum internis': English translation: *A Treatise of Oswaldus Crollius of Signatures of Internal Things; or a True and Lively Anatomy of the Greater and Lesser World* (London, 1669).

a complicate number, number is an unfolded unity' and, by analogy, he comes to the conclusion that 'the world (as I may say) is God unfolded'.

Debus underlines the fact that it is not easy to see a continuity of the theoretical ideas expressed in Croll's preface and the practical part of his works dedicated to the chemical pharmacopoeia.[109] The section on signatures, however, is a pharmacological application of the theory expounded in his preface. The science of signatures needed to be supported by a theoretical framework, outside which it was hardly sustainable. Tradition and common sense easily combined to reject it, as the herbalist Dodoens wrote in 1583: 'the doctrine of the Signatures of Plants has received the authority of no ancient writer who is held in any esteem: moreover it is so changeable and uncertain that, as far as science and learning is concerned, it seems absolutely unworthy of acceptance.'[110]

Conclusion

The different views on the use of medicinal plants expressed or implied in the sources examined above reveal that the *Nuovo ricettario fiorentino* offered only a partial view. Although it represented the current fundamental tenets of therapy, it furnished only a simplistic picture of the medical scene of the period. The need for order and unity on the basis of which it was first required could not but leave out all that might be the object of controversy, and what was new was accepted very cautiously. Its development, which marks some significant changes up to the 1560s (editions of 1499, 1550, 1567), was subsequently arrested. There were very marginal changes in the edition of 1597 compared with that of 1567, and that of 1623 was identical. This can be partially explained by the fact that the editions from 1567 onward were no longer drawn up by the Collegio dei Medici, but by a group of compilers directly appointed by the grand duke. It seems, therefore, that a stricter surveillance by the state resulted in greater caution in innovation. This is unsurprising from a political point of view, but it is in contrast to the fact that all new ideas and new therapies were accepted and sometimes even practised by the grand dukes themselves and members of their family and court.

Some of the texts and documents discussed in this chapter provide evidence that chemical preparations were known and more widely used than can be inferred from the Florentine pharmacopoeia. Certainly there is an apparent discrepancy between the *Ricettari* of 1597 and 1623 and the book entirely devoted to chemical preparations published by Antonio de' Medici at the

---

[109] Debus, *The Chemical Philosophy*, p. 124.

[110] Rembert Dodoens, *Stirpium historiae pemptades sex sive libri XXX*, Book I, ch. 11 (Antwerp, 1583). Quoted and translated by Arber, *Herbals*, p. 211.

Casino di San Marco in 1604. Even distillation, which was praised as 'la nuova via del curare' by the compiler of the manuscript from the *fonderia* of Cosimo I as early as 1556 was not given the importance one would expect to find in the *Ricettario*.

Our research shows that in the second half of the sixteenth century not only Paracelsian remedies, but also Paracelsian medical theories were known in Tuscany. Evidence of this is furnished by the great number of books by Paracelsus and by Paracelsians that appear in the inventory of the botanical garden in Pisa, and in that of the Casino di San Marco. Further evidence is provided by Adam von Bodenstein's long dedicatory letter of 1563 to Cosimo I, in which the medical ideas of Paracelsus are expounded at length. If Cosimo read Bodenstein's dedicatory letter, which is probable, given his great interest in medical matters, and circulated the book among the doctors of his circle, then evidently Paracelsus's ideas, certainly revolutionary in the field of medicine, did not cause a great sensation. We know that in the rest of Europe Paracelsus's theories had caused fierce controversies. In Italy, however, although Paracelsus's theories were known, they were taken into account quietly, making no particular stir. In other words, the fact that they challenged the traditional Galenic theory was not seen as something outrageous. This appears to reverse the current idea that Paracelsus's theories did not penetrate into the community of Italian learned doctors because their 'humanism' rendered them impermeable to any theory contrary to the humoral tradition.[111] If we assume that Paracelsus's ideas *did* penetrate into Italy and were known to learned physicians, and yet did not provoke any particular debate, we are led to the opposite conclusion that the humoral theory was no longer considered as an absolute authority.

This by no means implies a direct challenge to the theory of humours. All the prominent physicians of the time such as Mattioli, Falloppio, Cesalpino and Mercuriale refer to it as the basis of therapy in all their writings. Some practices or views such as distillation and the doctrine of signatures which have been often regarded as 'Paracelsian' and had a certain contiguity with actual Paracelsian methods or theories, could be shared and put into practice without contradicting the principles of the Galenic theory.

Distillation played a leading role in the second half of the sixteenth century and, although a characteristic method of Paracelsian therapy, was largely applied to herbal medicine, and partially transformed the way of using plants in medicinal preparations. It was considered perfectly compatible with traditional medical theory, and largely employed by non-paracelsians. As seen above, Della Porta maintains that the qualities of simples of hot, cold, dry and moist are better valued through distillation than by taste as the ancient authors did, but the theory underlying the whole system is not questioned. Letters, books, and collections

---

[111] Clericuzio, 'Chemical Medicine and Paracelsianism', p. 60.

of recipes of the time offer ample evidence of its use in Tuscany for remedies based on medicinal herbs, and, to a lesser degree, on chemical substances.

In contrast to distillation, which could be practised as a 'laboratory activity' without any theoretical implications, the doctrine of signatures was unsustainable, and even incomprehensible without a belief in a system of correspondences and sympathies between each part of the physical world. This belief was characteristic of the medical thought of Paracelsus as we have seen in his use of medicinal plants in therapy. The same belief in a macrocosm constantly mirrored by a microcosm, however, was shared by Della Porta who wrote an entire book on the signatures of plants, without referring to Paracelsus and without contradicting the humoral theory. Once the clever doctor had discovered the medical virtues hidden behind the outer aspect of plants, he could perfectly use them applying the Galenic principles. The doctrine of signatures per se did not challenge the theory of humours.

Seen from the broader view of the current understanding of plants in general, the theory of signs is a perfect exemplification of the belief that plants existed uniquely for the use of man. According to the doctrine of signatures, they were created by the mercy of God with the signs of their inner medical virtues stamped on their outer features, so that man could recognize them and use them as a remedy for his diseases. No doctrine could be further than this from the idea that plants could be studied in their own right. Oswald Croll's attack on herbalists, who were concerned only with the 'denominations' of herbs and their 'matter, substance, and corporeity' and were 'wholly occupied about the exterior bitter rind', is very significant.[112] The doctrine of signatures implied an understanding of plants that was diametrically opposed to that from which botany, as a discipline separate from medicine, at the same period, took its first steps.

---

[112]   Croll, preface of 'Signatures', p. 1.

Chapter 6
Theory and Practice

This chapter will examine the link between the theory and practice of therapy, in an attempt to shed some light on the actual use of medicinal plants at the time. My purpose is to investigate whether 'practical medicine', taught as a university subject to future doctors, and the practice of medicine actually adopted when they entered the profession were one and the same. To do so I will draw on a variety of sources dealing with therapy, from the texts prescribed for the subject of *Medicina practica* at the university, to medical *Consilia*, to letters describing specific treatments, to the medicinal ingredients sold by an apothecary's shop. An analysis of these different texts will allow me to discuss to what extent the principles and treatments expounded in the theoretical texts were actually put into practice, and which were the medicinal herbs actually prescribed and used.

In the university curriculum, medicine was traditionally divided into *theorica* and *practica*, and this distinction had generated interminable discussions on the definition and boundaries of the two branches, the core of which was whether medicine was to be numbered among *scientiae* or *artes*.[1] In the traditional hierarchic vision, theoretical medicine held the higher position, and was seen as a *scientia* bordering upon natural philosophy; practical medicine, on the other hand, was seen as the part that mingled with *ars*, even *ars mechanica*, according to the opinion of some authors. Practical medicine was nevertheless considered fundamental, as the ultimate purpose of medicine, the maintaining or restoring of health, could not be separated from practical intervention.

Medical Practice in the Faculty of Medicine

The two principal subjects taught in the faculties of medicine, however, did not involve this clear-cut distinction. Although they were called 'medical theory' and 'medical practice', they both dealt mainly with the reading of classical texts.

---

[1]   The basis for the discussion was the definitions that Avicenna had given in the first fen of the first book of his *Canon*. See Nancy Siraisi, *Avicenna in Renaissance Italy: The Canon and Medical Teaching in Italian Universities after 1500* (Princeton, NJ, 1987).

Practical medicine included the study of the various diseases, but it had nothing to do with what we would now call 'clinic'.[2]

The teaching of medical theory was considered the most important, and ordinary professors of medical theory enjoyed a higher prestige and even received a higher salary. In the second half of the sixteenth century, however, the teaching of practical medicine seems to have risen in esteem, and eminent professors, such as Andrea Cesalpino and Girolamo Mercuriale, held the chair of *Medicina practica* at the University of Pisa. Mercuriale even declared the superiority of practical medicine, on the grounds that it is on practice, and not on books, that the medical profession is based.[3]

The treatises that went under the name of *practica* were usually texts in which diseases 'from head to foot' (*a capite usque ad pedes*) were listed and described together with their treatments. Each disease was generally subdivided into different standard sections: name, definition, cause, diagnosis, prognosis, and therapy.[4] The models were Galen and Avicenna, but many university professors, and among them Cesalpino and Mercuriale, wrote their own books of *practica*.[5]

Apart from these, other works were of use in the practice or teaching of medicine. Herbals, collections of recipes, pharmacopoeias, and *consilia*, although different traditional genres, were all useful practical aids in support of the medical profession. Herbals listed and described all the plants known, and expounded their medicinal characteristics and use; Dioscorides's treatise on plants, as we have seen in the preceding chapters, was the textbook read for the new course of *Materia medica*. The commentary to it by Mattioli, and by the *lectores simplicium* at Pisa, were useful both for didactic and professional use. Books of recipes, notwithstanding all the difficulties of interpretation and nomenclature and contrasting information, were necessary tools of therapy; the new pharmacopoeias, introduced to restore some order in such muddled

---

[2]   See Jerome J. Bylebyl, 'The School of Padua: Humanistic Medicine in the Sixteenth Century', in C. Webster (ed.), *Health, Medicine and Mortality in the Sixteenth Century* (Cambridge, 1979), pp. 335–70. Bylebyl calls attention to the fact that students' education was complemented by bedside teaching in the hospital, carried out by professors of both theory and practice. This practice, developed in Padua by Gianbattista Da Monte (1498–1551), was customary in other universities as well. As far as Tuscany is concerned, see Henderson, *The Renaissance Hospital*, ch. 7.

[3]   Girolamo Mercuriale, *Medicina practica, seu de cognoscendis, discernendis, & curandis omnis humani corporis affectibus, earum causis indagandis, libri V* (Frankfurt, 1602), p. 443.

[4]   Andrew Wear, 'Explorations in Renaissance Writings on the Practice of Medicine', in A. Wear, R.K. French and I.M. Lonie (eds), *The Medical Renaissance of the Sixteenth Century* (Cambridge, 1985), pp. 118–45.

[5]   Mercuriale, *Medicina Practica*; Andrea Cesalpino, *Praxis uniuersae artis medicae* (Treviso, 1606).

literature, and provide pharmacists with some rules to which to conform, were also designed to play a key role in the practice of medicine.

These works, which were certainly valuable aids to early modern doctors, however, are not sufficient sources of evidence for the historian in search of information about the medical practice of the time. They provide a great deal of information about which treatment *should* be used for a particular disease, and about why and how it *should* be administered, but they do not tell us which remedies were actually prescribed in everyday practice, and which, among the recipes, sometimes very complex and containing a great number of medicinal plants, were most frequently prescribed.[6]

Even *consilia*, which are usually believed to be accounts of medical cases, and therefore samples of actual practice, on careful reading reveal unexpected aspects. *Consilia*, at least in the sixteenth century, were usually collections of counsels of an expert and authoritative physician on a single medical case. The patients about whom advice was requested (almost always by another physician and not by the patient himself) were usually from prominent families, and to be able to collect and publish one's own *consilia* was per se a sign of high status. A *consilium* was seldom written as a plain report, as it had to conform to fixed patterns as any other piece of medical literature.[7]

The authors of *consilia*, being learned physicians, had to demonstrate their knowledge of the classical writers, and had to justify their therapeutic advice on the grounds of theoretical principles. Mercuriale, for example, left us a great number of *consilia*, some of which were written when he was teaching at Pisa.[8] They are in the form of medical epistles in reply to a physician who asked an opinion about the illness of a particular patient. Given the great number of letters, written over a long period, the style is not always uniform. A great part of them, however, are little medical essays, with the usual display of erudition and frequent references to classical authors. The name of the patients are often but not always mentioned, and the reasons to mention or not to mention them (at least at a first survey) are not clear, and probably vary according to different circumstances. Often the purpose of the *consilium* seems to go beyond the single case, and there is an effort to render it an example, useful for similar cases. On the whole, Mercuriale's *consilia* can be considered, as many others of the same period, as texts halfway between theory and professional practice.[9]

---

6   Siraisi, *Medieval and Early Renaissance Medicine*.

7   John M. Riddle, 'Theory and Practice in Medieval Medicine', *Quid pro Quo: Studies in the History of Drugs* (Aldershot, 1992), pp. 157–84.

8   Hieronymi Mercurialis Foriliviensis, *Responsorum et consultationum medicinalium in duo volumina digesta* (Venice, 1589–90). Further on I will refer to the 1624 edition: Hieronymi Mercurialis, *Consultationes et responsa medicinalia* (Venice, 1624).

9   Jole Agrimi and Chiara Crisciani, *Les Consilia médicaux* (Turnhout, 1994), p. 119.

After this brief survey of the works that can be included in the branch of practical medicine, let us see which were the texts used to teach this subject at the university. Professors of practical medicine usually read and commented on part of a classical medical text on diseases. At the *Studio pisano*, the text prescribed for *Medicina practica* in the 1543 Statutes for first-year students, was the first *fen* of the fourth book of Avicenna's *Canon*, 'De febribus'.[10] The same book of Avicenna's *Canon* was also the text for this subject at Bologna and was maintained for all the rest of the century and beyond, in both universities. Avicenna's *Canon* was chosen as textbook because it was considered a comprehensive and well-organized summary of all Graeco-Arabic Medicine, based mainly on Hippocras, Galen and Rasis.[11] His 'De febribus' is a very lengthy and detailed book, divided into four 'treatises' (*tractati*), each one dealing with a particular kind of fever. Each *tractatus*, in its turn, is subdivided into a great number of chapters (145 in total). The Latin translators (Gerardo da Cremona and Andrea Alpago, in the edition I have consulted) provide us with very useful tables which give an idea of the complexity and sophistication of the content.[12]

Fevers, as Nancy Siraisi explains, were considered a fundamental part of pathology: 'Among conditions regarded as diseases of the whole body, fever, the paradigmatic example of a 'hot' disease, occupied a special place. The subject of fever came to constitute almost a separate branch of pathology.'[13] We have a great number of sixteenth-century treatises on fevers at our disposal. Almost all professors of practical medicine dealt with this subject, and both Cesalpino and Mercuriale, in their *practica*, devoted a substantial part to fevers. We therefore have a great deal of theoretical information about them and their treatment, and we know how this subject was taught.[14]

---

[10]   *Storia dell' Università di Pisa*, vol. 1, p. 131. Avicenna IV, I, was prescribed for the first year. The two books of the *Canon* that dealt with pharmacology, i.e. Book II 'On simples', and Book V, which contains an *antidotarium*, were never prescribed. For the second and third year the text was Book IX of Rhazes ad Almansorem *De curibus particularibus* (*From head to heart* the first year, *and from heart to the inferior parts* in the second). The same texts were prescribed for practical medicine *at Bologna*. When Mercuriale, assumed the teaching of *Practica* at Pisa, he was allowed, in his capacity of *supraordinarius* (1592–1605), to choose the authors and texts on which he wanted to lecture. We know that he lectured on Hippocrates's *Epidemics* (Books I and III), as we can see from the commentary contained in his *Praelectiones Pisanae*.

[11]   Siraisi, *Avicenna*, p. 20.

[12]   *Avicennae Arabum medicorum principis* [*Canon medicinae*] *ex Gerardi Cremonensis versione, et Andreae Alpagi Bellunensis castigatione* (Venice, 1595).

[13]   Siraisi, *Medieval and Early Renaissance Medicine*, p. 130.

[14]   See also I.M. Lonie, 'Fever Pathology in the Sixteenth Century: Tradition and Innovations', in W.F. Bynum and V. Nutton (eds) 'Theories of Fever from Antiquity to the Enlightenment', *Medical History*, Supplement 1 (1981), pp. 19–44.

Three Texts by Mercuriale on Quartan Fever

As usual, when it comes to practice, the problem is to find sources from which one can derive that kind of information. Fevers are a good starting point, as they were connected with various pathologies and were very common. As far as the Medici court and family are concerned, we have information about various cases of fever, above all 'quartan', now recognized as a malarial fever. Looking at the *Tractatus* 'De febribus putridis' of Avicenna's Canon (seventy-one chapters), for example, we see that these fevers are caused by a putrefaction (*putredo*) of the humours, and quartan in particular originates from the putrefaction of black bile. Apart from minor details, the theory at the basis of the cause of fevers is shared by all sixteenth-century authors who dealt with this topic, and the same can be said for each particular group of fevers and for each fever in particular.[15]

As a first step, in order to investigate the relationship between theory and practice, I tried to find a series of writings on the treatment of fevers by the same author, from the more general and theoretical to the more specific and practical. I concentrated on various texts written by Mercuriale on fevers, and more particularly on quartan. The first is in his *Medicina practica* (published also in his *Praelectiones Patavinae*); the second is among his *consilia*; the third is a small group of four letters giving an account of a quartan fever from which the grand duchess of Tuscany suffered in 1601.[16] We will consider first the theoretical text, then the *consilium* which is by definition halfway between theory and practice, and finally the letters which are the account of a real case. Following these sources from the more general to the more specific, I will make a first attempt to determine to what extent theoretical principles coincided with day-to-day practice.

The first source we are going to examine is the section on 'Putrid fevers' from the treatise 'De febribus' in Mercuriale's *Praelectiones Patavinae*. It is a learned account of all fevers, from which we learn that quartan is a fever with a hot *intemperies* recurring every fourth day; its immediate cause is the putrid melancholic (black bile) humour. After long disquisitions and distinctions between the various forms of this kind of fever, with constant reference to the classical authors, the section on treatment begins. Quartan is difficult to treat, Mercuriale explains, because the humour which causes it is dense, viscous

---

[15] See for example, Guido Guidi, *De febribus libri VII*, and Matteo Corti, *De febribus curandis*, published in the same volume (Padua, 1595).

[16] Mercuriale, *Praelectiones Patavinae, de cognoscendis, et curandis humani corporis affectibus* (Venice, 1606), Book 5, 'De Febribus', pp. 465–644, in particular, ch. 11, 'De febris quartanis', pp. 572–89; Mercuriale, *Consultationes et responsa medicinalia*, 'Consultatio LVIII – De Quartana', pp. 116–17.

and slow moving (*crassus, viscidus, tardus*) and therefore very hard to expel.[17] Moreover quartan fevers occur in autumn, or at the beginning of winter, and all diseases starting in these seasons are very persistent and lengthy.[18] Mercuriale then mentions a theoretical riddle he had already referred to in the section concerning putrid fevers in general.[19] While fever had a hot quality, and therefore required cold and moist remedies, the cause (black bile), being cold and dry, required hot and moist remedies. This was a point of divergence between Galen and Avicenna. Mercuriale's opinion is that when it comes to putrid fevers, the fundamental need is to remove the obstructions (*deobstruere*) and purge (*purgare*). The remedies which have the power to do so are hot, but one has to use them, not because of their hot faculty but because of their capacity to unclog and purge.[20] There is then a short section dealing with part of the non-naturals, with recommendations about the temperature of the air, sleep and waking, and about the exercise a patient suffering from quartan is allowed on the day of the onset of the fever, and on other days.

As far as remedies are concerned, the first rule that must be followed is to intervene in the early days of the illness with mild clysters, becoming gradually stronger. This advice, corroborated by Galen and Avicenna, is repeated in all the theoretical treatises that deal with this subject. The evacuation of the putrid humours must be prepared in a series of gradual steps. The first clysters are administered only as emollient to prepare the material that has to be evacuated. Here Mercuriale gives the recipes for four clysters with different levels of strength, and it must be noted that they are part of the general rules in a section dedicated to the non-naturals. A series of detailed rules on diet follows. If wine is allowed, and what kind; what kind of bread, meat, fish, spices, fruit and vegetables. Among the latter, borage, bugloss, and balm mint are the most advisable. As a general rule, any food which is dense, viscous or hard is to be avoided. The purpose is always to soothe, mollify and free all blockages, and to do so, Mercuriale continues, the most frequently used medicaments are 'mel rosatus lenitivus, myrabolani nigri, cassia, electuarium lenitivum hiera, diacatholicum'.

---

[17]   Another reason why quartan is difficult to treat is because bodies suffering from this fever are characterized by great 'astringency' so that they are not subject to perspiration; quartan also causes a weakness of the viscera, due to the accumulation of non-digested humours.

[18]   Mercuriale, *Praelectiones Patavinae*, pp. 575–6.

[19]   Mercuriale, *Practica*, p. 500.

[20]   The discussion is to be found in other texts concerning quartan fever. For example, in Cesalpino's *Praxis universae*, ch. 25, 'Curatio quartanae', p. 124, the same discussion is reported. While Avicenna was in favour of 'refrigerantia', Galen recommended 'calefacentia and humectantia'. This therapy contradicts the principle that opposites cure opposites. See also Giuseppe Donzelli, *Teatro farmaceutico dogmatico e spagirico* (Venice, 1704), p. III of the 1666 Dedication, who considers the question from a Paracelsian point of view.

Here he provides other recipes, this time under the form of *bolus* (a big pill) or *potus* (beverage) that must be administered in sequence. A beverage of rose honey, syrup of betony and fumitory; a *bolus* of hiera, myrabolani nigri and cassia; finally a syrup of rose honey *solutivus* and syrup of apples (de pomis).

After this preparation, it is time to start the treatment *par excellence* of the fever, that is to say bloodletting. The quality of the blood will determine the quantity that must be taken; if it is black and thick it must be let, otherwise the vain must be compressed and closed. After bloodletting, food must be reduced in quantity and must be lighter than before. After that, medicaments must be administered ('Post haec medicamentis agendum est'),[21] and it must be noted that this is the first time that Mercuriale uses the term *medicamenta*. The recipes provided so far were only preparatory. However, before taking the medicaments proper, once again the humours must be 'prepared' with syrup of fumitory, syrup of hop, syrup *byzantium*, syrup of apples, juice of borage, and some recipes are provided. Once the humours have been prepared, they can be expurgated, beginning with the most 'benign' medicaments, based on polypodium, epithyme, sena, root of black hellebore, rhubarb; among the composite syrups, syrup of polypodium and of apples, Confectio Hamech, and the like.[22] After this first *purgatio*, a few days' rest is advisable. However, as the melancholic humour is very persistent, its preparation and digestion must be continued with internal remedies (such as syrups) and external remedies (such as sponge-baths and ointments). After that, pills made of more powerful substances can be used, for example, pills of lapis lazuli, pills 'cochiarum' with hellebore, 'diagridium' and castor, etc.'[23] A discussion about vomit, and a short section on the use of theriac conclude the chapter.[24]

Let us now turn to the second source, 'Consultatio LVIII' in Mercuriale's second volume of *consilia*, where we can read what he recommended for a case of quartan fever from which a 'most illustrious man' was suffering. Here Mercuriale repeats the same observations about the length of autumn fevers, and the rules about air, exercise, sleep and diet. The only new recommendation, which appears to concern a specific habit of the person for whom this counsel was provided, is to avoid beer (*cervisia*), which should be substituted by a decoction of cinnamon and sugar. The first clysters, as in the theoretical text I have examined above, are considered part of the diet. Here, however, they are simply made of leaves of senna and mercorella (a very common plant which has the same laxative virtues as senna), while in the preceding text they were more complex and had to be administered one after the other according to their different strength. To prepare the body for

---

21   Mercuriale, *Praelectiones Patavinae*, p. 579.

22   Ibid., Polypodium, epithymus, sena, helleborus niger, are also listed among the simples that evacuate black bile in Gabriele Falloppio's *De simplicibus medicamentis purgantibus* (Venice, 1565), p. 202.

23   Ibid., p. 580.

24   Ibid., pp. 581–2.

the evacuation of the putrid melancholic humour, the *quaternarius* will have to take a lenient electuary mixed with leaves of senna and sugar before dinner. Then he will have to take a syrup made of borage, hop, balm mint, betony, raisins, etc., for seven consecutive days. Meanwhile the patient can be bled (from a vein in the left arm or from the haemorrhoids) taking six to eight ounces of blood. After the seventh day of syrup, a medicament of black hellebore, leaves of epythime, senna, mirabolani nigri, Damascene plums, flowers of cordalium can be administered. After that another compound made with rhubarb, agaric, cinnamon, Confectio Amech, rose honey, and manna. Once the body has been purged with these medicaments, on the day before the onset of fever, the patient will ingest a *bolus* of theriac, lapis lazuli, sugar, and borage. On the day of the onset, an ointment with oil of euphorbium, nard, sweet almonds, eau de vie and wax will be very useful.

On the whole, apart from the fact that the treatment seems simpler than that of the general exposition in the *Praelectiones Patavinae*, the sequence of medicaments and the ingredients of which they are composed, are more or less the same, with minor differences, which is only natural, given the different nature of the two texts. Although Mercuriale's *consilia* are very learned short essays on the topics they deal with, remedies had to be adapted, at least partly, to the particular patient.

The third source we will examine is four letters on the same subject written by Mercuriale in the autumn of 1601, when he was professor at Pisa.[25] The letters are addressed to Grand Duke Ferdinando I to inform him about a quartan fever from which his wife Cristina di Lorena was suffering while she was at the villa l'Ambrogiana, and are therefore an account of the treatment of a 'real' case. The first letter was written the day after an onset of the fever, and Mercuriale provides us with some medical details, such as that he had noticed a little catarrh, that the grand duchess's pulse was almost normal, and that she had only a slight fever. He records how she slept, spent her day, and ate her meals. The only treatment mentioned is a clyster, which had to be repeated the following day to take away that 'shadow of fever that usually appears towards the beginning of the day'.[26] The second letter describes another onset (*parocismo*) with cold and pallor. No medical preparation is referred to either in this, or in the other two letters. Not even bloodletting is mentioned. The letters provide details about the grand duchess's meals, sleep and exercise, and great emphasis is placed on her good character and disposition. The fact that Cristina faces her illness with cheerfulness ('alegrezza del animo') and merriment ('ilarità') is considered a very positive way to defeat these 'lengthy diseases' ('mali longhi').[27] The only remedies mentioned, however, are clysters.

---

[25]   Mercuriale was in correspondence with the grand dukes already before 1592, when he moved from Bologna to Pisa. See Gerolamo Mercuriale, 'Quattro lettere di sulla malattia della Granduchessa di Toscana nel novembre del 1601', published by Alessandro Simili, *Romagna medica* (Bollettino della Società Medico-chirurgica della Romagna), 8(6) (1956), p. 1.

[26]   A. Simili, 'Quattro lettere', p. 4.

[27]   Ibid., p. 5.

We know that the grand duchess recovered from this fever, which obviously did not turn into one of those malignant forms that were almost always lethal. Although one can assume that the actual treatment might be simpler than that described in the theoretical or semi-theoretical texts, one cannot draw any conclusive data on the basis of such a small group of letters. In his *Practica* Mercuriale, while speaking of the four kinds of medicaments required to cure putrid fevers (*lenientia, preparantia, purgantia and corroborantia*) points out that somebody maintains that these medicaments are not necessary, and that clysters are sufficient. He does not exclude this possibility, but only when, he underlines, the undigested humours to be expelled are all in the lower part of the intestine. Bloodletting, on the other hand, is considered fundamental by Mercuriale, as the patient will recover much more quickly ('adhibito hoc auxilio [sanguinis missio] multo citius liberantur aegri').[28] There are only few cases in which it is advisable to postpone bloodletting, and these do not seem to concern the grand duchess. The fact that we cannot find any mention of medicaments or bloodletting in these letters is surprising; however, they do not constitute enough evidence to allow us to jump to the conclusion that practical treatments were very different from the theoretical.

Some Other Cases of Fever in the Medici Family

As letters remain one of the best sources for exploring the link between books and everyday life, I will pursue my inquiry into fever and its actual treatment considering other cases associated with the Medici family.

Malaria was very frequent in Tuscany, and some areas, among which the Maremma, were marshlands where the disease was almost impossible to escape. We have evidence of very many cases of malaria in the Medici court, and among the Medici family itself. Three of the sons of Cosimo I, Giovanni, Garzia, and Ferdinando, contracted malarial fever after a trip to the Maremma with their father, and only Ferdinando survived. Gaetano Pieraccini also attributes to malaria the deaths of Francesco I and his second wife Bianca Cappello, although, despite the various exhumations, it is still debatable whether they died of natural causes or were poisoned. Among the reports of the various physicians of the Medici family, we find some accounts of intermittent fevers which were clear symptoms of malaria. Cosimo I himself suffered from quartan fevers between August and December 1544, and the evolution of this illness can be followed almost day by day through the letters that Lorenzo Pagni (one of the duke's secretaries) sent to Pier Francesco Riccio, *segretario intimo* to Cosimo.[29] Pagni

---

[28] Mercuriale, *Practica*, p. 502.
[29] ASF, vol. 1171, cc. 88–172. After c. 153 (162–72) the letters are from Christiano Pagni.

in his letters never refers to specific drugs: he confines himself to describing the course of Cosimo's fever, his mood, whether he slept, ate, went out, and whether he was strong enough or too weak to deal with *negozi*. Only once does he mention Cosimo's physician Andrea Pasquali, to say that the duke had decided to let himself be purged.[30] We can be sure that the fever was quartan, as Lorenzo Pagni in one of his letters reports that the grand duchess (Eleonora di Toledo, Cosimo's first wife), although asking for confirmation of the diagnosis from Andrea Pasquali, had told him 'not to spread the news that the *quartana* had come back, not to make the gossipers gossip'.[31] Moreover we know, from another letter, that Colonel Lucantonio Cuppano had sent a remedy for the duke's *quartana*.[32] We do not know anything about this remedy, but Cosimo was certainly willing to try it, as in a subsequent letter Pagni says that he was cutting, on his orders, some twigs of hazelnut, according to Lucantonio's instructions for its preparation. The only other reference to a remedy is not medical, but in Pagni's words 'nothing else but prayer'. This remedy was suggested by a Spanish relative, and the duchess herself saw to it, entrusting the prayers to the future Saint Caterina de' Ricci from the Monastery of Saint Vincent in Prato.[33]

As far as the medical treatment is concerned, these letters, like the ones written by Mercuriale about Cristina di Lorena's quartan, contain very little evidence. They are interesting because they too show the great attention paid to the non-naturals; in the case of Cosimo's disease, however, we must remember that they were not written by a physician. The two groups of letters seem to have in common a complete absence of references to medicines. In both cases not even bloodletting is mentioned. In this regard we have a very interesting letter of 1549 from Lorenzo Pagni to Pier Francesco Riccio that reports the opinion of Cosimo about the treatment of quartan fever. Cosimo thinks that it has to be treated with bloodletting from the outset, and 'he approves of this remedy of bloodletting as unique and true, and [considers] the medicines totally noxious for the body'.[34] He also adds that if when he suffered from that fever (he probably refers to his malarial fever of 1544) he had been bled at the beginning,

---

[30]   'Il Pasquali mi dice che si è risoluto di lassarsi purgare', ibid., c. 135 (letter of 9 October 1544).

[31]   Ibid., c. 99.

[32]   Colonel Lucantonio Cuppano, when he was under the command of Giovanni dalle Bande Nere, had transcribed, probably at his request, a famous book of recipes compiled by Caterina Sforza, mother of Giovanni and grandmother of Cosimo I. *Experimenti de la ex.ma s.ra Caterina da Forlj matre de lo Inllux.mo signor Giovanni de Medici*, ed. P.D. Pasolini (Imola, 1894). See De Vries, *Caterina Sforza and the Art of Appearances*, p. 211, and M.K. Ray, 'Experiments with Alchemy: Caterina Sforza in Early Modern Scientific Culture', in *Gender and Scientific Discourse in Early Modern Culture* (Aldershot, 2010), pp. 139–64.

[33]   ASF 1171, c. 268.

[34]   ASF 1175 (Inserto 6), c. 45.

the illness would not have lasted so long. Although the opinion on bloodletting is very similar to that of Mercuriale, it is very unlikely that Mercuriale or other doctors shared the grand duke's view of the absolute harmfulness of medicines, as it would contradict all the medical literature, and would undermine one of the fundamental prerogatives of the medical profession, jealously guarded from the apothecaries. One of the reasons why maybe bloodletting had not been prescribed in the cases discussed above might be that the forms that Cosimo and Cristina had developed, although long and debilitating, were not considered particularly serious, and anyway not life-threatening.

We have evidence that bloodletting was always practised in the serious cases of quartan, as we can read in the two letters Cosimo sent to his son Francesco describing the treatments prior to the deaths of his brothers Giovanni and Garzia, caused by malarial fever. In a letter of 21 November 1562 concerning Giovanni's death after only six days of 'malignant' fever, Cosimo refers to two bloodlettings of two 'libbre' of blood each, and adds 'we used all the other remedies that could be used, and that were never missing in our house'.[35] We do not know what these remedies might have been, but in the letter describing the illness and death of Garzia, the reference is again only to bloodlettings.[36]

In January 1563 Cosimo sent a letter to his eldest son Francesco which contains an account of the illness of Ferdinando, the only one of his three sons who survived the malarial fever contracted during their trip to Maremma. The letter is written after sixty days of a fever which was diagnosed as a type of quartan ('quartanario rinterzato'), but that now seemed to have become continuous. Given his age (12 years) Ferdinando is behaving very well, and takes all the remedies he is prescribed with a good disposition. However, the duke adds, the poor boy is very debilitated by the long disease, the frequent evacuations, and the incessant fever, which gives serious cause for concern. 'Even yesterday morning these physicians have taken about six ounces of blood with leeches, and although he seemed better, and yesterday evening he was relieved and had a good meal, during the night the fever never left him ...'.[37]

---

[35] The letter is reported in Guglielmo Enrico Saltini, *Tragedie medicee domestiche* (Florence, 1898), pp. 125–8. Quoted in part in Gaetano Pieraccini, *La stirpe de' Medici di Cafaggiolo: Saggio di ricerche sulla trasmissione ereditaria e dei caratteri biologici* (Florence, 1924–25), vol. 2, p. 113.

[36] Saltini, *Tragedie medicee*, pp. 136–42. Quoted in Pieraccini, *La stirpe de' Medici*, vol. 2, p. 122.

[37] Pieraccini, *La stirpe de' Medici*, vol. 2, pp. 293–5. Bloodletting is considered the right remedy also in another case of quartan fever, that from which suffered Eleonora de' Medici, Duchess of Mantua, mentioned in a letter of 23 April 1588. ASF, MdP, 4681(Medici Archive project).

Cosimo I's Illness in 1572

Among the manuscripts kept at the Archivio di Stato of Florence, an entire volume of 104 *carte* is devoted to the account of an illness of Grand Duke Cosimo in 1572, while he was in Pisa.[38] The pathology here is more complex, as Cosimo, a couple of years before, had suffered an apoplectic fit on the left side, and had been stricken with temporary paralysis. He recovered, but he remained debilitated, and his speech was slightly impaired. The illness from which he suffered between March and September 1572 was characterized by fever, catarrh, and a leg ulcer caused by gout. Most of the letters are written by the physician Baccio Gatteschi (usually called 'lo Strada') to Cosimo's son Francesco to keep him informed about his father's health. Some of them are signed jointly by both of Cosimo's physicians at that time, Baccio Baldini and Baccio Gatteschi.[39]

The first letter of Baccio Gatteschi to Francesco contains a description and explanation of Cosimo's disease. The cause was to be found in the phlegmatic and undigested humours in his head, which were naturally descending towards the lower parts of the body. This material, being putrefied, caused a slight fever. The same humours were also at the origin of the *podagra* and his leg ulcer. In order to cure these ailments, the head had to be drained, to prevent the passage of material to the lower organs. Only at this point could a cautery be considered. Many remedies can be employed, Baccio Gatteschi explains, but it will not be possible to administer them all. He will try to give the grand duke some pills or other medicines to facilitate the evacuation. In this case the fever from which Cosimo is suffering is not quartan, which we know is caused by black bile, but probably 'quotidiana' which is caused by phlegm.

The following letters about Cosimo's state of health, which were sent to Francesco daily, provide invaluable information about the regimen he followed, and the treatment he received. As always, the account of the non-naturals is very meticulous, and we are informed about how the grand duke spent his days and nights. Great attention is paid to his state of mind and his attitude to the treatments he was given. Baccio Gatteschi repeats over and over again that one of the reasons why he did not get better was that he was not willing to follow his doctors' recommendations, and refused some of the remedies prescribed. This was made worse by his low spirits, which were partly imputed to his second wife Cammilla, who seemed to be universally disliked. Anyway the impression one gets from these letters is that Cosimo's illness involved both the body and the mind.

---

[38]   ASF 642/A. 'Ragguagli di medici e altri della malattia di Sua Altezza mentre era in Pisa'. I am grateful to Alessio Assonitis for drawing this *filza* to my attention.

[39]   The physician Baccio Gatteschi (usually called 'lo Strada') had been asked to stay and follow Cosimo's illness. Some other letters of the volume are sent by the secretary Antonio da Montalvo to Duke Francesco, some others by Baccio Gatteschi to the secretary Bartolomeo Concino.

The accounts of Baccio Gatteschi, unlike those of Lorenzo Pagni, contain a great number of references to medical remedies. There is hardly any letter which does not mention the treatment the grand duke was receiving. While in the first month the gout and the ulcer seem to be the main concern, in the following months more attention is paid to the general state of the grand duke's health.[40] The accounts of his defecations are almost obsessive, and we are often told by which medicaments they were induced, and how often they produced an effect. We know that he was administered syrups, then enemas and pills. Unfortunately we are not told of which simples or substances the syrups or the enemas were composed, but we can assume they were made of standard emollient and laxative ingredients. On one occasion, Gatteschi mentions a clyster of 'chicken broth and egg yolk', 'to comfort and moisten the bowels'.[41] The sort of pills used, on the other hand, is specified, and we know that their main ingredient was 'castoreum', a substance extracted from a beaver's gland, which is described both in the *Ricettario fiorentino* and in Mattioli's *Discorsi*.[42] The bloodletting was practised using leeches (*mignatte*) and apparently was very moderate. Among the external remedies, frictions and ointments were one of his usual treatments.

On 13 December a medical consultation took place in order to decide whether it was the right time to employ a cautery. On this occasion, the doctors recommended that the grand duke should take water of guaiacum (*acqua del legno*) for ten to twelve days.[43] This *acqua del legno* is very often mentioned in the subsequent letters, and we learn that the grand duke used to drink it daily with his dinner, even in place of wine. At least once, when he had refused his usual syrup, laxative substances were surreptitiously added to the water. Here the *cura del legno* is not the kind of remedy used in the cases of the French disease and described in the medical literature as an extremely strong, and difficult to bear treatment.[44] The water of guaiacum administered to Cosimo was a decoction

---

[40] In the letter of 28 December the secretary Antonio da Montalvo reports to Francesco that the ulcer in the leg had cicatrized ('la piaga si è saldata').

[41] c. 28.

[42] In Mattioli's *Discorsi* (1568) pp. 352–4, there is a beautiful description of the beaver. Mattioli explains that the medicinal substance in use was not taken from testicles, as it was believed, but from a particular gland. Both in Mattioli and in the *Ricettario fiorentino* is reported that the duke had brought two beavers from Germany. 'Castor' was used mainly in the cases in which a hot remedy was required.

[43] Guaiacum, which was introduced into Europe from the New World as a cure for the French disease, was very fashionable at the time, and was often administered to patients who did not suffer from it. Mercuriale, for example, prescribes 'acqua del legno' for a patient who had stomach disorders. We have evidence of this also from many letters where guaiacum is mentioned as a remedy for various ailments. Mercuriale explains that guaiacum was good for any disease where a hot and dry remedy had to be used. See also Mattioli, *Discorsi* 1568, pp. 199–200.

[44] Arrizabalaga, Henderson and French, *The Great Pox*.

apparently used for the most disparate cases.[45] In a consultation for a patient with a stomach ailment for example, Mercuriale recommends a decoction of guaiacum, and adds: 'this medicament is very efficient for its particular quality of producing heat and dissipating exhalations'.[46] Because of this quality, it was prescribed for many different diseases, and several letters of the period provide evidence that it was widely used.[47] Apart from these recurring remedies, some other drugs are occasionally mentioned. In a letter of 19 January, Baccio Gatteschi reports to secretary Concino that the grand duke took a little 'electuary Alchermes' in the mornings. This electuary, which appears in the *Ricettario fiorentino* under the name 'Lattovaro Alchermes di Mesue', was made of rare and costly ingredients such as scarlet silk dyed with kermes, boiled in rose and apple water with amber, lapis lazuli, white pearls, gold leaf, and musk. ('seta scarlatta tinta con Alkermes, bollita in acqua di rose e di pomi con ambra, lapislazzuli, perle bianche, fogli d'oro, muschio'.)[48] As seen, this electuary was also recommended by Mercuriale, in a compound with other medicinal plants, for the treatment of quartan. After a few days, following a temporary aggravation of Cosimo's general condition, and of his difficulty of speech in particular, the physicians administered to him a 'masticativo' to help him evacuate the phlegmatic humours from his head. On this occasion, in addition to the usual enemas, leeches, ointments, and pills, mithridate was added.[49]

There is a letter, sent by Baccio Gatteschi to the grand duke's secretary Bartolomeo Concino, that describes some days of Cosimo's illness, which can be useful to provide a general idea of the treatment he was given, and of the physicians' main concerns.

> Wednesday evening we gave up syrup because he [Cosimo] did not want to take it anymore. Instead of it we administered a clyster which was very effective, he dined ... and drank his water of holy wood. That night he slept quite well and at 11 hours he took the pills which at 14 hours moved his bowels vigorously ... Then at 15 once again, and before lunch which was at 18 hours a further two times, to the great satisfaction of His Highness and myself ... The day went by ... In the morning [of Thursday] he drank a little wine to take his pills and he did not like it very much, so

---

[45]   Pietro Andrea Mattioli in his *Discorsi* of 1568, p. 200, explains how he had rendered the treatment much more tolerable, and gives a recipe of 'wine of guaiacum'. He points out the 'faculties of guaiacum', and lists the diseases that can be treated with it.

[46]   Italo Paoletti, *Gerolamo Mercuriale e il suo tempo, Studio eseguito su 62 lettere e un consulto inediti del medico forlivese giacenti presso l'Archivio di Stato di Parma* (Lanciano, 1963), p. 63.

[47]   In a letter of 4 October 1567, for example, Giordano Orsini (Isabella de' Medici's husband), is said to be taking *acqua del legno* to lose weight. ASF, vol. 3080, Folio 154 (Medici Archive Project).

[48]   Corradi, *Le prime farmacopee*, p. IX.

[49]   c. 14.

in the evening he drank only water of holy wood. He had a modest dinner and slept as usual. Friday morning he had another good motion; he got up very relieved, had a good meal, and drank a little wine, and after lunch, as it seemed a nice day, he went as far as the garden by coach ... Saturday morning he had two motions, was very relieved, had a good lunch and went for a ride by coach for about an hour. Yesterday [Sunday] morning he did not have a motion but urinated a great deal and his left eye was very red but did not ache ... He went out with no support but his stick, had a modest lunch with his usual wine, remained at home the whole day and walked with Colonel Simone ... and with Signor di Piombino talking about business, so that yesterday evening he said that he was tired, however he had quite a good dinner with his usual water [of holy wood] ... He will continue for some days to drink water of holy wood in the evening, and in the mornings he will take a little electuary Alchermes, and other medicaments are now no longer needed and therefore Vostra Signoria will be so kind as to ask the Prince whether he thinks that I could leave because here I do not have anything more to do.[50]

However, in this letter as well as in the other ones concerning Cosimo's disease of 1572, we do not get much information about the medicinal substances used in everyday practice. Medicinal herbs or substances are very seldom directly referred to. The recipes mentioned, moreover, are no more than half a dozen.[51]

To pursue this kind of information we have to search for different sources, such as the record of the substances a pharmacy actually sold over a particular period of time.

The Account Books of the Speziale al Giglio

In order to obtain more specific data about the medicinal plants most frequently used, I have chosen to examine, as my case study, the account books of a Florentine apothecary shop, the speziale al Giglio, kept at the Archive of the Ospedale degli Innocenti in Florence.[52] These books are an invaluable source of

---

50   Letter of 19 January 1572, c. 12r and 12v.

51   In the letters of 1572 about Grand Duke Cosimo's illness, the names of some generic preparations such as syrups, enemas, pills, '*pittime*', ointments, '*masticativi*' (medicines to help expectoration), and electuaries, are often mentioned. The specific recipes mentioned, however, are only pills or electuaries of *castoreum*, water of holy wood, rose honey, julep of citron, electuary alkermes and mithridate.

52   Firenze, Archivio dell'Ospedale degli Innocenti, Fondo Estranei, Serie 144, 904–906 covers the period between 1537 and 1545. The accounts of 1545 are contained in n. 906 'Questo libro è dell'erede di Tommaso di Giovanni Speziali al Giglio in sul quale si scriveranno tutte le robe date all'Illustrissimo Signore Duca Cosimo de' Medici e chiamasi libro verde ed è segnato C'. The years between 1546 and 1568 are contained in Serie 144, n. 592–4.

information as they record the date, the substances sold, the name of the person to whom they were sold, the quantity, the container used to take them home, and the cost. They sometimes also record the kind of medicament they were for (a decoction, an infusion, a pill, etc.), although they never indicate the disease they were to cure.

A very detailed and comprehensive study of the account books of the Giglio, and in particular the ones relating to 1494, has been made by James Shaw and Evelyn Welch. It considers all aspects and all the products sold by the shop.[53] The books I am considering are of a later period, and concern only the supply of medicines to the Medici court. My purpose is to find which were the substances actually used in daily practice, and which recipes were actually prescribed; thus I will concentrate on medicinal products. The books that record the medicines sold to the Medici court were kept by the speziale al Giglio between 1537 and 1568. It is important to note that, as was inscribed on the first page of the books, all the purchases were made at the expense of the *Illustrissimo Signore Duca Cosimo de' Medici*. The grand duke, in other words, provided medicines for his relatives and for all the members of the court personnel. In fact, the customers recorded in the books vary from the members of the Medici family and their guests, to various people of different ranks and functions. I have considered the account books of 1566, 1567 and 1568, and I have concentrated in particular on 1568, as this year offers a great deal of contemporary material for comparison and observation. A new edition of the *Ricettario fiorentino* was published (1567), as well as a new edition of Mattioli's *Discorsi* (1568); in this year, moreover, an inventory of the Giglio was taken.[54]

Between April and February 1568 (ten months), there are 440 entries, and the number of people mentioned is forty-seven;[55] in some entries, it is specified that the person who collects the medicine is not the same for whom the medicine was prescribed, and in that case both persons are mentioned in the books. In very rare cases the physician who had prescribed the recipe or the substance sold is also recorded. A substantial number of purchases is made for the grand-ducal workshop (sixty-five), and usually collected by the *maestro di fonderia*. Treatments were usually repeated and protracted, and there are few customers mentioned only once. Customers are sometimes entered with their names and surnames, but more often with a name or nickname. Some are defined by their relationship with the Medici family, but most of them according to their role or profession within the court.

---

[53]   Shaw and Welch, *Making and Marketing Medicine*.

[54]   *Il Ricettario Medicinale necessario a tutti i Medici, & Speziali* (Florence, 1567); Mattioli, *Discorsi* 1568; AOI, Processi antichi, Processo 20.

[55]   According to the Florentine calendar the year began on 25 March, the day of the Annunciation. The book of the speziale al Giglio of 1568 begins on 1 April and ends on 9 February, with the death of the *speziale* Lorenzo Lapini.

Table 6.1   Customers of the speziale al Giglio (April–February 1568).
Names, role or profession, number of purchases

Members and relatives of the Medici family		
Sua Eccellenza	Cosimo I	26
Signore don Petrino	Pietro de' Medici	2
Signora Leonora[1]	Leonora de Toledo	2
Puttino da Pitti[2]	Don Giovanni de' Medici	3
Functionaries of the State		
Vergilio Carnesecchi[3]	*Camarlingo* of Pietrasanta	36
Household administrators		
Giovanni Ghori	major-domo	4
Papa	di *guardaroba*	22
Cesari	di *guardaroba*	1
Meo	di *credenza*	8
Spagnolo	di *dispensa*	2
Luca	di *tinello*	7
Pages		
Pompilio paggio	page	15
Luigi Guarzoni paggio[4]	page	9
Ridolfo paggio	page	3
Signor Pirro paggio[5]	page	29
Silla paggio	page	19
Aniballe paggio	page	1
Bernardino Feo paggio	page	1
Marcantonio paggio	page	1
Gentlemen (role unspecified)		
Piero Barbino[6]		11
Francesco Busi		14
Geremia Foresi		4
Other personnel		
Luca canonaro	pipe fitter	3
Michele	cook	17
Chimenti mulatere	muleteer	1
Benedetto legnaiolo	carpenter	3
Meo	dwarf	1
Balia del putino[7]	wet nurse	3

Medical practitioners[8]		
Lorenzo Venturini	surgeon	19
Baccio Baldini	physician	1
Felice Gattai[9]	barber	2

Artists		
Gianico[10]	assistant of Niccolò Santini	3
Giulio commessore di pietre	Artist of *pietre dure*	2

Religious orders		
Sandrina in San Cremente[11]	Agostinian nun	3

Ducal *Fonderia*		
Berghamo di *fonderia*	Master of the *fonderia*	55
Giuliano Chiavacci	Role unknown	10

Notes: [1] Leonora de Toledo, cousin and wife of Don Pietro de' Medici, youngest son of Cosimo and Eleonora, who married her in 1571. He strangled her in 1576 at Cafaggiolo. In the entry of 10 September it is specified 's.ra Leonora di don Petrino ill.mo', although they were not yet married, not to be confused with Eleonora de Toledo, first wife of Cosimo, who had died in 1562, or with Eleonora degli Abizi, lover of Cosimo, and mother of Don Giovanni de' Medici.

[2] Don Giovanni de Medici (born in 1567), natural son of Duke Cosimo and Eleonora degli Albizi.

[3] The Carnesecchi were a prominent Tuscan family. Giovanni Cinelli says that the angel of Santi di Tito's Annunciation in Santa Maria Novella is a portrayal of Virgilio Carnesecchi. Francesco Bocchi and Giovanni Cinelli, Bellezze della città di Fiorenza (Florence, 1677), p. 240.

[4] Luigi Guarzoni is mentioned by Cosimo I as 'mio creato' in a letter of May 1572. He was one of the several gentlemen of Cosimo's entourage who served on the Florentine galleys during the 1572 naval campaign of the Holy League in the Mediterranean (Medici Archive Project).

[5] Probably Pirro Barbolani di Montatuto (18 years old in 1568). In 1557 Cosimo bought from him (he was then 7 years old and his father was dead) some properties in Portoferraio (Medici Archivi Project). In this book he is usually called s.re Pirro paggio.

[6] The name of Piero Barbino is mentioned in a letter of Cosimo I of 31 January 1566 (Medici Archive Project).

[7] Nurse of Don Giovanni de Medici. In the book is mentioned in the first entry (14 September) as 'balia della s.ra Leonora ill.ma' (Eleonora degli Albizi), and in another entry (26 October) as 'balia del putino di Sua Eccellenza'.

[8] They were the medical staff of Duke Cosimo in that period. They usually collected the medicines at the apothecary shop.

[9] Felice Gattai, was Cosimo's barber. In 1572 he sends letters to Francesco to inform him about his father's illness. He is in Lisbon with Don Pietro de' Medici in 1579–82.

[10] Niccolò Santini was a goldsmith active at the Medici court in this period. He is mentioned in Cellini's Vita and in various letters between 1565 and 1570 (Medici Archive Project). See Marco Collareta, 'Per Niccolò Santini, orefice fiorentino del Cinquecento', Prospettiva, 14 (1978), pp. 65–7.

[11] Sandrina (we do not know her family name) was an Agostinian nun in the Convent of San Clemente in the via San Gallo, which was under the protection of the Medici. Her name appears in two letters (of 1571 and 1572) sent by Cosimo I to authorize payments to the convent on her behalf (Medici Archive Project).

On the whole, the 1568 customers of the speziale al Giglio represent a good cross-section of the Medici court. Looking at the table above, however, one immediately notes that women are almost absent. There is mention of only three women, a nun (Sandrina in San Cremente), a wet nurse (balia del putino di Sua Eccellenza), and a noblewoman, a relative of the family (Leonora de Toledo).[56] Women are almost absent also in the account books of the preceding years.[57] It is evident that, apart from the relatives of the Medici or their guests, only the functionaries and personnel of the court, i.e. the *salariati*, but not their families, had the right to purchase medicines at the duke's expense.

Simples

From examining the purchases of the account books of the speziale al Giglio we can get a rough idea of the medicinal plants most frequently used in everyday practice. I say 'rough' because the plants included in the account books are not always easily identified, and therefore an exact number is not obtainable. The plants and herbs purchased are not always mentioned directly. Sometimes only the name of a recipe is mentioned, and one has to find out of what it is composed. For example if *diacodion* is mentioned, one must know that it is a sort of electuary whose principal ingredient is poppies. However, in the *Ricettario fiorentino* of 1567 there are two recipes of *diacodion*, one is the *diacodion semplice* of Galen, the other the *diacodion composto* of Mesue. While the first contains only poppies, water and honey, the latter is obviously more complex and contains many more ingredients.[58] One therefore can seldom be sure which are the ingredients used to compose a particular recipe. A similar problem, but much more frequent, arises when a preparation based on a particular plant is mentioned, for example 'syrup of chicory'. In a composite syrup, besides sugar or honey, which are the basic components, there can be many more ingredients than the one mentioned. Very often,

---

[56] Eleonora di Toledo appears twice (10 and 14 September). The nun appears several times in the period between 1 and 13 April; the wet nurse appears twice, on 14 September and 26 November.

[57] In the first six months of 1567, for example, only one woman (Lucrezia in San Martino, probably a nun) is mentioned.

[58] *Ricettario* 1567, p. 142 and p. 143.

moreover, the reference is to very generic preparations such as '*decozione di più erbe fresche*' (decoction of several fresh herbs) or '*una presa di sciroppo usato*' (a portion of the usual syrup) and these are formulas repeated over and over again. A decoction was usually used to dilute laxatives or enemas. A *Decozione comune magistrale da stemperare le medicine* can be found in the same edition of the Florentine pharmacopoeia, and similar recipes are reported for the same function.[59] Looking at the *Ricettario fiorentino* of 1567 and Mattioli's *Discorsi* of 1568 we can find which herbs were normally used in the kind of decoctions or syrups defined as 'common' or simple, and learn that ten vegetable substances were contained in a 'common decoction' to dilute a medicine.[60]

The ingredients most frequently mentioned in the account book of 1568 appear to be sugar (forty), honey (twenty-eight), and roses. Roses are directly mentioned seven times (always red roses, which were thought to be purgative), but the word '*rosato*', that is to say containing roses, or made out of roses, appears 85 times. Sugar and honey, although they were believed to have some medicinal virtues themselves, were mainly used for conservation and to render the taste of medicaments more pleasant. These products are very often substances regularly added to some medicaments and do not appear directly in the account books. We know, for example, that sugar and/or honey will be one of the ingredients every time a syrup is mentioned.

Apart from these 'basic' ingredients, the medicinal plant most sold is cassia which appears 21 times in 1568. Cassia, an exotic plant unknown to Dioscorides, was one of the most widely used laxative drugs. 'Cassia fistula' in particular had mild purgative properties and was very often part of the 'preparatory' treatment. It appears in the account book in diverse forms. Sometimes it is only 'cassia', at other times 'cassia comune' or 'olio di cassia' or 'diacassia', which was a preparation made from cassia pulp, senna, tamarinds, rhubarb, violets, polypody, aniseed, liquorice, 'penniti'. Besides cassia, there are only four plants mentioned more than ten times: chicory (eighteen), camomile (sixteen), almonds (fourteen), and senna (twelve). Chicory was very often used in the form of a syrup (*sciroppo di cichorea*), or 'water' (*acqua di cichorea*), or as one of the components of a decoction used to dilute various preparations.[61] It was defined by Dioscorides as wild endive, and the same definition is maintained in Mattioli's *Discorsi*. It is cold and dry in the second grade, and is suitable for curing ailments of the

---

[59]   Ibid., pp. 124–5.

[60]   'Decoz. Comune Magistrale da stemperare le medicine', ibid., p. 124.

[61]   In the *Ricettario* of 1568, the 'sciroppo di cicorea semplice' (p. 133) is made from chicory juice and sugar, while the 'sciroppo di cicorea composto' (pp. 134–5) contains twenty-two ingredients.

liver.[62] Camomile, again according to Mattioli, is hot and dry in the first grade and had many medicinal virtues, among which was the calming effect for which it is still used. It is composed of 'subtle parts' and has digestive and soothing properties. It is analgesic, reduces inflammation, and cures some types of fever, especially those caused by an excess of yellow and black bile. Almonds helped to expectorate the viscous humours from the chest and lungs, freed all blockages of the liver, and alleviated pain from the spleen and loins, and that caused by colics.[63] Senna (or sena) was not included in Dioscorides and Galen's treatises, but only in those of Arab authors, such as Mesue and Serapion. As is said in the *Ricettario fiorentino*, it was of two sorts, the Oriental and the local. The best one came from Mecca, had purgative properties but no unpleasant side effects. Mattioli devotes a long section to 'senna', in which he points out the mistakes made by contemporary authors. He maintains that senna was very common in Tuscany, and 'that he had sown almost an entire field with senna in order to experiment on its pods', to see whether they should be used green, or dry.[64] He agrees with the compilers of the Florentine Pharmacopoeia that the best was imported from the Orient. Senna, as well as cassia, was one of the plants most frequently used in purgative compounds.[65]

Beyond these, however, there are many other plants, mentioned a few times or just once. There are 102 vegetable ingredients mentioned in the account book of 1568.

[62] Mattioli, *Discorsi* 1568, ch. 121, pp. 535–6.

[63] Ibid., ch. 140, pp. 292–3.

[64] Mattioli, *Discorsi* 1568, ch. 79 ('Del Delphinio'), pp. 825–9.

[65] 'Diacatholicon', the best-selling purgative drug at the Giglio in 1493–94 contained both senna and cassia. See Shaw and Welch, *Making and Marketing Medicine*, p. 245. Diacatholicon is never mentioned in the 1568 book of the Giglio, and it is mentioned only once in 1567 (30 August).

Table 6.2   Medicinal plants mentioned in the 1568 Account Book of the speziale al Giglio for the Medici court[66]

Abezzo	4	Acanto	1	Acetosa	7
Agarico	1	Aloe	9	Altea	7
Aneto	4	Anici	8	Appio	3
Assaro	3	Assenzio	8	Balausti	2
Bengui	1	Betonica	9	Bistorta	2
Borrana	1	Calcanto	1	Camomilla	16
Cannella	9	Cassia	21	Cedro	3
Cerusa	2	Cicoria	15	Comino	1
Consolida	1	Coriandoli	2	Cotognato	3
Datteri	6	Enula campana	1	Epatica	1
Erbina	4	Fave	1	Feghetella	2
Fiengreco	4	Finocchio	2	Fumosterno	3
Garofani	2	Geriaco	2	Ghalbano	1
Gromma	10	Iera	8	Incenso	6
Indivia	3	Ireos	2	Lattuga	1
Legno santo (guaiaco)	1	Lentisco	1	Limoni	6
Linseme	5	Logorizia	1	Lupini	3
Madreselva	1	Malva	2	Mandorle	14
Mandragola	1	Mastice	7	Mele (miele)	31
Melograne	1	Menta	3	Mirra	1
Mortella-mortine	3	Muscho-muschato	6	Nenufaro	1
Noci moscate	1	Lauro	1	Orzo	4
Papaveri	5	Pece greca	1	Pepe	1
Piantaggine	5	Pimpinella	5	Pinoli	2
Prezzemolo	1	Puleggio	1	Rabarbaro	3
Radicchio	1	Ragia	2	Rapa	1
Regolizia	4	Riso	1	Romice	3
Rose-rosato	102	Ruta	2	Salvia	1
Sangue di drago	4	Sapa	1	Senapa	3
Senna	12	Sercocolla	1	Spigo	1
Spigonardo	2	Squinanti	3	Storace	2
Susine	1	Terebinto	2	Timo	5
Trementina	7	Vino	7	Zafferano	2
Zucca	1	Viole-violato	4	Zucchero	40

---

[66]   The number indicates how many times the plant is mentioned.

We know that the *Nuovo Ricettario Fiorentino*, already in its first edition of 1498, included more than 400 medicinal plants.[67] Even if not all the substances contained in the recipes of the Giglio account books are named, the discrepancy between the numbers suggests that the remedies used in practice might be less numerous, and the compounds less complex than those reported in the pharmacopoeia.

Table 6.3   Animal substances mentioned in the 1568 Account Book of the speziale al Giglio for the Medici court

Burro	1	Cappone	1	Cera	11
Lombrichi	3	Pollo	6	Scorpioni	1
Spugne	4				

The animal substances mentioned are only seven. We know that chickens and capons were the basis of the usual diet of the sick;[68] their broth was also used to dilute medicines. Sponges were used as a means to apply the various substances of external remedies, because of their great absorbency. They were sometimes burned and the ash obtained formed an ingredient of some recipes. Earthworms and scorpions were believed to be real medicinal substances, the latter being the principal ingredient of scorpion oil, a recipe of Mesue adapted and produced by the grand dukes themselves.[69]

As to minerals, which are sometimes considered to be the new discovery of European pharmacology, they do not appear to be frequently used in the medical practice of the day.

Table 6.4   Mineral substances mentioned in the 1568 Account Book of the speziale al Giglio for the Medici court

Allume	3	Argento vivo	2	Bolio	3
Cerusa	2	Cinabro	1	Piombo	4
Ranno	1	Sale	5	Salnitro	2
Silicato	1	Tuzia (polvere di zinco)	13	Zolfo	1

---

[67]   Huguet-Termes, *Approximacion historico-farmacologica*, pp. 88–100.

[68]   An extract of chicken and capon was distilled in the 'kitchen' of the apothecary shop of the hospital of S. Maria Nuova in Florence, to be given 'to the seriously ill both in the hospital and outside it'. Henderson, *The Renaissance Hospital*, p. 294.

[69]   See Chapter 1, p. 58 and ibid., note 78.

In the account book of 1568 only twelve mineral substances are recorded, of which *tuzia* (zync oxide), usually to be found in ointments and oils for external therapy, is the most frequent.

In addition to these, however, we have to consider 'triafarmaco', an ointment containing litharge (called by Dioscorides 'silver foam'), for curing ulcers, a recipe by Mesue for external use, which is recorded four times. Vergilio Carnesecchi, the most assiduous client of the Giglio in the sample year, was prescribed both medicaments; these, however, were very ancient recipes that cannot be numbered with the new discoveries. There is, therefore, no doubt that minerals were still very few compared to vegetable substances, and there is no sign that the new principles of iatrochemistry were being adopted. The only 'modern' recipe of note containing a mineral substance is the 'quicksilver ointment', also prescribed to Vergilio Carnesecchi, which suggests that he might have been suffering from syphilitic ulcers. It also demonstrates that mercury, although not even mentioned in the 1567 *Ricettario Fiorentino*, was actually in use at least as an external therapy.

Medicines

These are the simples mentioned in the 1568 account book of the speziale al Giglio. But how were they used, and which kind of recipes were they for? The records show that they were very seldom sold separately, as ingredients of a recipe to be processed at home by the patient. It is interesting to note that the major part of the sales of individual simples were on behalf of the ducal *fonderia*, which was a pharmaceutical laboratory itself, and where new recipes were experimented on. The account books show that simples were usually sold in the form of a ready-made product, or of ready-made drugs that could be simply assembled to obtain the remedy for which they were intended. If compared with those of 1494, the purchases of 1568 reveal a much less standardized use of the ingredients. Only very few of the traditional electuaries which constituted the top ten drugs in 1494 appear among the sales of 1568.[70] Diarrhodon abbatis, a sweet electuary (115 sales in 1494), is mentioned three times in 1568.[71] Diaphoenicon (141 sales in 1494) appears only once.[72] Diacatholicon, the best-selling drug at the Giglio in 1494 (171 sales), does not appear at all in our sample year, and appears only once in 1567.[73]

---

[70]   Shaw and Welch, *Making and Marketing Medicine*, p. 245.

[71]   *Ricettario* 1567, p. 149.

[72]   Ibid., p. 165.

[73]   Ibid., p. 164.

Apart from Diarrhodon abatis and Diaphoenicon only very few of the drugs recorded in the *Ricettario fiorentino* are mentioned in the Giglio account book of 1568, and very seldom. They are Diacassia (two), Diacodion (one), Diagridio (one), and Diapalma (two).

Sometimes peculiar or relatively complex recipes are described, but they appear to be special prescriptions by the patient's doctor. Vergilio Carnesecchi, for example, was prescribed a drug made out of butter cooked in a big turnip.[74] Franceschino staffiere was prescribed an enema composed of 'eight cyclamens [bulbs] well grated put in an infusion of two *fiaschi* of Greek wine and then boiled until they are reduced to three 'mezette' [quarters] and then divided into three parts of one 'mezetta' each and to each part a glass of urine of a small child and two of common honey were added ...'.[75]

The two most prestigious electuaries of the ancients, theriac and mithridate, are almost absent from the records of the speziale al Giglio. We know that theriac was so complex that only a few *speziali* were licensed to produce it. Its shelf life, on the other hand, was incredibly long (at least twenty years), and any apothecary could buy it and keep it in his shop.[76] In the letters we have examined, only mithridate is mentioned once, when it was prescribed to old Cosimo in 1572 after the administration of purgative medicines.[77] In the 1568 account book of the Giglio theriac only appears once, and is completely absent in that of 1567. Sometimes theriac and mithridate were not prescribed on their own, but as part of other compounds; we have seen, for example, that Mercuriale, in his *consilium* about a case of quartan fever recommends that the patient should take a *bolus* of theriac, lapis lazuli, sugar, and borage on the day before the onset of the fever.[78] Theriac and mithridate were also ingredients of the famous scorpion oil and the *elixir vitae* produced by the grand dukes in their *fonderie*.[79] Even though there had been extensive research in order to identify and re-establish all the ingredients that made up the theriac of the ancients, and to restore it to its original potency, and although theriac was often mentioned in the books of *practica*, the impression is that it was seldom prescribed, at least on its own.[80]

---

[74] 'Adi 19 novembre per vergilio carnesechi d. 2 di bituro fresco messo in una rapa grossa e dipoi messa nel fuoco tanto sia cotta e dipoi cavatone il burro e un albo di vetro.'

[75] 'Per Franceschino staffiere per otto pamporcini grattugiati bene infusi in due fiaschi di vingreco di suo per spazio di ore 24 e poi fatti bollire tanto che tornino tre mezette e poi fattone tre parti d'una mezetta l'una e ciascuna mezetta agiugni un bicchiere di orina di fanciullo picolo e due di mele comune per un serviziale e farne tre serviziali e tre pentole (19 gennaio).'

[76] *Ricettario* 1567, p. 108.

[77] ASF, Medici del Principato, vol. 642, c. 18.

[78] See above, p. 235.

[79] However, 1 pound of ready-made oil of scorpions is collected on 17 December 1568 by Giuliano Chiavacci for the *fonderia*.

[80] See for example, Mercuriale, *Praelectiones Patavinae*, libro V, 'De febribus', p. 581.

At the Giglio there was a separate area where all the substances for the production of theriac (*ordinate per la teriaca*) were stored.[81] The making of theriac involved a very long procedure, and some of its ingredients had to undergo a process of seasoning for months, before being introduced into the compound. In addition, we do not know if the *speziale* Lorenzo Lapini was among the few *speziali* licensed to produce it. It is therefore difficult to know if the substances for the production of theriac would have been sold to other apothecaries, or were there to be used by the speziale al Giglio itself. Certainly theriac could not be prepared on the spot when prescribed, but it had to be already made. Probably, as James Shaw and Evelyn Welch suggest, to be able to gather and keep in the shop the 'true' ingredients of theriac (the inventory lists almost fifty substances) was per se a sign of professional skill and prestige.[82] As far as the demand of the Medici court was concerned, it remains a fact that theriac was sold only once in two years.[83]

It is surprising that guaiacum, which in this period was considered the best remedy for the French disease, and was also used for many other ailments, was sold only once in 1568 (on the last day of the account book) and was requested by the ducal *fonderia*. In the account books of 1566 and 1567 we see that it is mentioned more frequently, and is often associated with sarsaparilla, the other American drug used for the French disease.[84] It does not seem, however, to have been prescribed for other ailments, as it appeared from the *acqua del legno* regularly taken by old Cosimo, or in other letters where it is clearly prescribed for reasons that had nothing to do with syphilis.[85] A large quantity of *legno santo*, in different forms, appear on the inventory which was taken on 9 June 1568, after the death of the *speziale* Lorenzo Lapini. The inventory records almost 480 lbs of guaiacum, and a further thirty-three already ordered.

It is very likely that large quantities of the above mentioned substances were stored at the Giglio which acted as an intermediary for supplying communities such as hospitals and monasteries. We know that only few hospitals had a pharmacy of their own, and therefore ordered simples and ready-made preparations from external apothecaries. The same can be said for convents and monasteries which sometimes were able to produce some of the medicines they needed, but very rarely all of them.[86] As far as guaiacum is concerned, we know, for example, that it was required in large amounts by the Florentine '*Incurabili*

---

[81] Inventory of 1568, cc. 93v–94r. See Shaw and Welch, *Making and Marketing Medicine*, p. 297.

[82] Ibid., p. 299.

[83] See above, p. 256.

[84] In 1567, for example, *legno santo* is recorded a dozen times, for three people (one of whom was Vergilio Carnesecchi), the same for whom salsaparilla was prescribed.

[85] See above, p. 242.

[86] Strocchia, 'The nun apothecaries of Renaissance Florence', pp. 627–47.

hospital' of SS. Trinita, where the patients suffering from French disease were treated.[87]

The tables below show the groups of medicinal products and the number of times they were sold in 1568.

Table 6.5   Medicinal products for internal use sold by the speziale al Giglio in 1568

Sciroppi	176	Elettuari (unspecified)	5
Acque	50	Datteri	8
Decozioni	22	Morselletti	2
Pillole	9	Sopposte	1
Giulebbi	9	Madaleoni	1
Serviziali	7	Miele rosato solutivo	15
Diarrhodon abbatis	3	Diaphoenicon	1
Diacassia	2	Diapalma	2
Diagridion	1	Diacodion	1

Table 6.6   Medicinal products for external use sold by the speziale al Giglio in 1568

Oli	43	Cerotti	4
Unguenti	31	Bagni	2
Fumenti	9	Impiastri	1

As one can see, the medicament by far the most mentioned is syrup. In the account book of 1568 (which records the purchases between 1 April and 9 February)[88] syrup is sold 176 times in about ten months, on an average of more than 17 sales per month. The majority of these sales (152 – more than 85 per cent) is recorded with the same wording, that is to say 'one dose of the usual syrup'.

---

[87]   Henderson, *The Renaissance Hospital*, p. 110. The 1574 Statutes of SS. Trinita established that 'people having need to take the wood' could be admitted into the hospital.

[88]   In the Florentine calendar the year began on 25 March. The account book of 1568 terminates on 9 February, probably when the apothecary Lorenzo Lapini died.

Table 6.7   Syrups sold by the speziale al Giglio in 1568

Sciroppi 'usati'	152	Sciroppo di betonica	3
Sciroppo rosato	13	Sciroppo di fumosterno	3
Sciroppo di cicorea	4	Sciroppo di jera	1

The 'usual' syrups were very probably simple syrups made of honey or sugar and water, maybe rose water, which were prescribed after a purge or between two purges.[89] Syrup was considered very useful for preparing or keeping soft the material to be expelled. Falloppio in his book about purges heaps praise on syrups;[90] we have seen that Mercuriale in his *consilium* about a case of quartan fever recommends syrups every day for a long period. All the customers that appear several times in the books of the speziale al Giglio, without exception, are recorded as taking 'one dose of the usual syrup' before, after, or between treatments. One can follow, for example, the case of Vergilio Carnesecchi who is the most assiduous customer in the year under study.[91] He is in frequent need of drugs and, given the different medicaments he is prescribed, seems to be suffering from a serious disease, not easily cured. His purchases, between May and December 1568, are thirty-six of which fourteen (that is to say more than one-third) are 'doses of the usual syrup'. The same proportion is found for other customers, for example, for Signor Pirro, a page who appears on the book twenty-eight times between 10 August and 7 September, nine of which to collect a 'dose of the usual syrup'. Although the disease is not mentioned, sometimes one can recognize the procedure to expel the humour which causes it by the sequence of medicines prescribed to the same customer; at first the mild ones for the preparation, often in the form of syrups or enemas, and then the stronger, in the form of pills, electuaries, or composite syrups.

The most frequently sold medicinal products after syrups were waters. Waters were divided into natural waters (rain water, wells and springs, thermal baths)[92] and artificial waters, which were waters of herbs processed by distillation.[93] The

---

[89]   The types of syrup of the account book are very few in comparison with those that appear in the 1568 inventory of the speziale al Giglio. Here long lists of syrups are recorded. The 'sciroppo usato' could be that named 'fresh rose syrup' (*sciroppo rosato fresco*). AOI, Processo 20, cc. 62r–62v, 77r–78v, and *passim*.

[90]   Falloppio, *De simplicibus medicamentis purgantibus*, p. 170.

[91]   The highest number of purchases is on behalf of the ducal *fonderia* (55 purchases collected by Berghamo, master of the fonderia, and ten collected by Giuliano Chiavacci).'

[92]   The thermal baths mentioned are: La Porretta, Montecatini, Acqua, San Filippo, Santa Maria, La Villa. *Ricettario fiorentino* 1573, p. 6.

[93]   Ibid., pp. 6–7.

waters mentioned in our sample year are fifty, ten of which are thermal, and forty made from seventeen different plants. They were necessary to prepare liquid remedies (above all purges) and to dilute them, but at the same time they were used to reach the desired balance between hot-cold-dry-humid qualities. Waters, moreover, unlike decoctions, which had to be made on the spot, had a shelf life of one year. This explains the great variety of waters that apothecaries shops had in stock. The 1568 inventory of the Giglio records waters of thirty-four different medicinal plants.[94] The table below lists the kind of waters that were sold in our sample year.

Table 6.8   Waters sold by the speziale al Giglio in 1568

Acqua di betonica	4	Acqua di cannella	3
Acqua di rosa	5	Acqua di epatica (feghetella)	2
Acqua di sena	5	Acqua d'orzo	1
Acqua di cicorea	4	Acqua di fumosterno	1
Acqua di piantaggine	4	Acqua di Malva	1
Acqua di finocchio	2	Acqua di acetosa	1
Acqua pettorale[1]	2	Acqua di luppoli	1
Acqua di gramigna	3	Thermal waters[2]	10
Acqua di camomilla	1	Acqua di nenufaro	1

Notes: [1] The main ingredient of acqua pettorale (water *for the chest) was usually liquorice.*
[2] Mainly acqua del tettuccio *(Montecatini) and acqua della Villa.*

Decoctions could not be preserved, and had to be made freshly by the *speziale*, which explains why they are not mentioned in the inventory of 1568. They had the same function as waters and were used to dilute medicaments; as waters they could also have some medicinal property themselves. In the account books of the Giglio decoctions appear twenty-one times of which fifteen under the wording 'decoction of several fresh herbs' ('decozione di più erbe fresche'), and three with the wording 'common decoction'. Only three times is a decoction of sena *magistrale* recorded, which was a purgative compound containing sena and a few other ingredients.

    Another category of medicinal drugs was that which included various forms of 'pills', such as *pillole, datteri, morselletti, madaleoni, boli*. They were not ready-made pills but rather medicinal compounds dried and compressed, which could

---

    [94]   AOI, Processo 20, cc. 66r–66v.

be rendered soft with a syrup, a water or a decoction and then transformed in pastilles, tablets, or lozenges to be swallowed.

Among the external drugs, oils were the most used. They were applied to various parts of the body, often to the stomach, the head or the feet. They were also the usual ingredients of almost all other compounds for external use, such as ointments, plasters and cerates. Oils, like syrups, decoctions, and waters could be made of almost all the plants which were considered to have medicinal properties. Oils could be extracted from plants by distillation, but usually were infusions of herbs in olive oil.[95]

Table 6.9   Oils sold by the speziale al Giglio in 1568

Olio di linseme	3	Olio di trementina	4
Olio rosato	6	Olio mirtino	1
Olio laurino	1	Olio melino	1
Olio di cassia	6	Olio di lombrici	1
Olio di camomilla	1	Olio di lentisco	1
Olio di ruta	1	Olio 'fine'	1
Olio di mandorle amare	1	Olio di abezo	2
Olio di mandorle dolci	7	Olio di scorpioni	1
Olio di gigli	1	Olio di spigonardo	1
Olio di assenzio	1	Olio malvato	1

Conclusion

Considering the information and data gathered from the sources I have examined, we should speak of two different levels of conclusion, rather than of a single conclusion.

The general scheme of humoral theory implied a set pattern of therapy, although sophisticated and many-sided. The widespread use of purges that was typical of the accounts of the physicians or the apothecary's books may seem surprising, as we are used to attributing only one function to purgative substances. Purgative medicaments, at that time, were simply all the medicinal plants or the preparations that, in various ways, were used to drain away the humours that had to be eliminated to restore health. As this was the principle at the basis of therapy, it is obvious that the great majority of the internal remedies were *medicamenti purgantes*. Examining the pharmacology of purgatives one realises how the theoretical framework was

---

[95]   See Chapter 5, p. 205.

refined and studied in minute detail, and according to which criteria the theory was translated into practice. For this reason it is useful to look at works specifically devoted to the simples performing that function. In Gabriele Falloppio's work on this subject, for example, one discovers that, as Hippocrates had said, 'each purgative medicament evacuates a certain humour'.[96] That is to say that some simples evacuate only the yellow bile, others only the black bile, and others only the serum (phlegm).[97] For example, if we administer scammony (a kind of convolvulus) to a patient, only the yellow bile will be evacuated; if hellebore, only the black bile. The way in which the *purgans* drug acts on the humour is by way of an attraction based on the similarity of their substances, and (according to Galen) through a 'digestion' (*coctio*). The *umor peccans* can be removed via all the orifices and pores of the human body (*per vomitum, per intestina, per palatum, per nares, per uterum*, etc.). As well as this general theoretical scheme, (which is much more complex than in my résumé), Falloppio provides us with a detailed account of the different levels of 'strength' of the various substances, and their different functions in the progress of the evacuation, with a vast vocabulary of 'technical' terms.[98] From this account it is clear that the final evacuation is the result of gradual steps, and that it must be prepared carefully. At the end of the treatise a series of chapters explains which simples are to be used for the draining of the different humours.[99] Chapters XXVI–XXXI deal with the quantities of the drugs that must be administered, and the kind of preparation (pills, syrups, etc.), with particular attention to enemas. Chapters XXXII–LXIX provide us with a list of the simples (about forty) used as purgatives. As therapy hinged on the evacuation of bad humours, it is not surprising that in the numerous medical works that deal with fevers, the section on therapy is a repetition, with some adjustments, of treatises about *purgantes* like the one considered above. For example, as quartan fever is said to originate from the putrefaction of black bile, the cure will be the evacuation of black bile, according to the same prescriptions of Gabriele Falloppio's treatise on purges.

Even if the data we can gather from the sources so far taken into account does not seem always to conform with the specific treatments expounded in the theoretical texts, the fundamental principles at the basis of therapy were constantly observed. If one thought of the theory of humours as a framework devoid of any real function, these texts provide evidence that, on the contrary, it is the real pivot on which all the operations connected with therapy revolved. There is ample evidence that the collateral but essential tenets of the theory were

---

[96]   Falloppio, *De simplicibus medicamentis purgantibus*, p. 30.

[97]   It is debatable if blood can be evacuated through some sort of drug or only through bloodletting.

[98]   For example, in ch. 19, 'Per intestina', the medicaments are divided into three sections according to their strength. Falloppio, *De simplicibus medicamentis purgantibus* p. 168.

[99]   For example, in ch. 25, pp. 200–202, all the simples for black bile are listed. Ibid., p. 202.

also believed in and followed. There cannot be any doubt about the importance attributed to the non-naturals in maintaining or regaining health. The other fundamental general rule of the Galenic medical system, that treatments had to be modified and adapted each time to the patient, according to his complexion, age, sex, season, etc., is also proven to have been constantly put into practice.[100] The same physicians, who had expounded the treatment of a certain disease in their theoretical or pseudo-theoretical works, reserved the right to change the therapy according to a particular patient. Conformity to this rule is probably the simplest explanation to account for the fact that in some of the letters examined above the remedies we had expected to find were not mentioned, as in the case of young Cosimo (1544), or of the Grand Duchess Cristina's quartan fevers (1601).

The first, very general level of conclusion is, therefore, that there was undoubtedly a very close correspondence between the theoretical framework and the practical application of therapy.

At a second level, however, that of the actual use of the remedies which appear in the works of *Practica* written by university professors, in the pharmacopoeias, and often in the *consilia*, the correspondence is much less evident. Simples, that is to say single medicinal plants, although dealt with in famous treatises (first of all Dioscorides's and Mattioli's commentary) and also forming the subject of university courses on *materia medica*, were hardly ever used by themselves and were always part of more or less complex compounds. Each was classified as having particular properties, but a combination with others was considered necessary in order to achieve the right effect in terms of hot/cold, dry/humid faculties and other sophisticated parameters. Very often they were said to be appropriate to cure certain ailments (almost always many and disparate ones), but they were usually not thought to be a specific to a particular disease, in the sense we think of remedies today. As it clearly appears from the texts we have seen, they were often believed to be effective through an 'indirect' process, based on evacuation, and according to the principle that opposites cure opposites.[101] The function of simples is not easily understood. They are used in a way which renders their properties hardly discernible in practice. In the case of fevers, for example, the property required is the capacity to drain a certain humour which is the root cause of that particular fever. Black hellebore which is appropriate for the draining of the black bile which causes quartan fever, is taken after a long preparatory sequence of other preparations, and always in a compound,

---

[100]   Siraisi, *Medieval and Early Renaissance Medicine*, p. 120.

[101]   Guaiacum, for example, was thought to be effective for French disease, but it too, acted through evacuation and sweating. A clear example is that regarding the therapy of quartan fever which, as seen, was based on a gradual process of evacuation, and changed completely when a specific (Peruvian bark, from which quinine was extracted), was discovered.

together with other simples. It is thus very difficult to gauge the particular virtue of black hellebore.[102]

That simples were very seldom used separately, at least by learned physicians, is immediately apparent from the Florentine pharmacopoeia, where the great majority of the recipes reported were compounds of ancient medical authors.[103] As was declared in the 'Prohemio' of the first edition of the *Nuovo ricettario fiorentino*, the intention of the Florentine *Collegio dei Medici* was not to adopt new recipes, but to keep to those written by the most prominent Arab and Greek authors.[104] The *Ricettario* was compiled for practical reasons, and the sections concerning the internal layout of the apothecary shop, or the rules for the gathering of herbs and their conservation, could certainly be profitably put into practice. Paradoxically, it is the section of the *antidotarium*, i.e. the collection of recipes proper, that raises questions about the correspondence between theory and practice.

When reading the first edition of the *Ricettario* (1498), one is struck by the fact that the compilers often added whether a particular recipe was in use or not. Some long and elaborate recipes are reported even if it is declared that they were not used. For example, Dyrodon, a recipe described both by Mesue and Nicholao, appears in the *Ricettario*, even if it is said not to be in use (*non si usa*); the same can be said for 'Lactovaro di Re', 'Lactovaro resumptivo', 'Saxinea', 'Dyamorte', etc.[105] Sometimes the compilers offer an explanation. With reference to the 'Lactovaro di gemme' ('Electuary of precious stones'), for example, they say that the recipe is included although not in use, 'because of its nobility'.[106] In the edition of 1567, the words 'in use' or 'not in use' no longer appear, but the 'Electuary of precious stones' is still there.[107]

From the sources examined there is evidence that it was very rare to encounter in practice prescriptions of the very complex 'electuaries' transcribed in the books,

---

[102] As far as fevers are concerned, the medicinal plants mentioned by Dioscorides for their treatment are very often mentioned with doubtful words. Some of them are to be used as amulets or associated with magic formulas. See for example 'teasle', III, 11 (2): p. 183: 'The worms contained within the head, wrapped up and worn around the neck or arm are said to cure quartan fevers.' Or 'plantain', II, 126 (4), p. 146: 'Three roots ... help with tertian fever. Four roots ... help with quartan fever.' Or 'treacle clover', III,109 (2), p. 231: Some give three leaves or three seeds in wine for tertian fever and four for quartan fever, on the assumption that they stop the periodic fever.' Or 'holy vervain', IV, 60 (2): 'The third joint from the ground with the surrounding leaves is given to people who have tertian fever, and to those who have quartan fever, the fourth.' In Pedanius Dioscorides of Anarzabus, *De materia medica*, translated by Lily Y. Beck (Hildesheim, Zurich and New York, 2005).

[103] Huguet-Termes, *Approximacion historico-farmacologica*, p. 80, note 194.

[104] See Chapter 5, pp. 188–9.

[105] *Ricettario fiorentino* 1498, Book II, 'De Lactovari dolci'.

[106] 'This lactovaro is after Mesue & is not in use: it is reported for its nobility'. Ibid.

[107] *Il Ricettario Medicinale necessario a tutti i Medici, & Speziali* (1567), p. 152.

even for the wealthy members of the Medici family and their court. Apart from mithridate (which anyway was mentioned only once), the only electuary of that sort that can be found among the preparations administered to old Cosimo in 1572 is 'lattovaro alchermes', prescribed by the physician Baccio Gatteschi, after he had tried every possible means of restoring Cosimo's health. From the account books of the *spetieria* and the letters we have examined, which are the documents closest to actual practice, we get the impression that the medicines used in practice were usually simpler than the ones written in the books. Other studies, such as that carried out by John Henderson on the recipe book of the hospital of Santa Maria Nuova in Florence, that of James Shaw and Evelyn Welch on the sales of the speziale al Giglio in 1494, or that of Giovanni Silini on the recipes prescribed by the doctors of a small village in Piedmont, seem to confirm this view.[108] The fact that the Giglio book of 1568 records very few 'ancient' electuaries in comparison with 1494 suggests that there had been an evolution towards a freer use of the ingredients and simpler remedies. Probably many of the complex electuaries of the ancient authors were simply 'not in use', as had already been declared for some of them in the first edition of the *Ricettario fiorentino*. In the medical books, however, even in those that dealt with the practice of therapy, the humanistic approach to the classics and the importance attributed to them still carried enormous weight, and still came first. As for the 'electuary of precious stones' included in the *Ricettario fiorentino*, the 'nobility' of the recipe was more important than its actual use. One of the reasons is that, as seen above, physicians did not consider themselves obliged to follow literally the classic recipes. On the other hand, it is clear, as has already been said with regard to *consilia*, that a display of erudition, and adherence to the classics, was a necessity for the prestige and the status of university doctors. The same purpose of prestige, although the criterion is different, is apparent in the case of the collection of recipes compiled by the learned apothecary Stefano Rosselli. Stefano wrote a book of 'secrets' in order to leave them to his sons, but the choice of the preparations he included is, above all, an act of homage to the Medici family. The preparations in fact are those used or produced by the grand dukes, like the famous scorpion oil, or otherwise reveal, in the title or in the text, some sort of link with the Medici.[109] We know that Stefano, who belonged to a well-known

---

[108] Henderson, *The Renaissance Hospital*, pp. 297–335; Shaw and Welch, *Making and Marketing Medicine*, p. 245; Silini, *Umori e farmaci*. It is significant that in Santa Maria Nuova, the hospital personnel (above all the *medici di casa*), although they had at their disposal the recipes of prominent medical authors, often wrote their own recipes to treat their patients. See Henderson, *The Renaissance Hospital*, pp. 299–302.

[109] The recipes are published in Stefano Francesco di Romolo Rosselli, *Mes secrets à Florence au temps des Médicis 1593*, ed. Rodrigo de Zayas (Paris, 1996). Some titles: 'Modo di fare l'olio contro a velenj del Serenis.mo Gran Duca di Toscana Cosimo Medicj', p. 212; 'Modo di fare il vino composto aromatico detto hypoclas, avuto dalla Ill.ma et Ex.ma Dogna Isabella Medicj Orsina', p. 217; Unguento da nervj di S.A.S.ma Cosimo Medici', p. 218; 'Olio

Florentine family, owned an apothecary shop (the 'Speziale al San Francesco'), at the Canto del Giglio, opposite that of the Lapini, and that he took on the supply of medicines to the Medici court after Lorenzo Lapini's death.[110]

Practical medical literature went well beyond practical therapy; part of it, which included the recipes of ancient classical authorities, was crystallized in a parallel life of its own which served a different kind of practice. It was governed by a series of conventions and unwritten rules that had to be rigorously observed by physicians who aspired to be counted among the restricted number of doctors of the élite. Being closely associated with the profession, it was seen as a vehicle by which to acquire and maintain authority and fame, be competitive in the most promising sectors of the marketplace, and be chosen as physicians by princes and prominent courtiers.

---

da stomaco del Gran Duca Ferdinando', p. 220; 'Acqua da pietra del Gran Duca Cosimo, che la insegnò a Reverendo Romitj di Camaldolj, et ancor oggi s'usa in fonderia di S.A.', p. 222; 'Preparazione dello acciaio che usava il Duca Francesco per farlo potabile; et ancora ridotto in pasta, cosa utilissima per l'opilazione, et oggi è molto in uso in nostra botega', p. 222.

[110] Shaw and Welch, *Making and Marketing Medicine*, p. 304.

Conclusion

This study brings to the fore the variety of views, beliefs, customs and practices that were associated with sixteenth-century plants. Its purpose was to bring together all these elements in a picture where plants would regain the place they occupied in sixteenth-century Tuscany, and thus identify the routes which led to the development of the new disciplinary field which later came to be called botany. The picture that emerged is far from static, and if we were to choose a feature to describe it, it would be the enormous intellectual and practical ferment that it displays.

In very general terms, we can observe that medicine still occupied the major part of the space, as plants maintained, through the whole period under discussion, a pre-eminent role in therapy. The traditional theory of humours was still the conceptual scheme that directed all medical activity. What clearly emerges, however, is that it was flexible enough to allow the physician to decide how to apply it. The vegetable substances that were still the basis of almost all remedies appeared in the Florentine pharmacopoeia according to the ancient recipes, but our investigation reveals that only a part of them were the current herbs sold by an apothecary shop for standard treatments. The ancient authors were still revered, and we have seen how all literary medical works, from herbals to *Consilia* and pharmacopoeias, paid homage to them and pursued credibility through their authority. At the same time emancipation from ancient authors is often demonstrated, in direct or indirect ways, and it is apparent that although the *antiqui* were still the starting-point for pharmacological research, they were no longer unquestioned authorities. Even the radical and iconoclastic ideas of Paracelsus had penetrated the circle of the Medici and Florentine intellectuals without creating any particular scandal.

The categories where plants were usually accommodated, the Hippocratic-Galenic system for medicine, and Aristotelianism combined with a Christian Neo-Platonic vision for natural philosophy, were not the static and heavy chains that have often been described as obstacles to the liberation from ignorance and superstition, and hindrances to scientific progress. They were rather large-meshed nets, which allowed to encompass and reconcile what we would now consider irreconcilable. The same person could be both a 'man of science' and a believer in magic and occult forces. Cesalpino used observation and even carried out experiments on plants, which can be seen as very close to a scientific approach, but also wrote about demons and amulets. Mattioli in the preface to his *Discorsi* mocks the simple and the superstitious who utter prayers or spells when using herbs and roots, 'as if the virtues and faculties of medicaments could be augmented, diminished or assimilated through words', but a few pages further on maintains that a crown of bay will prevent one from being struck by lightning.[1] Alchemy and pharmacology used the same methods and were often indistinguishable from one another. In gardens, plants were used to develop allegorical and symbolic programmes, but were also monitored carefully during their growth, and chosen for being beautiful and exotic.

Drawing on a diverse range of visual and documentary evidence, we have seen how natural objects were part of a world that appears larger than ours, where belief in occult sympathies and magic could coexist with the trends that we now attribute to scientific thought.

But how did plants take the independent route that led them to become the subject of a new discipline?

The impact of humanism was certainly fundamental in this process, as first-hand investigation of medicinal plants was brought into sharp relief by most ancient medical authorities, and above all by Galen and Dioscorides. In our study we have seen how this new approach to pharmacology was institutionalized with a new chair of *materia medica* in the medical faculty of the *Studio pisano*, which was complemented by a botanical garden, and how a series of new methods were devised and spread by Luca Ghini and his circle, to organize and record the results of first-hand investigation. Here we can recognize a point of contact and an overlap between medicine and natural philosophy, as a different attitude towards nature was at stake. It was through these new procedures and techniques that plants began to be studied and researched in their own right. We can see with our own eyes how the development of this particular branch of medicine gradually led to the study of plants for themselves and we can acknowledge what Agnes Arber calls 'the incalculable debt which Botany owes to Medicine'.[2] This debt, however, is not to be ascribed only to the fact that, as she says, 'an overwhelming majority of the herbalists were physicians who were led to the study of botany on account of its connection with the arts of healing', but also to the fact that this development involved a different attitude towards the natural world. Knowledge of nature was now regarded as something to pursue through observation and the study of empirical data rather than just through philosophical speculation.

This general framework provides the context for the encounter with the vast number of new plants from the New World which, though they did not change substantially the pharmacopoeia, were welcomed with great enthusiasm by naturalists, irrespective of their utility. The discovery of a whole new flora enlarged enormously the vegetable kingdom, and brought about the unsettling idea that God's creation did not coincide at all with the orderly natural world the ancients had described. This constant increase of plants, which could not be kept under control, presented naturalists with problems that had nothing to do

---

[1]   Mattioli, *Discorsi* 1568, p. 5, and p. 16.
[2]   Arber, *Herbals*, pp. 221–2.

with medicine. Andrea Cesalpino tried to cope with this problem by building a rational system of classification; he was able to do so by applying philosophical thought to a comparison of the plants that he had collected in his herbarium, and through careful observation in the field. Before embarking on his attempt at classification, Cesalpino assessed which were the 'accidental' and which the inherent qualities of a plant, establishing with certainty that medicinal properties belonged with the 'accidental'.

In the overlapping area of pharmacology and natural history, what emerges is a new way of looking at the physical world. This shift in natural philosophy, that appears clearly in our study, has been described many times by historians, and historians of science, as a necessary condition of what has been called the 'scientific revolution'.

That this new attitude could still arouse disapproval is attested by the words of Falloppio, who reproves Aldrovandi for leaving the teaching of natural philosophy and Aristotle's more speculative works to take up the teaching of *materia medica* and what were considered Aristotle's lesser works.[3] In Falloppio's letter, we recognize the traditional separation between the theoretical and the practical spheres of knowledge. Observation and description were not considered by Falloppio to be a dignified intellectual pursuit, or a way to acquire new knowledge. But his letter, in the light of our research, represents an opinion which is already anachronistic. Our study, in fact, reveals the opposite. The new approaches to the analysis of the physical world, implied a series of pragmatic activities which were considered necessary, and put into practice, not only at Pisa, where they were probably initiated, but also in other European Universities. But it is not only the academic milieu which provides evidence for our assertion that the contempt for empirical activities attested by Falloppio was no longer the general view. The descriptions of the grand dukes working in their *fonderie* or following the rooting and development of plants in their gardens, testify to a very different attitude. What is striking, when reading of the grand dukes producing medicaments 'with their own hands', is not only that one would not expect that particular activity from a prince, but also that this behaviour was usually described by contemporaries with admiration, and not just by obliging courtiers. The same thing can be said of the extraordinary practical attention the grand dukes devoted to plants and gardens. While their gardens contained many allegorical and symbolic elements, the personal interest demonstrated by their correspondence with their gardeners and secretaries attests to a new kind of interest. These 'scientific' activities, along with other more traditional issues of their cultural policy, were seen as new credentials contributing to their personal prestige, and adding lustre to the new state. They became an example for the next generations as the botanist Paolo Boccone declared in his *Museo di fisica e di esperienze* (1697): 'I observed that in Florence,

---

³ See Chapter 2, pp. 85–6.

in imitation of their ruler, all the Nobles are enamored of the studies of physic and of experiences'.[4]

The new approach to nature was reflected in the realistic and meticulous illustrations which began to appear in sixteenth-century herbals. Their role, after the advent of the printing press, which allowed a fundamental standardization of texts and images, has been widely discussed, and some historians have attributed to them an important role in the history of science.[5] However, it is interesting to note how this attention to natural objects had already been revealed by the visual arts long before the first herbals containing realistic botanical illustrations were printed. In this connection, we cannot leave out the role that art played in the early stages of natural history. It is significant that Benedetto Varchi, a convinced advocate of 'experience' as opposed to erudition, admired and considered the illustrations of Fuchs's herbal on a par with the paintings of Bacchiacca in the Palazzo Vecchio.[6] What would now be seen as something scarcely comparable was then unified by the same ability to reproduce in detail natural objects. This leads us to a more general reflection on the coincidence of art and 'science' in a period when science (as we now regard it) had not yet arrived on the scene. Historians of science and historians of art have both called attention to this subject. Herbert Butterfield (1950), the historian who coined the very expression 'scientific revolution', envisaged Renaissance naturalism in art 'as a chapter in the history of science'.[7] Erwin Panofsky, in a famous article, traced a parallel between science and art which advanced 'on a united front', and wondered whether we should not consider 'some of the achievements of the arts to be vital contributions to the progress of the sciences'. The Renaissance, Panofsky argues, broke down 'the barriers between theoretical insight, which was supposed to be a matter of the pure intellect, and practical pursuit ...', and it 'bridged the gap which had separated the scholar and thinker from the practitioner'.[8]

The new attitudes towards nature which produced a shift in natural philosophy, while bringing to the fore 'experience', by no means cancelled the importance of erudition. Investigation of nature was now complemented by first-hand observation, but classical authors, although sometimes contradicted or challenged, could by no means be ignored.

---

[4]   Paolo Boccone, *Museo di fisica e di esperienze* (Venice, 1697), p. 267. Quoted in Findlen, *Possessing Nature*, p. 9.

[5]   See Baroncini, 'Note sull'illustrazione scientifica', pp. 527–43; Renzo Baldasso, 'The role of visual representation in the scientific revolution', pp. 69–88; Kusukawa, *Picturing the Book of Nature*.

[6]   See above, Chapter 3, p. 131.

[7]   Herbert Butterfield, 'Renaissance art and modern science', *University Review*, 1(2) (1954), pp. 25–37, p. 33. Quoted in Baldasso, 'The Role of Visual Representation', pp. 71–2.

[8]   Erwin Panofsky, 'Artist, Scientist, Genius: Notes on the "Renaissance-Dämmerung"', in Wallace K. Ferguson et al. (eds), *The Renaissance: Six Essays* (New York, 1962), pp. 128, 131, 135–6.

The meaning and definition of the term 'observation' is of course under discussion, as well as the textual or visual description that it produces. As has long been understood, it cannot account for 'truth' or 'reality' *tout court*, since we observe things by using a conceptual system which is that of our age, if not our own. Brian Ogilvie, reflecting on the impulse that prompted the development of natural history in the sixteenth century, concludes that its prime motivation was aesthetic.[9] Undoubtedly the aesthetic approach played an important role, and it is not difficult to share this view when thinking how often beauty, singularity and rarity were adopted as a criterion for the choice of plants to grow in the botanical garden, or for a botanical drawing, or for inserting a new specimen in a herbal. Gardens and flowers had always been considered lovely and pleasant, and in the literature of the preceding centuries it is easy to find passages which celebrate their beauty. But beauty for the naturalists and amateurs of this period seems to have acquired a less generic meaning. It refers to particular natural objects and is closely associated with the desire to know and to possess. The apparently frivolous gesture of Francesco I who picks up a flower and looks at it with meticulous care, and the enthusiastic description of the American aloe in Cesalpino's herbal reveal the same attitude. One can easily separate this kind of aesthetic approach from the link with utility, while retaining a cognitive purpose.

These are some observations that can be drawn looking at the grand duchy of Tuscany and the Medici court in the period under study. Through the lens of plants we have pointed out some salient features that characterized the intellectual endeavours and practices in that particular social and cultural environment, and we have found how some routes branched off from the study of medicine and led to the emergence of botany and natural history.

The great dynamism that characterizes our picture of that time naturally remained active beyond the period under consideration. Shortly afterwards, the new understanding of plants was sanctioned by a new genre of books, completely distinct from herbals, usually called *flora* or *florilegia*, which eschewed any reference to the utilitarian qualities of plants. One of the best examples is *De florum cultura* of the Sienese Jesuit Giovan Battista Ferrari (1584–1655) which came out in 1633.[10]

It was the first book dedicated exclusively to flowers and ornamental plants. It contained allegorical drawings of mythological fables and beautiful naturalistic pictures, but also the very first printed botanical illustration made with the aid of a microscope (Figure C.1).[11]

---

[9]   Olgivie, *The Science of Description*, pp. 265–9.

[10]   Giovan Battista Ferrari, *De florum cultura*, Book IV (Rome, 1633; Italian translation, *Flora overo cultura di fiori*, Rome, 1638; facsimile reprint, Florence, 2001).

[11]   See David Freedberg, *The Eye of the Linx: Galileo, his Friends, and the Beginnings of Modern Natural History* (Chicago, IL, 2002), pp. 38–53.

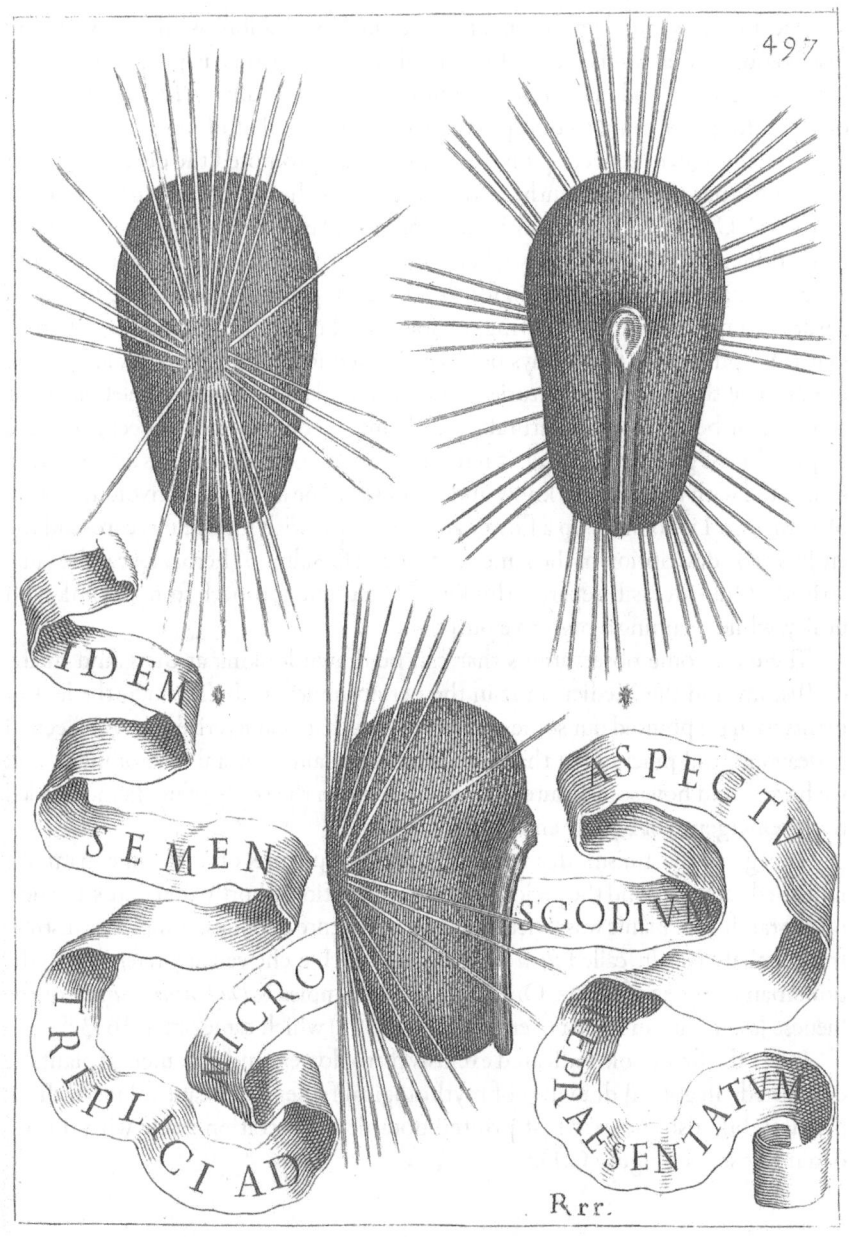

Figure C.1   Giovan Battista Ferrari, a seed of hibiscus seen through a
microscope. *Flora overo cultura di fiori*, Florence: Olschki, 2001

Bibliography

Primary Sources (manuscript)

Abbreviations

AOIF   Archivio dell'Ospedale degli Innocenti di Firenze.
ASF   Archivio di stato di Firenze.
BNCF   Biblioteca Nazionale Centrale di Firenze.
BUB   Biblioteca dell'Università di Bologna.
MdP   Medici del Principato.

***

AOIF, Fondo Estranei, Serie 144, 904–906.
AOIF, Fondo Estranei, Serie 144, 592–94.
AOIF, Processi Antichi, 20, cc. 56v–61v.
ASF, MdP, 1175 (Inserto 6), c. 45.
ASF, MdP, 642/A, 'Ragguagli di Medici et d'altri della malattia di S. A. Mentre era in Pisa'.
ASF, MdP, 642, c. 18.
ASF, MdP, 1171, cc. 88–172.
ASF, Guardaroba Medicea, 399, c.3r, 'Inventario di tutto quello che si è ritrovato in diverse stanze nel Palazzo de il Casino dell'Illustrissimo e Eccellentissimo Sig. Don Antonio Medici alla sua morte seguita il di 2 di maggio 1621'.
BNCF, Magliab. XIV, 8, *Leonhardi Thurneisseri Historia sive descritione plantarum*.
BNCF, Magliab. XIV, 9, *Breve compendio e transunto d'intorno la descrizione di tutte le piante de i semplici tanto nostrali, quanto d'altri Paesi data in luce a comune utilità da Lionardo Turneissero Medico Ordinario dell'Elettore di Brandemburgh. Opera Tradotta di Lingua Latina in Vulgare da P. Jacopo Carpi cappellano fiorentino.*
BNCF, Banco Rari, 119 – Di Pedacio Dioscoride Anazarbeo *Libri cinque della istoria & materia medicinale tradotti in lingua volgare Italiana da M. Pietro Andrea Matthiolo Sanese Medico*, (Venice: Bascarini, 1544) – (notes by Cosimo I in the margin).
BNCF, Magliab. XIII, 34 Giovanni Cinelli, 'Bozze delle bellezze di Firenze'.

BNCF, Magliab. XIII, 36 'Appartamenti principali di Palazzo de Pitti di S.A.S. fatto da me D.M. Marmi', c. 10r.

BNCF, XVI, 63. *Apparato della Fonderia dell'Illustrissimo et Eccellentissimo Sig. D. Antonio Medici. Nel quale si contiene tutta l'arte spagirica di Teofrasto Paracelso et sue medicine e altri segreti bellissimi.*

BNCF, Magliab. XV, 140, *Segreti sperimentati dall'Ill.mo et Ecc.mo Sig. Principe D. Antonio de' Medici nella sua fonderia del Casino di S. Marco.*

BNCF, MS Palatinus 1139 [*Li*]*bro nel quale si scriveranno esperimenti e cose certe per mano del duca di Fiorenza o vero in sua presentia, né ci sarà su cosa che non sia certissima per utile comune* (1556).

BNCF, MS Targioni Tozzetti 56, vols 1–3, Agostino del Riccio, *Agricoltura sperimentale.*

BUB, MS Aldrovandi 136, vol. 14 'Catalogus omnium plantarum quae erant in horto publico studiorum tempore Luca Ghini qui publice profitebatur lectionem simplicium, et horti studiorum praefectus erat. Numerus autem eo tempore plantarum erat 620. Hic tamen describam ex hillo horto pulchriora simplicia et rariora, in quibusdam vero eius opinio apparebit'.

BUB, MS Aldrovandi 98, vol. 2, cc. 53v–55r, 'Catalogo delli Semplici che mi manchano da mettere nel Dioscoride perché non li conosco'.

BUB, MS Aldrovandi 98, vol. 2, cc. 33r-53r, 'Clarissimi atque Excellentiss. Lucae Ghini in celebri Pisana Academia materiae medicae professoris doctissimi. De quibusdam simplicibus placita ad Andream Mathiolum senensem celeberrimum medicum conscripta, idibus Octobris an. LI – Pisis'.

BUB, MS Aldrovandi 98, vol. 2, cc. 69v-148r, 'Ex lectionibus D. L. Ghini in Academia Pisana legentis collecta'.

Printed Primary Sources

Aldrovandi, Ulisse, 'Discorso naturale', in Sandra Tugnoli Pattaro (ed.), *Metodo e sistema delle scienze nel pensiero di Ulisse Aldrovandi* (Bologna: Clueb, 1981).

Aldrovandi, Ulisse, 'La vita d'Ulisse Aldrovandi cominciando dalla sua natività sin' a l'età di 64 anni vivendo ancora', in R. Simili (ed.), *Il teatro della natura di Ulisse Aldrovandi* (Bologna: Editrice Compositori, 2001).

Antidotarii Bononiensis sive de usitata ratione componendorum, miscendorumque medicamentorum epitome (Bologna: Apud Joannem Rossium, 1574).

Avicenna, *Avicennae Arabum medicorum principis* [*Canon medicinae*] *ex Gerardi Cremonensis versione, et Andreae Alpagi Bellunensis castigatione* (Venice: Giunta, 1595).

Baldini, Baccio, *Vita di Cosimo I Granduca di Toscana* (Florence: Bartolomeo Sermatelli, 1578).

Belon, Pierre, *Les Remonstrances sur le default du labour & culture des plantes & de la cognoissance d'icelles* (Paris: G. Cauellat, 1558).

Belon, Pierre, *De neglecta cultura stirpium* (Antwerp: Christophe Plantin, 1589).

Bencivenni Pelli, Giuseppe, 'Descrizione della Galleria di Filippo Pigafetta', in *Saggio istorico della Real Galleria di Firenze* (Florence: Gaetano Gambiagi, 1779).

Biringuccio, Vannoccio, *De la pyrotechnia (1540)* (Milan: Edizioni il Polifilo, 1977).

Boccone, Paolo, *Museo di fisica e di esperienze, variato, e decorato di osservazioni naturali* (Venice: Zuccato, 1697).

Bocchi, Francesco and Giovanni Cinelli, *Bellezze della città di Fiorenza: ora da M. Giovanni Cinelli ampliate ed accresciute* (Florence: G. Gugliantini, 1677).

Brunfels, Otto, *Herbarum vivae icones, ad naturam imitationem, summa cum diligentia et artificio effigiatae* (Strasbourg: apud Johannem Schottum, 3 vols, 1530, 1532, 1536).

Calvi, Giovanni, *Commentarium inserviturum Historiae Pisani Vireti Botanici Academici* (Pisa: Fratelli Pizzorni, 1777).

Calzolari, Francesco, *Il viaggio di Montebaldo* (Venice: Valgrisi, 1566).

Carletti, Francesco, *Ragionamenti di Francesco Carletti Fiorentino sopra le cose da lui vedute nei suoi viaggi si dell'Indie occidentali, e orientali come d'altri paesi* (Florence: Giuseppe Manni, 1701).

Caruel, Théodore, *Theodori Caruelii Illustratio in hortum siccum Andreae Caesalpini: Rudimentum ex plantis libro Agglutinatis vigere scio in testimonium eorum, quae in hoc volumine a me dicuntur* (Florence: Le Monnier, 1858).

Cei, Galeotto, *Viaggio e relazione delle Indie*, ed. Francesco Surdich (Rome: Bulzoni, 1992).

Cellini, Benvenuto, *La vita*, ed. G. Davico Bonino (Turin: Einaudi 1973).

Cesalpino, Andrea, *Andreae Caesalpini Aretini Peripateticarum quaestionum libri quinque* (Venice: Giunta, 1571).

Cesalpino, Andrea, *Daemonum investigatio peripatetica in qua investigatur locus Hippocratis si quid divinum in morbis habetur* (Florence: Giunta, 1580).

Cesalpino, Andrea, *De plantis libri XVI* (Florence: apud Georgium Marescottum, 1583).

Cesalpino, Andrea, *Andreae Caesalpini Aretini De medicamentorum Facultatibus* (Venice: Giunta, 1593).

Cesalpino, Andrea, *De metallicis libri tres* (Rome: Luigi Zannetti, 1596).

Cesalpino, Andrea, *Appendix ad libros De plantis et Quaestiones peripateticae* (1603), published in Paolo Boccone, *Museo di piante rare della Sicilia, Malta, Corsica, Italia, Piemonte e Germania* (Venice: Battista Zuccato, 1697).

Cesalpino, Andrea, *Praxis uniuersae artis medicae, generalium aeque, ac particularium humani corporis praeter naturam affectuum dignotionem, iuditium & curam omnium uberrime complectens, summo labore, et studio concinnata, & unum recenter in volumen coniecta* (Treviso: Roberto Meietti, 1606).

Cesalpino, Andrea, 'Al R.mo Monsignore il S.or Alfonso vescovo de Tornabuoni' (Dedicatory letter of his herbarium) in Théodore Caruel, *Illustratio in hortum siccum Andreae Caesalpini: Rudimentum ex plantis libro Agglutinatis vigere scio in testimonium eorum, quae in hoc volumine a me dicuntur* (Florence: Le Monnier, 1858).

Clusius, Carolus (Charles de L'Ecluse), *Antidotarium, sive de componendorum miscendorumque medicamentorum ratione libri tres ex Graecorum, Arabum & recentiorum medicorum scriptis collecti. Nunc vero primum ex Italico sermone Latini facti* (Antwerp: Christophe Plantin, 1561).

Colombo, Cristoforo, *The Spanish Letter of Columbus to Luis de Sant'Angel* (London: Bernard Quaritch, 1891).

Colombo, Cristoforo, *Giornale di bordo (1492–93)* (Milan: Bompiani 1968).

Corti, Matteo, *De febribus curandis* (Padua: Paolo Meietti, 1595).

Croll, Oswald, *Oswaldi Crollii Basilica chymica: pluribus selectis et secretissimis propria manuali Experentia approbatis Descriptionibus, et Usu Remdiorum chymicorum selectissimorum* (Geneva: Chouet, 1643).

Croll, Oswald, *A Treatise of Oswaldus Crollius of Signatures of Internal Things: Or, a True and Lively Anatomy of the Greater and Lesser World* (London: Printed for John Starkey at the Mitre in Fleet Street, and Thomas Passenger at the Three Bibles upon London Bridge, 1669).

Del Migliore, Leopoldo, *Firenze città nobilissima illustrata* (Florence: Stamp. Della Stella, 1684; facsimile reprint, Bologna: Forni, 1968).

Delicado, Francisco, *El modo di adoperare el legno di India Occidentale, salutifero rimedio a ogni piaga & mal incurabile* (Venice: sumptibus vener. Presbyt. Francisci Delicati Hispani, 1529).

Della Porta, Giambattista, *Physiognomonia* (Vico Equense: Giuseppe Cacchi, 1586).

Della Porta, Giambattista, *Phytognomonica octo libris contenta. In quibus nova, facillimaque affertur methodus, qua plantarum, animalium, metallorum, rerumquedenique omnium ex prima extimae faciei inspectione quivis abditas vires assequatur* (Naples: Orazio Salviani, 1588).

Della Porta, Giambattista, *Magiae naturalis libri viginti* (Frankfurt: heirs of A. Wechel, 1591).

Della Porta, Giambattista, *De distillationibus Libri IX* (Strasbourg: Lazarus Zetzner, 1609).

Della Porta, Giambattista, *Natural Magick* by John Baptista Porta (London: Thomas Young and Samuel Speed, 1658).

Dioscorides Pedanius of Anarzabus, *De materia medica*, translated by Lily Y. Beck (Hildesheim, Zurich and New York: Georg Olms Verlag, 2005).

Dodoens, Rembert, *Stirpium historiae pemptades sex sive libri XXX*, Book I, ch. 11 (Antwerp: Christophe Plantin, 1583).

Donzelli, Giuseppe, *Teatro farmaceutico dogmatico e spagirico* (Venice: A. Bortoli, 1704).

Durante, Castore, 'Compendiosa narratio de usu & praxi radicis Mechoacan', in Giles Everard (ed.), *De herba panacea, quam alii tabacum, alii petum aut nicotianam vocant, brevis commentariolus* (Antwerp: J. Bellerus, 1587), pp. 57–73.

Evelyn, John, *Diary and Correspondence*, ed. William Bray (London: Routledge and Sons, 1906).

Fabbrucci, Stefano Maria, 'De Pisano Gymnasio sub Cosmo Primo Mediceo feliciter renovato', in A. Calogierà (ed.), *Nuova Raccolta d'opuscoli scientifici e filologici*, vol. 6 (Venice: Simone Occhi, 1709), pp. 1–137.

Fabroni, Angelo, *Historia academiae pisanae*, 3 vols (Pisa: 1791–95; reprint, Bologna: Forni, 1971).

Falloppio, Gabriele, *De simplicibus medicamentis purgantibus* (Venice: Giordano Ziletti, 1565).

Falloppio, Gabriele, *De morbo gallico liber absolutissimus* (Venice: Egidio Regazzola, 1574).

Falloppio, Gabriele, 'Tractatus de morbo gallico', *Opera quae extant omnia* (Frankfurt: heirs of A. Wechel, 1584), pp. 770–848.

Falloppio, Gabriele, *De morbo Gallico, Opera Omnia* (Venice, 1606).

Fantuzzi, Giovanni, *Memorie della vita di Ulisse Aldrovandi* (Bologna: Lelio Della Volpe, 1744).

Ferrari, Giovan Battista, *De florum cultura libri IV* (Rome: Stefano Paolini, 1633; Italian translation, *Flora overo cultura di fiori*, Rome, 1638; facsimile reprint, Florence: Olschki, 2001).

Filippo da Firenze, *Compendio della facultà de' semplici di tutte quelle cose, che sono più in uso nell'arte della medicina, con le ordinationi nuovamente fatte da riformatori, poste a' proprii capitoli di detti semplici* (Florence: Giorgio Marescotti, 1572).

Fiumi, Fabrizia and Giovanna Tempesta, 'Gli "experimenti" di Caterina Sforza', *Caterina Sforza, una donna del cinquecento: storia e arte tra Medioevo e Rinascimento* (Imola: La Mandragora, 2000).

Fuchs, Leonhart, *Errata recentiorum medicorum* (Haguenau, 1530).

Fuchs, Leonhart, *De historia stirpium commentarii insignes* (Basel: in officina Isingriniana, 1542).

Fuchs, Leonhart, *Paradoxorum medicinae libri tres* (Paris, 1546).

Fuchs, Leonhart, *Sessanta errori dei medici contemporanei con l'aggiunta delle confutazioni*, Italian translation and commentary by A. Morricone and V. Pedicino (Rome, 1963).

Galluzzi, Riguccio, *Istoria del Granducato di Toscana sotto il governo di casa Medici* (Florence: Gaetano Gambiagi, 1781).

Ghini, Luca, *Placiti*, in Gian Battista De Toni (ed.), 'I Placiti di Luca Ghini', *Memorie del Reale Veneto Istituto di Scienze Lettere e Arti*, 27 vols (Venice 1902–1907), vol. 8, pp. 3–49.

Ghini, Luca, *Morbi Gallici curandi ratio perbrevis*, in Luigi Sabbatani, *Morbi Gallici curandi ratio perbrevis: la cura del morbo gallico nelle lezioni di Luca Ghini* (Venice: Ferrari, 1921).

Ghini, Luca, 'Morbi Gallici curandi ratio perbrevis', in G. del Guerra e Pier Luigi Mondani (ed.), *I primi documenti quattrocenteschi sulla sifilide e le lezioni pisane di Luca Ghini* (Pisa: Casa Editrice Giardini, 1970), pp. 93–127.

Guidi, Guido, *De febribus libri VII* (Padua: Paolo Meietti, 1595).

Heikamp, Detlef, 'Agostino del Riccio: Del giardino di un re', in Giovanna Ragionieri (ed.), *Il giardino storico italiano* (Milan: Olschki, 1981), pp. 59–64.

Il Ricettario Medicinale necessario a tutti i Medici, & Speziali (Florence: nella stamperia de i Giunti, 1567).

L'Ecluse, Charles de (Carolus Clusius), *Antidotarium, sive de componendorum miscendorumque medicamentorum ratione libri tres ex Graecorum, Arabum & recentiorum medicorum scriptis collecti. Nunc vero primum ex Italico sermone Latini facti* (Antwerp: Christophe Plantin, 1561).

La fonderia dell'Ill.mo et ecc.mo Sig. Don Antonio Medici Principe di Capistrano – Nella quale si contiene tutta l'arte spagirica di Teofrasto Paracelso, & sue medicine. Et altri segreti bellissimi (Stampato nel Palazzo del Casino di S. E: Illustrissima in Fiorenza, 1604).

Lapini, Agostino, *Diario fiorentino di Agostino Lapini: dal 252 al 1596, ora per la prima volta pubblicato da G.O. Corazzini* (Florence: Sansoni, 1900).

Le lettere spirituali e familiari di S. Caterina De' Ricci Fiorentina Religiosa domenicana in S. Vincenzo di Prato (Prato: Ranieri Guasti, 1861).

Luisini, Luigi, *De Morbo Gallico omnia quae extant apud omnes medicos cujusque nationis ... in unum hoc corpus redacta* (Venice: Giordano Ziletti, 1566–67).

Mainetti, Mainetto, *Commentarius mire perspicuous ... in librum Aristotelis De sensu & sensibus* (Florence: Lorenzo Torrentino, 1555).

Mattioli, Pietro Andrea, *I discorsi di Pietro Andrea Mattioli sanese, medico cesareo, et del serenissimo Principe Ferdinando Archiduca d'Austria & c. Nelli sei libri di Pedacio Dioscoride Anazarbeo della materia medicinale. Hora di nuovo dal suo stesso autore ricorretti e aumentati. Con le figure grandi tutte di nuovo rifatte, & tirate dale naturali e vive piante, & animali, & in numero molto maggiore che le altre per avanti stampate* (Venice: Valgrisi, 1568).

Mercuriale, Girolamo, *Medicina practica, seu de cognoscendis, discernendis, & curandis omnis humani corporis affectibus, earum causis indagandis, libri V* (Frankfurt: Johan Theobald Shonwetter, 1602).

Mercuriale, Girolamo, *Praelectiones Patavinae, de cognoscendis, et curandis humani corporis affectibus* (Venice: Giunta, 1606).

Mercuriale, Girolamo, *Consultationes et responsa medicinalia* (Venice: Giunta, 1624).

Mercuriale, Gerolamo, 'Quattro lettere di sulla malattia della Granduchessa di Toscana nel novembre del 1601', in Alessandro Simili (ed.), *Romagna medica* (Bollettino della Società Medico-chirurgica della Romagna), 8(6) (1956), pp. 1–8.

Monardes, Nicolas, *Delle cose che vengono portate dall'Indie occidental pertinenti all'uso della medicina. Raccolte, & trattate dal dottor Nicolò Monardes, medico in Siviglia, parte prima [- seconda]. Novamente recata dalla spagnola nella nostra lingua italiana* (Venice: Giordano Ziletti, 1575).

Monardes, Nicolas, *Primera y segunda y tercera partes de la historia medicinal de las cosas que se traen de nuestras India Occidentales que sirven en medicina* [1565–74]. (Facsimile edn, Seville: Padilla libros, 1988; English translation, John Frampton, *Joyfull Newes Out of the Newe Founde Worlde*, London: E. Allde, by the assigne of Bonham Norton, 1596).

Montuus, Sebastianus, *Annotatiunculae S Montui in errata recentiorum medicorum per L. Fuchsium* (Lyon, 1533).

Montuus, Sebastianus, *Dialexeon medicinalium Libri duo* (Lyon, 1537).

Nuovo Receptario composto dal famosissimo chollegio degli eximii doctori della arte et medicina della inclita cipta di Firenze, Impresso Nella inclyta ciptà di Firenze per la compagnia del Dragho (1948).

Paracelso, 'The *Herbarius* of Paracelsus: Translated with an introduction by Bruce T. Moran', *Pharmacy in History*, 35(3) (1993), pp. 99–127.

Paracelso, *Contro i falsi medici: Sette autodifese*, ed. Massimo Luigi Bianchi (Bari: Laterza, 1995).

Pliny the Elder, *Natural History*, translated by W.H.S. Jones (Loeb Classical Library) (Cambridge, MA: Harvard University Press, 1956).

Redi, Francesco, 'Esperienze intorno alla generazione degli insetti', *Opere* (Milan, 1810).

Relazione del clarissimo messer Andrea Gussoni Ambasciator ritornato da Fiorenza l'anno 1576, *Relazioni degli Ambasciatori veneti al Senato* (Bari: Laterza, 1916).

Relazione di Firenze di Messer Vincenzo Fedeli tornato da quella corte l'anno 1561, *Relazioni degli Ambasciatori Veneti al Senato*, Raccolte, annotate ed edite da Eugenio Alberi, Series 2, Vol. 1 (Florence: Tipografia all'Insegna di Clio: 1839).

Rosselli, Stefano Francesco di Romolo, *Mes secrets à Florence au temps des Médicis 1593*, ed. Rodrigo de Zayas (Paris: Editions Jean-Michel Place, 1996).

Scaligero, Giulio Cesare, *In libros duos, qui inscribuntur de plantis, Aristotele autore, libri duo* (Paris: ex officinal Michaelis Vascosani, 1556).

Scaligero, Giulio Cesare, *Iulii Caesaris Scaligeri Commentarii, et animaduersiones, in sex libros De causis plantarum Theophrasti* (Lyon: G. Rovilium, 1566).

Sforza, Caterina, *Experimenti de la ex.ma s.ra Caterina da Forlj matre de lo Inllux.mo signor Giovanni de Medici*, ed. P.D. Pasolini (Imola: Tip. d'Ignazio Galeati e figlio, 1894).

Taegio, Bartolomeo, *La villa* (Milan: Stampa di Francesco Moscheni, 1559).

Targioni Tozzetti, Giovanni, *Notizie sulla storia delle scienze fisiche in Toscana* (Florence: Biblioteca Palatina, 1852).

The Earliest Printed Literature on Syphilis: Being Ten Tractates from the Years 1495–1498, in complete facsimile. With an introduction and other accessory material by Karl Sudhoff; adapted by Charles Singer (Florence: Lier, 1925).

Theophrastus, *Historia plantarum*, translated into French by Suzanne Amigues (Paris: Editions Belin, 2010).

Thurneysser, Leonhart, *Historia sive descriptio plantarum omnium, tam domesticarum, quam exoticarum* (Berlin: Michael Hentzsche, 1578).

Varchi, Benedetto, *Questione sull'alchimia* (Florence: Stamperia Magheri, 1827).

Varchi, Benedetto, *Lezzione nella quale si disputa della maggioranza delle arti e qual sia la più nobile, la scultura o la pittura* (1546). In *Trattati d'arte del Cinquecento fra Manierismo e Controriforma*, 3 vols (Bari: Laterza, 1960).

Vasari, Giorgio, 'Ragionamenti', *Le opere di Giorgio Vasari*, vol. 8, ed. G. Milanesi (Firenze: Sansoni, 1882), pp. 9–225.

Vasari, Giorgio, *Il Carteggio di G. Vasari dal 1563 al 1565*, ed. Karl Frey (Arezzo: Zelli, 1941).

Vasari, Giorgio, *Le vite dei più eccellenti pittori, scultori e architettori* (Novara: Istituto geografico De Agostini, 1967).

Vesalio, Andrea, *De humani corporis fabrica. Libri septem* (Basel: Giovanni Oporino, 1543).

Vieri, Francesco de, *Delle meravigliose opere di Pratolino e d'Amore* (Florence, 1586), in Paola Barocchi and Giovanna Gaeta Bertelà (eds), *Collezionismo mediceo e storia artistica* (Florence: SPES, 2002), vol. 1, pp. 284–302.

Welsch, Georg Hieronymus, *Georgii Hieronymi Velschii Exotericarum curationum et observationum medicinalium Chiliades duae* (Ulm, 1676).

Printed Secondary Sources

AA. VV., *Livorno e Pisa: due città e un territorio nella politica dei Medici* (Pisa: Nistri-Lischi e Pacini, 1980).

Acidini Luchinat, Cristina, 'Niccolò Gaddi collezionista e dilettante', *Paragone*, 359–61 (1980), pp. 141–75.

Ackerman, James S., 'The Involvement of Artists in Renaissance Science', in J.W. Shirley and F.D. Hoeniger (eds), *Science and the Arts in the Renaissance* (London and Toronto: Associated University Presses, 1985), pp 94–129.

Adams, Michael, Wandana Alther, Michael Kessler et al., 'Malaria in the Renaissance: Remedies from European Herbals from the 16th and 17th Century', *Journal of Ethnopharmacology*, 133(2) (2011), pp. 278–88.

Agamben, Giorgio, *Signatura rerum: Sul Metodo* (Turin: Bollati Boringhieri, 2008).

Agrimi, Jole and Chiara Crisciani, *Edocere Medicos* (Naples: Guerini e Associati, 1988).

Agrimi, Jole, and Chiara Crisciani, *Les Consilia médicaux* (Turnhout: Brepols, 1994).

Alchimia e le arti (L') – La fonderia degli Uffizi da laboratorio a stanza delle meraviglie (Florence: Sillabe, 2012).

Ames-Lewis, Francis, 'Fra Angelico, Fra Filippo Lippi, and the Early Medici', *The Early Medici and their Artists* (London: Birkbeck College, University of London, Department of History of Art, 1995).

Amigues, Suzanne, *Theophraste, Recherche sur les plantes: A' l'origine de la botanique* (Paris: Editions Belin, 2010).

Anguillara, Luigi, *Semplici dell'eccellente M. Luigi Anguillara, liquali in più pareri à diversi nobili huomini scritti appaiono* (Venice: Valgrisi, 1561).

Arber, Agnes, *Herbals: Their Origin and Evolution. A Chapter in the History of Botany 1470–1670* (Cambridge: Cambridge University Press, 1912).

Arber, Agnes, 'Review: B. Hryniewiecki, *Anton Schneeberger (1530–1581), ein Schüler Konrad Gesners in Poland*', *New Phitologist*, 37(5) (1938), p. 480.

Arber, Agnes, 'The Colouring of Sixteenth Century Herbals', *Nature*, 145 (1940), pp. 803–804.

Arcangeli, Letizia and Peyronel, Susanna (eds), *Donne di potere nel Rinascimento* (Rome: Viella, 2008).

Arrizabalaga, Jon, John Henderson and Roger French, *The Great Pox: The French Disease in Renaissance Europe* (New Haven and London: Yale University Press, 1997).

Ashworth, William B. Jr., 'Natural History and the Emblematic World View', in David C. Lindberg and Robert S. Westman (eds), *Reappraisals of the Scientific Revolution* (Cambridge: Cambridge University Press, 1980), pp. 303–32.

Atran, Scott, *Cognitive Foundations of Natural History: Towards an Anthropology of Science* (Cambridge, Cambridge University Press, 1990).

Azzi Vicentini, Margherita (ed.), *L'arte dei Giardini: Scritti teorici e pratici dal XIV al XIX secolo* (Milan: Edizioni il Polifilo, 1999).

Bacci, Mina and Anna Forlani (eds), *Mostra di disegni di Jacopo Ligozzi (1547–1626)*, Gabinetto disegni e stampe degli Uffizi (Florence: Olschki, 1961).

Baldasso, Renzo, 'The role of visual representation in the scientific revolution: A historiographic inquiry', *Centaurus*, 48 (2006), pp. 69–88.

Barocchi, Paola and Giovanna Gaeta Bertelà, *Collezionismo mediceo – Cosimo I, Francesco I e il Cardinale Ferdinando – Documenti 1540–1587* (Modena: Panini, 1993).

Barocchi, Paola and Giovanna Gaeta Bertela', *Collezionismo mediceo e storia artistica* (Florence: Studio per Edizioni scelte, 2002).

Baroncini, Gabriele, 'Note sull'illustrazione scientifica', *Nuncius*, 11(2) (1996), pp. 527–43.

Barrera, Antonio, 'Local Herbs, Global Medicines: Commerce, Knowledge, and Commodities in Spanish America', in Paula Findlen and Pamela Smith (eds), *Merchants and Marvels: Commerce, Science, and Art in Early Modern Europe* (New York: Routledge, 2002), pp. 163–81.

Battisti, Eugenio, *L'antirinascimento* (Milan: Feltrinelli, 1962).

Bénézet, Jean-Pierre, *Pharmacie et médicament en Méditerranée occidentale* (XIIIe-XVIe siècles) (Paris: Honoré Champion, 1999).

Beretta, Ilva, 'Illustration and Representation: Botany in the Renaissance', in F. Meroi, C. Pogliano (eds), *Immagini per Conoscere: Dal Rinascimento alla Rivoluzione scientifica* (Florence: Olschki, 2001).

Bernabeo, Raffaello A., 'Il 'De morbo gallico' di Luca Ghini', *Museologia scientifica*, 8 (1991–92), pp. 237–43.

Berti, Luciano, *Il principe dello studiolo: Francesco I dei Medici e la fine del Rinascimento fiorentino* (Florence: Edam, 1967).

Bianchi, Massimo Luigi, *Signatura rerum: Segni, magia e conoscenza da Paracelso a Leibnitz* (Rome: Edizioni dell'Ateneo, 1987).

Bianchi, Massimo Luigi, 'The Visible and the Invisible', in P. Rattansi and A. Clericuzio (eds), *Alchemy and Chemistry in the 16th and 17th Centuries* (Dordrecht and London: Kluwer Academic Publisher, 1994), pp. 17–50.

Blair, Ann, 'Natural Philosophy', *The Cambridge History of Science*, vol. 3: *Early Modern Science*, ed. K. Park and L. Daston (Cambridge: Cambridge University Press, 2006).

Bleichmar, Daniela, 'Books, Bodies, and Fields: Sixteenth-Century Transatlantic Encounters with New World *Materia Medica*', in Londa Schiebinger and Claudia Swan (eds), *Colonial Botany: Science, Commerce and Politics in the Early Modern World* (Philadelphia, PA: University of Pennsylvania Press, 2005), pp. 83–99.

Blunt, Wilfrid, *The Art of Botanical Illustration* (London: Collins, 1951).

Blunt, Wilfrid and Sandra Raphael, *The Illustrated Herbal* (London: Frances Lincoln, n.d.).

Bolzoni, Lina, 'L'invenzione dello stanzino di Francesco I', *Le arti della memoria* (Florence: SPES, 1980).

Boxer, Charles Ralph, *Two Pioneers of Tropical Medicine: Garcia d'Orta and Nicolas Monardes* (London: Hispanic and Luso-Brazilian Councils, 1963).

Bremekamp, C.E.B., 'A re-examination of Cesalpino's classification', *Acta Botanica Neerlandica*, 1 (1953), pp. 580–93.

Brogan, Roy, *A Signature of Power and Patronage: The Medici Coat of Arms 1299–1492* (New York: Peter Lang, c.1993).

Burke, Peter, *A Social History of Knowledge* (Cambridge: Polity, 2000).

Burke, Peter, *What is Cultural History* (Cambridge: Polity, 2004).

Butterfield, Herbert, *The Origins of Modern Science, 1300–1800* (London: Bell, 1950).

Butterfield, Herbert, 'Renaissance art and modern science', *University Review*, 1(2) (1954), pp. 25–37.

Butters, Suzanne, 'Le Cardinal Ferdinand de Médicis', pp. 170–96; 'Ferdinand et le jardin du Pincio', pp. 350–410; 'Ammannati et la Villa Médicis', pp. 257–316, in André Chastel and Philip Morel (eds), *La villa Médicis*, 5 vols (Rome: Académie de France; Ecole Française, 1989–2010), vol. 2.

Butters, Suzanne, *The Triumph of Vulcan: Sculptors' Tools, Porphyry, and the Prince in Ducal Florence*, 2 vols (Florence: Olschki, 1996).

Butters, Suzanne, 'Pressed Labor and Pratolino: Social Imagery and Social Reality in a Medici Garden', in Mirka Beneš and Dianne Harris (eds), *Villas and Gardens in Early Modern Italy and France* (Cambridge: Cambridge University Press, 2001), pp. 61–87, 347–61.

Bylebyl, Jerome, 'The School of Padua: Humanistic Medicine in the Sixteenth Century', in C. Webster (ed.), *Health, Medicine and Mortality in the Sixteenth Century* (Cambridge: Cambridge University Press, 1979), pp. 335–70.

Bylebyl, Jerome, 'The Manifest and the Hidden in the Renaissance Clinic', in W.F. Bynum and Roy Porter (eds), *Medicine and the Five Senses* (Cambridge: Cambridge University Press, 1993), pp. 40–60.

Calvi, Giulia and Spinelli, Riccardo (eds), *Le donne Medici nel sistema europeo delle corti (XVI–XVIII secolo)* (Florence: Edizioni Polistampa, 2008).

Caneva, Giulia, *Il mondo di Cerere nella loggia di Psiche* (Rome: Fratelli Palombi, 1992).

Cantù, Francesca (ed.), *I linguaggi del potere nell'età barocca: Politica e religione* (Rome: Viella, 2009).

Cartwright, Julia, *Italian Gardens of the Renaissance* (London: Smith, Elder & Co., 1914).

Caruel, Théodore, *Theodori Caruelii Illustratio in hortum siccum Andreae Caesalpini: Rudimentum ex plantis libro Agglutinatis vigere scio in testimonium eorum, quae in hoc volumine a me dicuntur* (Florence: Le Monnier, 1858).

Castiglione, Baldassarre, *Il libro del Cortegiano* (Milan: Rizzoli, 1993).

Cavallo, Sandra, *Artisans of the Body in Early Modern Italy: Identities, Families and Masculinities* (Manchester and New York: Manchester University Press, 2007).

Cellai, G., L. Fantoni and P. Luzzi, 'Intorno all'origine del giardino dei semplici di Firenze: Il Monastero di S. Domenico in Cafaggio', in *Atti e memorie dell'Accademia toscana di Scienze e Lettere la Colombaria* (Florence: Olschki, 2009), pp. 80–97.

Chiappelli, Fredi (ed.), *First Images of America: The Impact of the New World on the Old* (Berkeley and Los Angeles, CA, and London: University of California Press, 1976), vol. 1.

Ciasca, Raffaele, *L'arte dei medici e speziali nella storia e nel commercio fiorentino dal secolo XII al XV* (Florence: Olschki, 1927).

Clark, Mark E. and Kirk M. Summers, 'Hippocratic medicine and Aristotelian science in the *Daemonum investigatio peripatetica* of Andrea Cesalpino', *Bulletin of the History of Medicine*, 69(4) (1995), pp. 527–41.

Clericuzio, Antonio, 'Chemical Medicine and Paracelsianism in Italy, 1550–1650', in M. Pelling and S. Mandelbrote (eds), *The Practice of Reform in Health, Medicine, and Science, 1500–2000: Essays for Charles Webster* (Aldershot: Ashgate, 2005).

Cogliati Arano, Luisa, *The Medieval Health Handbook: Tacuinum Sanitatis* (New York: George Braziller, 1976).

Cohen, Floris H., *The Scientific Revolution: A Historiographical Inquiry* (Chicago, IL: University of Chicago Press, 1994).

Collareta, Marco, 'Per Niccolò Santini, orefice fiorentino del Cinquecento', *Prospettiva*, 14 (1978), pp. 65–7.

Collins, Minta, *Medieval Herbals: The Illustrative Traditions* (London: The British Library, 2000).

Conticelli, Valentina, '*Guardaroba di cose rare e preziose*': lo studiolo di Francesco I de' Medici. Arte, storia e significati* (Lugano: Agorà, 2007).

Conticelli, Valentina, 'Una storia di storie. La fonderia del granduca: laboratorio, wunderkammer e museo farmaceutico', in *L'alchimia e le arti: la fonderia degli Uffizi da laboratorio a stanza delle meraviglie* (Florence: Sillabe, 2012), pp. 9–33.

Corradi, Alfonso, 'L'acqua del legno e le cure depurative nel Cinquecento', *Annali Universali di Medicina e Chirurgia*, 269 (1884), pp. 49–82.

Corradi, Alfonso, *Le prime farmacopee italiane, ed in particolare: Dei Ricettari Fiorentini. Memoria* (Milan: Fratelli Rechiedei Editori, 1887).

Covoni, Pierfilippo, *Il Casino di S. Marco costruito dal Buontalenti ai tempi medicei* (Florence: Tipografia cooperativa, 1892).

Covoni, Pierfilippo, *Don Antonio de Medici al Casino di S. Marco* (Florence: Tipografia cooperativa, 1892).

Cristofolini, Giovanni, 'Luca Ghini a Bologna: la nascita della scienza moderna', *Museologia Scientifica*, 8 (1991–92), pp. 207–21.

D'Arienzo, Luisa, 'I Toscani sulla via delle Indie all'epoca di Cristoforo Colombo', *Rivista Geografica Italiana*, 100 (1993), pp. 321–43.

Dacos, Nicole, 'Alle fonti della natura morta italiana, Giovanni da Udine e le nature morte nei festoni', in *La natura morta in Italia* (Milan: Electa, 1989) pp. 55–68.

Dami, Luigi, *Il giardino italiano* (Milan: Casa editrice d'arte Bestetti e Tumminelli, 1924).

Daston, Lorraine and Katharine Park, *Wonders and the Order of Nature 1150–1750* (New York: Zone Books, 1998).

Dear, Peter, *Revolutionizing the Sciences: European Knowledge and its Ambitions, 1500–1700* (Basingstoke: Palgrave, 2009).

De Toni, Gian Battista, 'I Placiti di Luca Ghini', *Memorie del Reale Veneto Istituto di Scienze Lettere e Arti*, 27 vols (Venice, 1902–1907), vol. 8, pp. 3–49.

De Toni, Gian Battista, 'Spigolature Aldrovandiane: Le piante dell'antico Orto Botanico di Pisa ai tempi di Luca Ghini', *Annali di Botanica*, 5(3) (1907), pp. 421–40.

Debus, Allen G., *The Chemical Philosophy: Paracelsian Science and Medicine in the Sixteenth and Seventeenth Centuries* (Mineola, NY: Courier Dover Publications, 2002).

De Vivo, Filippo, 'Pharmacies as centres of communication in early modern Venice', *Renaissance Studies*, 21(4) (2007), pp. 505–21.

De Vries, Joyce, *Caterina Sforza and the Art of Appearances* (Aldershot: Ashgate, 2010).

Dezzi Bardeschi, Marco et al., *Lo stanzino del principe in Palazzo Vecchio: I concetti, le immagini, il desiderio* (Florence: Le lettere, 1980).

Di Pietro, Pericle (ed.), *Epistolario di Gabriele Falloppia* (Ferrara, 1970).

Eamon, William, 'Court, Academy, and Printing House: Patronage and Scientific Careers in Late Renaissance Italy', in Bruce T. Moran (ed.), *Patronage and Institutions: Science, Technology, and Medicine at the European Court 1500–1750* (Rochester, NY: Boydell, 1991), pp. 25–50.

Eamon, William, 'Medical self-fashioning, or how to get rich and famous in the Renaissance medical marketplace', *Pharmacy in History*, 45 (2003), pp. 123–9.

Eamon, William, *The Professor of Secrets: Mistery, Medicine and Alchemy in Renaissance Italy* (Washington, DC: National Geographic, 2010).

Edelstein, Bruce L., 'La fecundissima Signora Duchessa: The Courtly Persona of Eleonora di Toledo and the Iconography of Abundance', in K. Eisenbichler (ed.), *The Cultural World of Eleonora di Toledo, Duchess of Florence and Siena* (Aldershot: Ashgate, 2004).

Edgerton, S.Y., 'The Renaissance Development of Scientific Illustration', *Science and the Arts in the Renaissance*, in J.W. Shirley and F.D. Hoeniger (eds) (London and Toronto, 1985).

Evans, R.J.W., 'The Court: A Protean Institution and an Elusive Subject', in R.G. Asch and A.M. Birke (eds), *Princes, Patronage and the Nobility* (Oxford: Oxford University Press, 1990).

Evelyn, John, *Diary and Correspondence*, ed. William Bray (London: Routledge and Sons, 1906).

Ewan, Joseph, 'The Columbian Discoveries and the Growth of Botanical Ideas with Special Reference to the Sixteenth Century', in F. Chiappelli (ed.), *First Images of America, the Impact of the New World on the Old* (Berkeley and Los Angeles, CA, and London: University of California Press, 1976).

Fantoni, Marcello, *La corte del Granduca: Forma e simboli del potere mediceo fra Cinque e Seicento* (Rome: Bulzoni Editore, 1994).

Findlen, Paula, *Possessing Nature: Museums, Collecting and Scientific Culture in Early Modern Italy* (Berkeley, CA: University of California Press, 1994).

Findlen, Paula, 'The Formation of a Scientific Community: Natural History in Sixteenth-Century Italy', in Anthony Grafton and Nancy Siraisi (eds), *Natural Particulars: Nature and the Disciplines in Renaissance Europe* (Cambridge, MA: MIT Press, 1999), pp. 369–400.

Fiorentino, Francesco, 'Vita ed opere di A. Cesalpino', in *Studi e ritratti della Rinascenza* (Bari: Laterza, 1911).

Fissell, Mary E., 'Women, health, and healing in early Modern Europe', *Bulletin of the History of Medicine*, 28 (2008), pp. 1–17.

Forbes, Robert James, *A Short History of the Art of Distillation: From the Beginnings up to the Death of Cellier Blumenthal* (Leiden: E.J. Brill, 1970).

Foucault, Michel, *Les mots et les choses* (Paris: Gallimard, 1966).

Fracastoro, Girolamo, *Syphilis sive morbus gallicus* (Verona, 1530).

Franchini, Dario A. et al. (eds), *La scienza a corte: Collezionismo eclettico, natura e immagine a Mantova fra Rinascimento e Manierismo* (Rome: Bulzoni, 1979).

Frati, Lodovico, *Catalogo dei manoscritti di Ulisse Aldrovandi* (Bologna: Zanichelli, 1907).

Freedberg, David, *The Eye of the Linx: Galileo, his Friends, and the Beginnings of Modern Natural History* (Chicago, IL: University of Chicago Press, 2002).

Galassi, N., 'Luca Ghini, una vita per la scienza', *Museologia Scientifica*, 8 (1991–92), pp. 187–206.

Galluzzi, Paolo, 'Il mecenatismo mediceo e le scienze', in C. Vasoli (ed.), *Idee, Istituzioni, scienza ed arti nella Firenze dei Medici* (Florence: Giunti-Martello, 1980).

Galluzzi, Paolo, 'La rinascita della scienza', *La corte, il mare, i mercanti: La rinascita della scienza. Editoria e societa'. Astrologia, magia e alchimia* (Florence: Electa, 1980).

Galluzzi, Paolo, 'Motivi paracelsiani nella Toscana di Cosimo II e di Don Antonio dei Medici: alchimia, medicina 'chimica' e riforma del sapere', in *Scienze, credenze occulte, livelli di cultura* (Florence: Olschki, 1982).

Garbari, Fabio, Lucia Tongiorgi Tomasi and Alessandro Tosi, *Giardino dei Semplici: L'orto botanico di Pisa dal XVI al XX secolo* (Pisa: Pacini, 1991).

Garbari, Fabio, 'Luca Ghini a Pisa, cardine della cultura botanica del XVI secolo', *Museologia Scientifica*, 8 (1991–92), pp. 223–36.

Gavitt, Philip, 'Charity and State Building in Cinquecento Florence: Vincenzo Borghini as administrator of the Ospedale degli Innocenti', *Journal of Modern History*, 69(2) (1997), pp. 230–70.

Gentilcore, David, *Healers and Healing in Early Modern Italy* (Manchester: Manchester University Press, 1998).

Gentilcore, David, *Medical Charlatanism in Early Modern Italy* (Oxford: Oxford University Press, 2006).

Gentilcore, David, *Pomodoro!: A History of the Tomato in Italy* (New York and Chichester: Columbia University Press, 2010).

Gentilcore, David, *Italy and the Potato: A History 1550–2000* (London: Continuum, 2012).

Gentile, Sebastiano, 'Il ritorno di Platone, dei platonici e del Corpus ermetico: Filosofia, teologia e astrologia nell'opera di Marsilio Ficino', in Cesare Vasoli (ed.), *Le filosofie del Rinascimento* (Milan: Bruno Mondadori, 2002).

Gerbi, Antonello, *Nature in the New World* (Pittsburgh, PA: University of Pittsburgh Press, 2010).

Giannarelli, Elena (ed.), *Cosma e Damiano: Dall'Oriente a Firenze* (Florence: Edizioni della Meridiana, 2002).

Grande, Stefano, 'Le relazioni geografiche fra Pietro Bembo, Gerolamo Fracastoro, Giovanni Battista Ramusio e Giacomo Castaldi', *Memorie della Società Geografica Italiana*, 12 (1905), pp. 93–197.

Grant, Edward, 'Aristotelianism and the longevity of the medieval world view', *History of Science*, 16 (1978), pp. 93–106.

Greene, Edward Lee, *Landmarks of Botanical History* (Stanford, CA: Stanford University Press, 1983).

Grell, Ole Peter, Andrew Cunningham and Jon Arrizabalaga (eds), *Centres of Medical Excellence? Medical Travel and Education in Europe 1500–1789* (Aldershot: Ashgate, 2010).

Grendler, Paul F., *The Universities of the Italian Renaissance* (Baltimore, MD, and London: The Johns Hopkins University Press, 2002).

Harvey, Barbara F., *Living and Dying in England, 1100–1540: The Monastic Experience* (Oxford: Clarendon Press, 1995).

Heikamp, Detlef, *Mexico and the Medici* (Forence: Editrice Edam, 1972).

Heikamp, Detlef, 'Agostino del Riccio: Del giardino di un re', in Giovanna Ragionieri (ed.), *Il giardino storico italiano* (Milan: Olschki, 1981).

Henderson, John, *The Renaissance Hospital: Healing the Body and Healing the Soul* (New Haven, CT, and London: Yale University Press, 2006).

Henderson, John, 'Fracastoro, il legno santo e la cura del "mal francese"', in A. Pastore and E. Peruzzi (eds), *Girolamo Fracastoro: fra medicina, filosofia e scienze della natura* (Florence: Olschki, 2006), pp. 73–89.

Hobhouse, Penelope, *Plants in Garden History* (London: Pavilion Books 1977).

Hoeniger, F. David, 'How Plants and Animals Were Studied in the Mid-Sixteenth Century', in J.W. Shirley and F.D. Hoeniger (eds), *Science and the Arts in the Renaissance* (Washington, DC: Folger Shakespeare Library; London: Associated University Presses, 1985), pp. 131–48.

Huguet-Termes, M. Teresa, 'Approximacion Historico-farmacologica y studio comparativo de los codigos mas representativos de las primeras tendencias a la oficializacion en el contexto de la terapia preparacelsiana en Europa'. Doctoral thesis, Faculty of Pharmacy, University of Barcelona, 1998.

Huguet-Termes, M. Teresa, 'New World materia medica in Spanish Renaissance medicine: From scholarly reception to practical impact', *Medical History*, 45 (2001), pp. 359–76.

Jensen, Kristian, 'Description, Division, Definition: Caesalpinus and the Study of Plants as an Independent Discipline', in Marianne Pade (ed.), *Renaissance Readings of the Corpus Aristotelicum: Proceedings from the Conference held in Copenhagen, 23–25 April 1998*, (Copenhagen: Museum Tusculanum, 2001), pp. 185–206.

Kent, Dale, *Cosimo de' Medici and the Florence Renaissance, the Patron's Oeuvre* (New Haven, CT, and London: Yale University Press, 2000).

Kraye, Jill, 'La filosofia nelle Università italiane del XVI secolo', in Cesare Vasoli (ed.), *Le filosofie del Rinascimento* (Milan: Bruno Mondadori, 2002).

Kusukawa, Sachiko, 'Leonhart Fuchs on the importance of pictures', *Journal of the History of Ideas*, 58 (1997), pp. 403–27.

Kusukawa, Sachiko, 'Illustrating Nature', in Marina Frasca-Spada and Nick Jardine (eds), *Books and Sciences in History* (Cambridge: Cambridge University Press, 2000), pp. 90–113.

Kusukawa, Sachiko, *Picturing the Book of Nature: Image Text and Argument in Sixteenth-century Anatomy and Medical Botany* (Chicago, IL, and London: University of Chicago Press, 2012).

Lazzaro Claudia, *The Italian Renaissance Garden* (New Haven, CT, and London: Yale University Press, 1990).

Lensi, Alfredo, *Palazzo Vecchio* (Florence: Fratelli Alinari, 1911).

Lensi Orlandi, Giulio, *Il Palazzo Vecchio di Firenze* (Florence: Giunti-Martello, 1977).

Lensi Orlandi, Giulio, *Cosimo e Francesco de' Medici alchimisti* (Florence: Cardini, 1978).Leong, Elaine, 'Making medicines in the early modern household', *Bulletin of the History of Medicine*, 82 (2008), pp. 145–68.

Litchfield, R.B., *Florence Ducal Capital 1530–1630* (New York: ACLS E-book, 2008).

Lonie, I.M., 'Fever pathology in the sixteenth century: Tradition and innovations', in W.F. Binum and V. Nutton (eds), 'Theories of fever from antiquity to the enlightment', *Medical History*, Supplement 1 (1981), pp. 19–44.

López Piñero, José María and José Pardo Tomáš, *Nuevos materiales y noticias sobre la Historia de las plantas de Nueva España de Francisco Hernández* (Valencia: Universitat de Valencia-CSIC, 1997).

Luti, Filippo, *Don Antonio de' Medici e i suoi tempi* (Florence: Olschki, 2006).

Luzzi, P. and F. Fabbri, 'I tre giardini botanici di Firenze', in *I giardini dei semplici e gli orti botanici della Toscana* (Perugia: Quattroemme, 1993).

Marrara, Danilo, 'L'Università di Pisa come università statale nel granducato mediceo', *Rivista Giuridica della Scuola*, 8 (1965), pp. 7–40.

Marrara, Danilo, 'L'età medicea 1543–1737', *Storia dell'Universita di Pisa*, Commissione Rettorale per la storia dell'Università di Pisa, vol. 1 (Pisa: Edizioni Plus, 2000), pp. 79–187.

Marland, Hilary (ed.), *The Art of Midwifery* (London: Routledge, 1993).

Masson, Georgina, *Italian Gardens* (London: Thames & Hudson 1966).

Mattioli, Mario, *La scoperta della circolazione del sangue* (Naples: Edizioni scientifiche italiane, 1972).

Mayr, Ernst, *The Growth of Botanical Thought: Diversity, Evolution, and Inheritance* (Cambridge, MA, London: Harvard University Press, 1982).

McTavish, Lianne, *Childbirth and the Display of Authority in Early Modern France* (Aldershot: Ashgate, 2005).

Medici Archive Project – documents.medici.org/ (– Bia – The Medici Archive Project).

Meloni Trkulja Silvia, 'I Medici Santi', in Cristina Giannini (ed.), *Stanze segrete raccolte per caso. I Medici Santi – Gli arredi celati* (Florence: Olschki, 2003), pp. 25–42.

Menchini, Carmen, *Panegirici e vite di Cosimo I de' Medici* (Florence: Olschki, 2005).

Minelli, Alessandro (ed.), *The Botanical Garden of Padua 1545–1995* (Venice: Marsilio, 1995).

Moggi Guido, 'L'erbario di Andrea Cesalpino', in Chiara Nepi and Enrico Gusmeroli (eds), *Gli erbari aretini da Andrea Cesalpino ai giorni nostri* (Florence: Florence University Press, 2008).

Moran, Bruce T., 'The *Herbarius* of Paracelsus: Translated with an introduction by Bruce T. Moran', *Pharmacy in History*, 35(3) (1993), pp. 99–127.

Moran, Bruce T., *Distilling Knowledge: Alchemy, Chemistry and the Scientific Revolution* (Cambridge, MA: Harvard University Press, 2005).

Moran, Bruce T., 'Courts and Academies', *The Cambridge History of Science*, vol. 3: *Early Modern Science* (Cambridge: Cambridge University Press, 2006).

Morton, Alan G., *History of Botanical Science: An Account of the Development of Botany from Ancient Times to the Present Day* (London and New York: Academic Press, 1981).

Morton, Alan G., 'Marginalia to A. Cesalpino's work on botany', *Archives of Natural History* 10(1) (1981–82), pp. 31–6.

Multhauf, Robert, 'The significance of distillation in Renaissance medical chemistry', *Bulletin of the History of Medicine*, 30 (1956), pp. 329–46.

Munger, Robert S., 'Guaiacum, the holy wood from the New World', *Journal of the History of Medicine and Allied Sciences*, 4 (1949), pp. 169–229.

Nesselrath, Arnold (ed.), *Discorsi sulle piante e sugli animali: Il Dioscoride colorito e miniato da Gherardo Cibo per Francesco Maria II della Rovere Duca d'Urbino* (Rome: Edizioni dell'elefante, 1991).

Nissen, Claus, *Herbals of Five Centuries: A Contribution to Medical History and Bibliography* (Zurich: L'Art Auàen S.A. Antiquariat, 1958).

Novembri, Valeria, 'I Santi Cosma e Damiano e la tradizione manoscritta nella Firenze medicea', in Elena Giannarelli (ed.), *Cosma e Damiano: Dall'Oriente a Firenze* (Florence: Edizioni della Meridiana, 2002), pp. 66–74.

Ogilvie, Brian W., *The Science of Describing: Natural History in Renaissance Europe* (Chicago, IL, and London: The University of Chicago Press, 2006).

Olmi, Giuseppe, *L'inventario del mondo: catalogazione della natura e luoghi del sapere nella prima età moderna* (Bologna: Il Mulino, 1992).

Olmi, Giuseppe, 'Il collezionismo scientifico', in Raffaella Simili (ed.), *Il teatro della natura di Ulisse Aldrovandi* (Bologna: Università degli Studi di Bologna, Editrice Compositori, 2001).

Olmi, Giuseppe, 'Le raffigurazioni della natura nell'età moderna: "spirito e vita dei libri"', in M. Santoro and M.G. Tavoni (eds), *I dintorni del testo: approcci alle periferie del libro* (Rome: Edizioni dell'Ateneo, 2005).

Ongaro, Giuseppe and Elda Martellozzo Forin, 'Girolamo Mercuriale e lo studio di Padova', in A. Arcangeli and V. Nutton (eds), *Girolamo Mercuriale: Medicina e cultura nell'Europa del Cinquecento* (Florence: Olschki, 2008).

Pacht, Otto, 'Early Italian nature studies and the early calendar landscape', *Journal of the Warburg and Courtauld Institutes*, 13 (1950), pp. 13–47.

Pagallo, Giulio F., '*In confinio scientiae naturalis et artis medicae*: Medici e filosofi sul tema della *subalternatio* nello studio di Padova del "500"', in A. Arcangeli and V. Nutton (eds), *Girolamo Mercuriale: Medicina e cultura nell'Europa del Cinquecento* (Florence: Olschki, 2008), pp. 11–27.

Paganini, P., 'Statistica degli studenti pisani del secolo XVI', *Rivista critica della letteratura italiana*, 3 (1886–87), pp. 125–6.

Pagel, Walter, *Paracelsus, an Introduction to Philosophical Medicine in the Era of the Renaissance* (Basel and New York: S. Karger, 1958).

Palmer, Richard, 'Medical botany in northern Italy in the Renaissance', *Journal of the Royal Society of Medicine*, 78 (1985), pp. 149–57.

Panofsky, Erwin, 'Artist, Scientist, Genius: Notes on the "Renaissance-Dämmerung"', in Wallace K. Ferguson et al. (eds), *The Renaissance: Six Essays* (New York: Harper and Row, 1962), pp. 121–82.

Panofsky, Erwin, 'Galileo as a Critic of the Arts: Aesthetic Attitude and Scientific Thought', *Isis*, 47(1) (1956), pp. 3–15.

Paoletti Italo, *Gerolamo Mercuriale e il suo tempo, Studio eseguito su 62 lettere e un consulto inediti del medico forlivese giacenti presso l'Archivio di Stato di Parma* (Lanciano: Cooperativa Editoriale tipografica, 1963).

Pardo Tomáš, José, 'Obras Espanolas sobre historia natural y material medica americanas en la Italia del siglo XVI', *Asclepio*, 43(1) (1991), pp. 51–94.

Pardo Tomáš, José and Maria Luz López Terrada, *Las Primeras Noticias sobre plantas americanas en las relaciones de viajes y crónicas de Indias (1493–1553)* (Valencia: Universitat de Valencia-CSIC, 1993).

Pardo Tomáš, José and Maria Luz López Terrada, *La influencia Española en la introduccion en Europa de las plantas americanas (1493–1623)* (Valencia: Universitat de Valencia-CSIC, 1997).

Park, Katherine, *Doctors and Medicine in Early Renaissance Florence* (Princeton, NJ: Princeton University Press, 1985).

Partington, James R., *A History of Chemistry* (London: Macmillan, 1961–70).

Pasolini, Pier Desiderio, *Caterina Sforza* (Roma: Loescher, 1893).

Pasolini, Pier Desiderio (ed.), *Experimenti de la ex.ma s.ra Caterina da Forlj matre de lo Inllux.mo signor Giovanni de Medici,* (Imola: Tip. d'Ignazio Galeati e figli, 1894).

Pastore, Alessandro, 'Medicina, Scienza e storia in età moderna. Lo stato degli studi in Italia', in F. Chacòn et al. (eds), *Spagna e Italia in Età moderna: storiografie a confronto* (Roma: Viella, 2009), pp. 253–71.

Pavord, Anna, *The Naming of Names: The Search for Order in the World of Plants* (London: Bloomsbury, 2005).

Pender, Stephen and Nancy S. Stuever (eds), *Rethoric and Medicine in Early Modern Europe* (Farnham: Ashgate, 2012).

Perifano, Alfredo, 'Considerations autour de la question du Paracelsisme en Italie au XVIe siècle: les dédicaces d'Adam de Bodenstein au Doge de Venise et a Come Ier de Médicis', *Bibliothèque d'humanisme et Renaissance*, 62 (2000), pp. 49–61.

Perifano, Alfredo, *L'Alchimie à la Cour de Côme Ier de Médicis: savoirs, culture et politique* (Paris: Honoré Champion, 1997).

Pieraccini, Gaetano, *La stirpe de' Medici di Cafaggiolo: Saggio di ricerche sulla trasmissione ereditaria e dei caratteri biologici*, 3 vols (Florence: Nardini, 1924–25).

Pizzagalli, Daniela, *La signora del Rinascimento, vita e splendori di Isabella d'Este alla corte di Mantova* (Milan: Rizzoli BUR, 2013).

Plaisance, Michel, *L'Académie et le Prince: Culture et politique à Florence au temps de Côme Ier et de François Ier de Médicis* (Manziana: Vecchierelli Editore, 2004).

Ragazzini, Stefania, *I manoscritti di Pier Antonio Micheli conservati nella Biblioteca Botanica dell'Università di Firenze* (Florence: Giunta Regionale Toscana – Editrice bibliografica, 1993).

Ragionieri, Giovanna (ed.), *Il giardino storico italiano* (Florence: Olschki, 1981).

Rankin, Alisha, *Panaceia's Daughters: Noblewomen as Healers in Early Modern Germany* (Chicago, IL, and London: The University of Chicago Press, 2013).

Ray, John, *Methodus plantarum nova* (London: H. Faithorn & J. Kersey, 1682).

Ray, Meredith K., 'Experiments with Alchemy: Caterina Sforza in Early Modern Scientific Culture', in *Gender and Scientific Discourse in Early Modern Culture* (Aldershot: Ashgate, 2010), pp. 139–64.

Réau, Louis, *Iconographie de l'art crétien* (Paris: Presse universitaires de France, 1957).

Reeds, Karen, 'Renaissance humanism and botany', *Annals of Science*, 33 (1976), pp. 519–42.

Reeds, Karen, *Botany in Medieval and Renaissance Universities* (New York: Garland, 1991).

Repici, Luciana, *Uomini capovolti, le piante nel pensiero dei Greci* (Rome-Bari: Laterza, 2000).

Riddle, John M., 'Theory and Practice in Medieval Medicine', in *Quid pro Quo: Studies in the History of Drugs* (Aldershot: Variorum, 1992), pp. 157–84.

Risse, Guenter B., 'Transcending Cultural Barriers: The European Reception of Medicinal Plants from the Americas', in W.-H. Hein (ed.), *Botanical Drugs of the Americas in the Old and New Worlds* (Stuttgart: Wissenschaftliche Verlagsgesellschaft MBH, 1984), pp. 31–42.

Rotolo, V., 'La storia medica dello zucchero', *Rivista di storia della medicina*, 8(1) (1998), pp. 15–25.

Ruggiero, Guido, *The Renaissance in Italy: A Social and Cultural History of the Rinascimento* (Cambridge: Cambridge University Press, 2015).

Sabbatani, Luigi, *Lucae Ghini Morbi gallici curandi ratio perbrevis: la cura del morbo gallico nelle lezioni di Luca Ghini* (Venice: Ferrari, 1921).

Sabbatani, Luigi, *Morbi Gallici curandi ratio perbrevis: La cura del morbo gallico nelle lezioni di Luca Ghini* (Venice, 1921).

Sabbatani, Luigi, 'Di una supposta opera di Luca Ghini', *Archeion*, 5 (1924), pp. 37–40.

Sabbatani, Luigi, 'La cattedra dei semplici fondata a Bologna da Luca Ghini', *Studi e memorie per la storia dell'Università di Bologna*, 9 (1926), pp. 13–53.

Sachs, Julius, *History of Botany (1530–1860)* (Oxford: Clarendon Press, 1860).

Saltini, Guglielmo Enrico, *Tragedie medicee domestiche* (Florence: G. Barbera, 1898).

Sandri, Lucia and A.J. Grieco, 'Appunti per una storia dell'acquavite in Italia: da Taddeo Alderotti alla Fonderia Medicea di Palazzo Pitti (1280–1591)', in *Grappa e alchimia: un percorso nella millenaria storia della distillazione* (Rome: Agra, 1999), pp. 33–48.

Sandri, Lucia, 'Il Collegio medico fiorentino e la riforma di Cosimo I: origini e funzioni (secc. XIV–XVI)', in S.U. Baldassarri et al. (eds), *Umanesimo e università in Toscana (1300–1600)* (Florence: Le Lettere, 2012), pp. 183–213.

Saunders, Gill, *Picturing Plants: An Aanalytical History of Botanical Illustration* (Berkeley and Los Angeles, CA: University of California Press, 1995).

Sbrana, C. and Lucia Tongiorgi Tomasi, 'Una biblioteca scientifica Pisa durante il granducato mediceo: i libri del giardino dei semplici', in *Livorno e Pisa, due citta' e un territorio* (Pisa: Nistri-Lischi e Pacini, 1980).

Schiebinger, Londa and Claudia Swan (eds), *Colonial Botany: Science, Commerce and Politics in the Early Modern World* (Philadelphia, PA: University of Pennsylvania Press, 2005).

Schmitt, Charles B, 'The Faculty of Arts at Pisa at the time of Galileo', *Physis*, 14 (1972), pp. 243–72.

Schmitt, Charles B., 'Science in the Italian Universities in the Sixteenth and Early Seventeenth Centuries', in Maurice Crosland (ed.), *The Emergence of Science in Western Europe* (London: Macmillan, 1975).

Schmitt, Charles B., 'Recent Trends in the Study of Medieval and Renaissance Science', in Pietro Corsi and Paul Weindling (eds), *Information Sources in the History of Science and Medicine* (London: Butterworth, 1983), pp. 221–39.

Schmitt, Charles B., 'Aristotle among the Physicians', in Andrew Wear (ed.), *The Medical Renaissance in the Sixteenth Century* (Cambridge: Cambridge University Press, 1985), pp. 1–15.

Schmitt, Charles B., Esperienza ed esperimento: un confronto tra Zabarella e il giovane Galileo, in *Filosofia e scienza nel Rinascimento* (Milan: La Nuova Italia 2001), pp. 25–64.

Sebregondi, Ludovica, 'Cosma e Damiano. Santi Medici e Medicei', in Elena Giannarelli (ed.), *Cosma e Damiano: Dall'Oriente a Firenze* (Florence: Edizioni della Meridiana, 2002) pp. 75–105.

Seybold, S., 'Luca Ghini, Leonhard Rauwolff und Leonhart Fuchs. Uber die Erkunft der Aquarelle im Wiener Krauterbuchmanuskrpt von Fuchs', *Jahreshefte der Gesellschaft für die Naturkunde in Württemberg* (Stuttgart, 1990), 145, pp. 239–64.

Shaw, Elisabeth A., *Plants of the New World: The First 150 Years* (Cambridge, MA: Harvard University Press, 1992).

Shaw, James and Evelyn Welch, *Making and Marketing Medicine in Renaissance Florence* (Clio Medica 89 / The Wellcome Series in the History of Medicine) (Amsterdam and New York: Rodopi, 2011).

Signorini, Maria Adele, 'Sulle piante dipinte dal Bacchiacca nello scrittoio di Cosimo I a Palazzo Vecchio', *Mitteilungen des Kunsthistorischen Institutes in Florenz*, 37(2/3) (1993), pp. 396–407.

Silini, Giovanni, La cultura medica e farmaceutica', in G. Silini (ed.), *Herbe Pincte* (Gorle: Iniziative Culturali, 2000).

Silini, Giovanni, *Uomini e farmaci: terapia medica tardo-medievale* (Gandino: iniziative Culturali, 2001).

Siraisi, Nancy, *Taddeo Alderotti and his Pupils: Two Generations of Italian Medical Learning* (Princeton, NJ: Princeton University Press, 1981).

Siraisi, Nancy, *Avicenna in Renaissance Italy: The Canon and Medical Teaching in Italian Universities after 1500* (Princeton, NJ: Princeton University Press, 1987).

Siraisi, Nancy, *Medieval and Early Renaissance Medicine: An Introduction to Knowledge and Practice* (Chicago, IL, and London: The University of Chicago Press, 1990).

Siraisi, Nancy, *Medicine and the Italian Universities 1250–1600* (Leiden: Brill, 2001).Smith, Pamela H. and Paula Findlen, *Merchants and Marvels: Commerce, Science, and Art in Early Modern Europe* (New York and London: Routledge, 2002).

Stannard, Jerry, 'Dioscorides and Renaissance *Materia Medica*', in M. Florkin (ed.), *Materia medica in the XVI Century: Proceedings of a Symposium of the International Academy of Medicine*, (Oxford: Pergamon Press, 1966), pp. 1-21.

Stannard, Jerry, *Herbs and Herbalism in the Middle Ages and Renaissance* (Aldershot: Ashgate, 1999).

Stein Claudia, 'The Meaning of Signs: Diagnosing the French Pox in early modern Augsburg', *Bulletin of the History of Medicine*, 80(4) (2006), pp. 617–47.

Stern, William P., 'Master memorial lecture', *Journal of the Royal Horticultural Society*, August (1965), p. 326.

Storia dell'Università di Pisa, Commissione rettorale per la storia dell'Università di Pisa (Pisa: Edizioni Plus, 2000).

Strocchia, Sharon T., 'The nun apothecaries of Renaissance Florence: Marketing medicines in the convent', *Renaissance Studies*, 25(5) (2011), pp. 627–47.

Swan, Claudia, 'Lectura-imago-ostensio: The Role of the "Libri Picturati" A.18-A.30 in Medical Instruction at the Leiden University', in G. Olmi, L. Tongiorgi Tomasi and A. Zanca (eds), *Natura-Cultura: l'interpretazione del mondo fisico nei testi e nelle immagini* (Florence: Olschki, 2000) pp. 189–214.

Targioni Tozzetti, Antonio, *Cenni storici sulla introduzione di varie piante nell'agricoltura e orticoltura toscana* (Florence: Tipografia Galileiana, 1853).

Targioni Tozzetti, Giovanni, *Notizie sulla storia delle scienze fisiche in Toscana cavate da un manoscritto inedito* (Florence: Biblioteca Palatina, 1852).

Targioni Tozzetti, Ottaviano, 'Di alcune opere relative alle scienze composte in volgare o in esso tradotte sotto il regno di Cosimo I Granduca di Toscana. Lezione tenuta il 9 agosto 1825, *Atti dell'Imperiale e Reale Accademia della Crusca* (Firenze: Tipografia all'insegna di Dante, 1829), pp. 302–9.

Thorndike, Lynn, *A History of Magic and Experimental Science* (New York: Columbia University Press, 1923–58), 8 vols.

Tolaini Emilio, *Forma Pisarum: Storia urbanistica della città di Pisa. Problemi e ricerche* (Pisa: Nistri-Lischi, 1979).

Tomas, Natalie, *The Medici Women: Gender and Power in Renaissance Florence* (Aldershot: Ashgate, 2003).

Tongiorgi Tomasi, Lucia, 'Gherardo Cibo: Visions of landscape and the botanical sciences in a sixteenth-century artist', *Journal of Garden History*, 9 (1989), pp. 199–216.

Tongiorgi Tomasi, Lucia, 'Dall'essenza vegetale agglutinata all'immagine a stampa', *Museologia Scientifica*, 8 (1991–92), pp. 271–95.

Tongiorgi Tomasi, Lucia (ed.), *I ritratti di piante di Jacopo Ligozzi* (Pisa: Pacini, 1993).

Tongiorgi Tomasi, Lucia, 'L'Università e gli artisti', *Storia dell'Università di Pisa*, Commissione rettorale per la storia dell'Università di Pisa (Pisa: Edizioni Plus, 2000), pp. 659–89.

Tongiorgi Tomasi, Lucia, *The Flowering of Florence: Botanical Art for the Medici* (Washington, DC: National Gallery of Art, 2002).

Tosi, Alessandro (ed.), *Ulisse Aldrovandi e la Toscana: Carteggio e testimonianze documentarie* (Florence: Olschki, 1989).

Tugnoli Pattaro, Sandra, *Metodo e sistema delle scienze nel pensiero di Ulisse Aldrovandi* (Bologna: Clueb, 1981).

Ubrizsy Savoia, Andrea, 'Le piante pisane nei manoscritti di Aldrovandi', *Museologia Scientifica*, 9 (1992–93), pp. 363–80.

Ubrizsy Savoia, Andrea, 'The botanical garden of Padua in Guilandino's day', in Alessandro Minelli (ed.), *The Botanical Garden of Padua 1545–1995* (Venice: Marsilio, 1995), pp. 173–95.

Ubrizsy Savoia, Andrea, 'La biodiversità americana nell'opera di Aldrovandi', in A. Maiarino, M. Minelli, A.L. Monti and B. Negroni (eds), *L'erbario dipinto di Ulisse Aldrovandi: un capolavoro del Rinascimento* (Vernasca: Ace International, 1995), pp. 75–104.

Una Farmacia preindustriale in Valdelsa: La Spezieria e lo Spedale di Santa Fina nella città di San Gimignano secc. XIV–XVIII (San Gimignano, Cat. Ex., 1981).

Vaccari, Maria Grazia, *La guardaroba medicea dell'Archivio di Stato di Firenze* (Florence: Giunta regionale toscana, 1997).

Vignau-Wilberg, Thea, 'Devotion and Observation of Nature in Art around 1600', in G. Olmi, L. Tongiorgi Tomasi and A. Zanca (eds), *Natura-Cultura: L'interpretazione del mondo fisico nei testi e nelle immagini* (Florence: Olschki, 2000), pp. 43–57.

Viroli, Maurizio, *Dalla politica alla ragion di stato: La scienza del governo tra XIII e XVII secolo* (Rome: Donzelli, 1994).

Viviani, Ugo, *Vita e opere di Andrea Cesalpino* (Arezzo: Ugo Viviani Editore, 1922).

Volpi, Guglielmo, 'Intorno all'origine del Giardino dei semplici di Firenze', *Archivio storico italiano*, 9(1) (1922), pp. 81–90.

Walcott Emmart, Emily, *The Badianus Manuscript (Codex Barberini, Latin 241, Vatican Library): An Aztec Herbal of 1522* (Baltimore, MD: The Johns Hopkins University Press, 1992).

Wear, Andrew, 'Explorations in Renaissance Writings on the Practice of Medicine', in A. Wear, R.K. French and I.M. Lonie (eds), *The Medical Renaissance of the Sixteenth Century* (Cambridge: Cambridge University Press, 1985), pp. 118–45.

Wear, Andrew, *Knowledge and Practice in English Medicine, 1550–1680* (Cambridge: Cambridge University Press, 2000).

Welch, Evelyn, *Shopping in the Renaissance: Consumer Culture in Italy 1440–1600* (New Haven and London: Yale University Press, 2005).

Welch, Evelyn, 'Art on the edge: Hair, hats and hands in Renaissance Italy', *Renaissance Studies*, 23(3) (2009), pp. 241–68.

Worth Estes, J., 'The European reception of the first drugs from the New World', *Pharmacy in History*, 37(1) (1995), pp. 3–23.

Zangheri, Luigi, *Pratolino, il giardino delle meraviglie* (Florence: Gonnelli, 1987).

Zanier, Giancarlo, 'La medicina paracelsiana in Italia: Aspetti di un'accoglienza particolare', *Rivista di storia della filosofia*, 4 (1985), pp. 627–53.

Zemon Davis, Natalie, *The Gift in Sixteenth-Century France* (Madison, WI: University of Wisconsin Press, c.2000).

Zucchi, Luca, 'Brunfels e Fuchs: L'illustrazione botanica quale ritratto della singola pianta o immagine della specie', *Nuncius*, 18 (2003), pp. 411–65.

Index